Receptors and Recognition

General Editors: P. Cuatrecasas and M.F. Greaves

About the series

Cellular recognition — the process by which cells interact with, and respond to, molecular signals in their environment — plays a crucial role in virtually all important biological functions. These encompass fertilization, infectious interactions, embryonic development, the activity of the nervous system, the regulation of growth and metabolism by hormones and the immune response to foreign antigens. Although our knowledge of these systems has grown rapidly in recent years, it is clear that a full understanding of cellular recognition phenomena will require an integrated and multidisciplinary approach.

This series aims to expedite such an understanding by bringing together accounts by leading researchers of all biochemical, cellular and evolutionary aspects of recognition systems. The series will contain volumes of two types. First, there will be volumes containing about five reviews from different areas of the general subject written at a level suitable for all biologically oriented scientists (Receptors and Recognition, series A). Secondly, there will be more specialized volumes, (Receptors and Recognition, series B), each of which will be devoted to just one particularly important area.

Advisory Editorial Board

Receptors and Recognition

Receptors and
Recognition

Series B Volume 5

Taxis and
Behavior

Elementary Sensory Systems
in Biology

Edited by
G. L. Hazelbauer

The Wallenberg Laboratory,
University of Uppsala, Sweden

LONDON

CHAPMAN AND HALL

A Halsted Press Book
John Wiley & Sons, New York

First published 1978
by Chapman and Hall Ltd.,
11 New Fetter Lane, London EC4P 4EE

Typeset by C. Josée Utteridge-Faivre
and printed in Great Britain
at the University Printing House, Cambridge

ISBN 0 412 14880 3

Distributed in the U.S.A. by Halsted Press,
a Division of John Wiley & Sons, Inc., New York

Library of Congress Cataloging in Publication Data

Main entry under title:

Taxis and behavior.

(Receptors and recognition: Series B; v.5)
'A Halsted Press book.'
1. Taxes (Biology) 2. Chemotaxis.
I. Hazelbauer, G.L. II. Series.
QH514.T39   574.1'8   78–14931
ISBN 0–470–26483–7

Contents

Contributors

P. Brachet, Departement de Biologie Moleculaire, Institut Pasteur, Paris, France.

C. Kung, Department of Molecular Biology, University of Wisconsin, Madison, Wisconsin, U.S.A.

M. Darmon, Departement de Biologie Moleculaire, Institut Pasteur, Paris, France.

M.F. Goy, Department of Biochemistry, University of Wisonsin, Madison, Wisconsin, U.S.A.

K. Hansen, Zooloisches Intitut der Universität Regensburg, Regensburg, West Germany.

E. Hildebrand, Institut für Neurobiologie der Kernforschungsanlage, Julich, West Germany.

E. Kramer, Max-Planck Institut für Verhaltensphysiologie, Seewiesen über Starnberg, West Germany.

J.P. Mascarenhas, Department of Biological Sciences, State University of New York at Albany, New York, U.S.A.

D.L. Nelson, Department of Biochemistry, University of Wisconsin, Madison, Wisconsin, U.S.A.

M.S. Springer, Department of Biochemistry, University of Wisconsin, Madison, Wisconsin, U.S.A.

S. Ward, Department of Embryology, Carnegie Institution of Washington, Baltimore, Maryland, U.S.A.

P. Wilkinson, Department of Bacteriology and Immunology, Western Infirmary, Glasgow, U.K.

Preface

The topics considered here constitute a list of research areas in which mechanisms that mediate behavioral patterns are presently being studied, or in which such studies could reasonably be initiated in the near future. I would not want to claim either originality or comprehensiveness for the list, but would like to consider it an appropriate beginning for those researchers and students actively or passively interested in mechanisms basic to sensory systems and the behavior they mediate. A molecular biologist in search of a sensory system in which to ply his trade might profitably start here.

In each of the systems discussed, the sensory phenomenon and behavioral pattern can be defined with some precision. *What* happens is sufficiently elementary that questions about *how* things happen can be approached experimentally. Clearly, some areas are more advanced than others, but the common factor in all these systems is a promise of answers to questions about mechanisms.

In communicating with the authors about their projected chapters, I outlined my hopes for an approach and a style by suggesting a hypothetical situation: 'Imagine that one of your colleagues is seriously interested in learning about your area of research, perhaps with the idea of becoming involved in the field himself. He has a general biological/biochemical background with some interest in receptor systems, but little knowledge of the details, or even the attractions of your field. So consider that you are trying to describe the given area of research, with what introductory and 'historical' material as is necessary to define the problems and then emphasizing areas that fascinate you either because of what has recently come to light or because of the problems still unsolved. You find yourself in a position of trying to convey the interest and promise inherent in the area, partially because you would like to encourage this colleague to start working in it. Thus it is not out of place to describe your own models and ideas about how the available data can be organized, as well as your opinions of what should and could be pursued in the future.' The impressive degree to which the authors achieved this goal of informed and cogent presentations can be attested to by my laboratory and colleagues, who, in the past several months, have been unable to avoid listening to me explaining still more 'fascinating facts and ideas of sensory biology' that I learned from each chapter as it arrived in Uppsala.

Earlier volumes edited by Sorkin (*Chemotaxis: Its Biology and Biochemistry,* Karger, 1974) and by Carlile (*Primitive Sensory and Communication Systems: The Taxes and Tropisms of Micro-organisms and Cells,* Academic Press, 1975) review some of the subjects considered here as well as some related areas. The chapters concerned with bacterial chemotaxis (Goy and Springer) and with *Dictyostelium* taxis (Darmon and Brachet) have companion, complementary chapters in another volume of the RECEPTORS AND RECOGNITION series (*Microbial Interactions,* J. Reissig, ed.). In each case, both chapters ought to be read to obtain a complete description of the present state of the field.

Implicit in the concept of a volume covering a wide range of organisms is the idea that the unity of living things is not limited to the replication of hereditary material or the synthesis of macromolecules. The unique features of a particular organism or sensory system define experimental approaches that are advantageous or conceivable, but the basic mechanisms of reception, signal transduction and signal transmission that are being sought in the study of different systems ought to be few in number, probably even variations on a common theme. As indicated in many of the chapters, there is a rather wide concensus that controlled movement of ions across membranes would be included in such a theme, as would a special role for the calcium ion. There may well be a new candidate for inclusion, methylation and demethylation of carboxyl side-chains of specific proteins. Goy and Springer discuss in detail the role of carboxymethylation in bacterial chemo-taxis and also cite a report (O'Dea *et al., Nature,* **272**, 462 (1978)), published as the manuscripts for this volume were being submitted, that the same reaction is correlated with chemotaxis by mammalian leucocytes! Axelrod and others have documented the existence of carboxymethylation in a number of mammalian endocrine organs and neural tissues, so it is tempting to speculate that in the phylogenetic territory between bacteria and mammals (for example, between chapters 1 and 9 of this volume) the same reaction is used for similar sensory functions. If that would turn out to be the case, Monod's dictum about *E. coli* and elephants will have found a whole new aspect of applicability.

April, 1978   *Gerald L. Hazelbauer*

1 In Search of the Linkage between Receptor and Response: The role of a protein methylation reaction in bacterial chemotaxis

M. F. GOY and M. S. SPRINGER

Acknowledgements
The authors would like to gratefully acknowledge their indebtedness to Julius Adler for his continual support and encouragement.

Taxis and Behavior
(*Receptors and Recognition,* Series B, Volume 5)
Edited by G.L. Hazelbauer
Published in 1978 by Chapman and Hall, 11 New Fetter Lane, London EC4P 4EE
© Chapman and Hall

1.1 INTRODUCTION

Life has evolved in environments which are often hostile and nearly always in a state of flux. Therefore, most, if not all, organisms have mechanisms for gathering information about the conditions surrounding them and, in turn, utilizing that information to influence the way in which they are affected by the environment. A variety of such mechanisms exist ranging from the induction of an enzyme to the conscious control of motor activities. These sorts of interactions between the organims and its surroundings serve as the basis for what we call 'behavior'.

Behavior may be defined as the response of an organism to a stimulus. In multicellular organisms most of the behavioral phenomena we observe are the results of the co-operative interaction of many specialized cells, called neurons, that are arranged in what are often exceedingly complex networks. A study of the operation of such a nervous system can be approached from two levels. First, how do the individual neurons function and, second, how do the elements of the network interact to bring about behavior? We know that when an external stimulus is encountered by the organism it results in the production of an electrical response in a special type of neuron, commonly called a receptor cell. The process by which the external information is converted to an internal signal is known as sensory transduction. This signal is subsequently communicated from the receptor cell to other neurons by a process called synaptic transmission: a 'transmitter' chemical is released pre-synaptically, from the receptor cell, and acts at a sensitive site on a nearby neuron to produce a new electrical signal. The initiation of such a response in a post-synaptic neuron may itself be considered a form of sensory transduction, since it involves conversion of an extracellular signal (the released chemical) to an intracellular signal (the electrical response). Ultimately, after the information has been passed in this way from one cell to another, in the proper sequence, it can give rise to a change in the behavior of the organism.

Even this greatly simplified summary indicates that much remains to be learned about the operation of the nervous system. At the network level, our understanding of how neurons interact to process information is limited to those nervous systems, or parts of nervous systems, that are sufficiently simple for the intercellular connections to be analyzed in detail. At the cellular level, despite considerable knowledge of the ionic basis of the electrical signals, little is known about the underlying molecular events which generate and control these signals.

An approach often taken by biological scientists, when faced with a difficult problem in a complex system, is to find a simpler organism in which to study the phenomenon. This has been extremely fruitful in the past since, as a consequence of evolution, basic mechanisms are in general conserved. Thus the chemical organization of the simplest prokaryote, its metabolic pathways, and its hereditary mechanisms are basically the same as those of the most complex eukaryote. Furthermore, the ability to interact with the environment appears to be so crucial for survival that it is found even in extremely primitive organisms, such as the unicellular bacteria. It has been known for nearly a hundred years that bacteria exhibit motor responses to a variety of stimuli, including changes in light intensity (Engelmann, 1883), chemical concentration (Pfeffer, 1883) and temperature (Schenk, 1893). Therefore it seems plausible that prokaryotes might serve as model systems in which to study behavioral phenomena. In particular, these organisms offer great advantages for studying the biochemistry and genetics of sensory transduction at the cellular level. As will be described below, what we have learned only strengthens this belief, since there are striking analogies between the chemotactic behavior of bacteria and the sensory behavior of the receptor cells of higher organisms.

This article presents some recent developments in our understanding of the biochemical mechanisms that underlie sensory transduction in bacteria. To some extent it reflects the interests and prejudices of the authors and is not intended to be a comprehensive review of bacterial chemotaxis. The reader is urged to consult a number of other articles for different emphases and different points of view (Adler, 1975; Berg, 1975; Hazelbauer and Parkinson, 1977; Koshland, 1976, 1977; Parkinson, 1977).

1.2 A COMPARISON OF BACTERIAL BEHAVIOR WITH THE BEHAVIOR OF SENSORY NEURONS

Since a major reason for studying bacterial chemotaxis is the expectation that it will serve as a model in which to study the process of sensory transduction that occurs in sensory neurons, it is appropriate to ask how similar the two phenomena are. First, we will briefly describe the behavior of the eukaryotic receptor cell.

When the intensity of an environmental stimulus changes, a typical receptor cell first records the information as a change in some chemical property of the cell (for example, the bleaching of rhodopsin by light). This leads to a graded change in the electrical potential maintained across the cell membrane and, ultimately, to a change in the output of the cell, usually an increase or decrease in the frequency of action potentials. These changes in the electrical properties of the cell constitute its response to the stimulus, and we refer to the initiation of this response as sensory excitation. Subsequently, in many receptor cells, a phenomenon called sensory adaptation is observed. In this article we will define sensory adaptation as a gradual decline in the response of a receptor cell following the delivery of a stimulus, even though the stimulus, once given, is maintained continuously. However, upon removal of the stimulus, the cell will regain its sensitivity and will respond normally if the stimulus is delivered again. The latter process may be considered the inverse of adaptation and we refer to it as de-adaptation. Thus, at any given instant, the

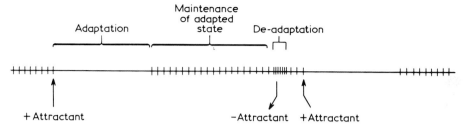

Fig. 1.1 Simplified schematic representation of temporal responses to an attractant. Each vertical line represents a tumble. These lines are drawn with regular spacing for the sake of convenience only, as the interval between tumbles is random. The attractant is added and removed as indicated by the arrows. The absence of vertical lines following addition of the attractant represents the complete supression of tumbling, while the increased frequency of lines following removal of the attractant represents continuous tumbling. Repellents have the opposite effect on behavior: addition of a repellent produces a transient period of continuous tumbling and removal of a repellent produces a transient period of suppressed tumbling.

behavior of such a receptor cell can be thought of as being determined by the balance between two processes: an excitational process that initiates responses to stimuli, and a slower adaptational process that extinguishes these responses.

At least qualitatively, the same phenomena are observed in *Escherichia coli.* These bacteria detect and respond to changes in the chemical composition of the environment, a process known as chemotaxis. When the concentration of a stimulatory chemical changes, the information is first represented by a change in the properties of specific chemoreceptor proteins located in the cell envelope (Aksamit and Koshland, 1974; Boos *et al.*, 1972; Hazelbauer and Adler, 1971; Hazelbauer and Parkinson, 1977; Zukin *et al.*, 1977). Some twenty different types of chemoreceptors have been identified, each type sensitive to a different class of structurally related compounds (Adler and Epstein, 1974; Adler *et al.*, 1973; Mesibov and Adler, 1972; Tso and Adler, 1974). In all cases where the chemoreceptor proteins have been isolated, it has been shown that they specifically bind the stimulatory compound to which they are sensitive (Adler and Epstein, 1974; Aksamit and Koshland, 1974; Hazelbauer, 1975; Hazelbauer and Adler, 1971; Spudich and Koshland, 1975). A change in degree of binding, which occurs when the concentration of the stimulatory chemical changes, constitutes the first step in the generation of the chemotactic response. This initiates a sequence of biochemical events, described in detail below, which appears to be accompanied by a perturbation of the membrane potential (Szmelcman and Adler, 1976). As a result, the output of the cell is modified.

The bacteria normally swim in smooth lines, interrupted at random intervals by a tumbling motion that abruptly alters the direction of travel (Berg and Brown, 1972; MacNab and Koshland, 1972). It is the frequency at which this tumbling occurs that is modified by the stimulus: addition of one class of stimulus, called attractants, leads to a dramatic suppression of tumbling (Brown and Berg, 1974; MacNab and Koshland, 1972), while addition of another class of stimulus, called repellents, leads to a dramatic enhancement of tumbling (Tsang *et al.*, 1973). Thus, as in eukaryotic receptor cells, sensory excitation involves a change in frequency, although not of action potentials since in this case it is the swimming behavior which is altered. Furthermore, as shown in Fig. 1.1, the change in tumbling frequency is transient; after some time passes the tumbling frequency returns to the pre-stimulus level, even though the stimulatory chemical is still present (MacNab and Koshland, 1972; Tsang *et al.*, 1973). These observations demonstrate that bacteria undergo sensory adaptation, in a manner analogous to that described above for eukaryotic receptor cells.

Once adaptation to a given chemical has occurred, the bacteria appear to have lost their sensitivity to its continued presence, although they are still sensitive to other chemicals detected by different chemoreceptors. These cells are referred to as being in the adapted state, and they will remain in this state for as long as the stimulatory chemical remains in the environment. This implies that some property of the sensory transduction machinery can undergo a long-term change, in order to produce and maintain the state of insensitivity. Furthermore, the change is not just qualitative, but quantitative as well. This is demonstrated by the observation that the magnitude of the response following a change to a new concentration of attractant is dependent on the initial concentration to which the cells have already adapted. For example, the length of response to a change in attractant concentration to 50 mM becomes progressively shorter if the cells have been previously adapted to 0, 0.5, or 5 mM of the same compound (Berg and Tedesco, 1975; Spudich and Koshland, 1975). In this example, pre-adaptation has produced a change in the cells' sensitivity to 50 mM attractant, and the extent of the change is related to the concentration of attractant used during the pre-adaptation period. This loss of sensitivity must be quantitatively reflected by a long-term change in some component of the sensory transduction machinery. However, any such long-term change must be readily reversible: when the attractant is removed the cell quickly regains its sensitivity to the chemical by the process of de-adaptation (Berg and Tedesco, 1975). Note from Fig. 1.1 that de-adaptation to an attractant is accompanied by a second behavioral response, a brief period of continuous tumbling (MacNab and Koshland, 1972). Similarly, cells adapted to a repellent respond to its removal with a transient period of smooth swimming (Tsang *et al.*, 1973).

A characteristic asymmetry in the properties of the bacterial transduction machinery should be pointed out here: adaptation to an attractant stimulus is slow, often requiring many minutes, whereas de-adaptation to the same stimulus is very rapid, being completed within a few seconds (Berg and Tedesco, 1975). Because the time required for de-adaptation is so short, it is difficult to determine whether there is any dependency of this interval on the magnitude of the stimulus. On the other hand, it is easily demonstrated that the time required for adaptation to an attractant is highly dependent on the magnitude of the stimulus: the larger the stimulus the longer the time required (Berg and Tedesco, 1975; Spudich and Koshland, 1975). In fact, the adaptation time is directly proportional to the change in the fraction of receptor binding sites occupied as a result of the stimulus (Spudich and Koshland, 1975). Furthermore, when two attractants are added simultaneously they act as one equivalent stimulus: the time required to adapt to such a stimulus usually approximates the sum of the adaptation times for the individual stimuli (Berg and Tedesco, 1975). However, when an attractant (which suppresses tumbling) and a repellent (which increases tumbling) are added simultaneously, the two tend to cancel each other's effects. In this case, whether the attractant or the repellent will dominate depends on the relative potency of the particular attractant and repellent chosen (Tsang *et al.,* 1973). Therefore, attractant and repellent signals appear to have opposite polarity. In a similar way, many eukaryotic neurons show responses which reflect either excitation or inhibition, depending on the type of stimulus, and can sum two or more excitatory and inhibitory inputs in order to produce a single integrated output.

1.3 BACTERIAL CHEMOTAXIS: ITS PHYSICAL BASIS

The data presented to this point indicate that bacteria such as *E. coli* are indeed able to gather information about the environment, and use this information to modify their behavior. When the concentration of a stimulatory chemical changes, which results in what we call a temporal gradient of the chemical, the cell can detect and respond to this change in much the same way as does a typical eukaryotic receptor cell. This ability is of considerable benefit, since it allows the cell to discriminate between chemically 'good' and chemically 'bad' environments. Thus, the organisms can vacate or avoid harmful, crowded, or nutritionally inferior environments and can seek out environments that are rich in metabolically useful compounds.

The problem for bacteria, as for other organisms that respond to environmental stimuli, is to use environmental information to control the direction in which they move. Bacteria swim by means of semi-rigid, helical flagella (Leifson, 1960). Each cell possesses about 6–8 flagella, which extend outward from random locations on the cell membrane (Leifson, 1960). These organelles develop the thrust to propel the bacterium through space by rotating (Berg and Anderson, 1973; Silverman and Simon, 1974): when they rotate in the counterclockwise direction* the flagella form a bundle at one end of the cell, work in unison, and the cell swims in smooth, gently curving lines; when they reverse and rotate clockwise, the bundle breaks apart, the flagella work independently, and the cell tumbles (Larsen *et al.,* 1974; MacNab, 1977; MacNab and Koshland, 1974). In a typical cell, the rotation of the flagellum is biased in the counterclockwise direction, so that the organism spends most of its time swimming smoothly. However, at intervals (averaging about one second in length) the direction of flagellar rotation spontaneously reverses for a brief instant, giving rise

---

* Viewed down the axis of the flagellum towards the cell body.

to a tumble (Berg and Brown, 1972; Larsen *et al.,* 1974). Each tumble serves to reorient the bacterium in a new direction for its next period of swimming (Berg and Brown, 1972).

Thus, the principal mechanism by which bacteria can actively alter their direction of travel is the tumble, and it is by control over the frequency of tumbling that bacteria control their movement through space. If the bacterium swims towards an increasing concentration of an attractant the sensory transduction machinery detects this increase (as described above) and modifies the behavior of the cell in such a way that the probability of tumbling is decreased (Berg and Brown, 1972). This leads to longer periods of swimming in the direction of increasing attractant concentration, and the cells gradually accumulate in the region of the gradient where the highest concentration of attractant is found. For repellents exactly the opposite is observed: when the cells swim toward a decreasing concentration of repellent the tumbling frequency is decreased (Berg and Brown, 1972; Tsang *et al.,* 1973). Thus, when presented with a spatial gradient of repellent, the cells tend to avoid the region of highest concentration and accumulate instead in regions where the concentration is low.

This type of behavioral control offers several advantages to the bacterium. First, it is based on the regulation of a single parameter: the frequency of tumbling. Hence, the mechanics of the process are extremely simple. The cell need only be concerned with regulating the transition between two behavioral states: clockwise and counterclockwise rotation of the flagella. Second, the use of a temporal sensing mechanism to measure the spatial gradient permits a great amplification of the stimulus (MacNab and Koshland, 1972). Rather than an instantaneous comparison of the concentration differential from one end of the cell to the other, which would be extremely inaccurate due to the small size of the organism (MacNab and Koshland, 1972), the cell can rely on comparisons made over distances many body lengths apart. Third, the incorporation of sensory adaptation into the behavioral response allows the organism to emphasize *changes* in the environment, without losing information about steady-state conditions. In a world where unpredictable changes can quickly produce lethal effects, a mechanism of this type seems particularly useful.

1.4 BEHAVIORAL MUTANTS

Our study of the mechanism of sensory transduction in *E. coli* has been greatly facilitated by the techniques of modern bacterial genetics which have led to the selection and characterization of a large number of behavioral mutants. These mutants fall into four broad classes. The first category consists of mutants that fail in the detection of any one stimulus, the second of mutants which are defective in response to more than one but not all stimuli, the third of mutants which are defective in response to all stimuli, and the fourth of mutants which have lost the ability to swim. The groupings of these mutants suggest that there is a great deal of convergence of information during the processing of chemotactic stimuli, from the initial stimulus detection events, where each different class of stimulus interacts with a different chemoreceptor, to the final effect of the stimuli on the flagella, by which point all the different signals have been processed and combined to produce a single integrated behavioral output. In a sense, one can trace the path of information flow during chemotaxis by studying the properties of the different types of mutants.

1.4.1 Stimulus-detection mutants

This category consists of mutants that have normal motility and normal responses to most stimuli, but are unable to respond to a specific compound or group of structurally related compounds. The lesions in these strains all lie in genes that code for individual chemoreceptors (specific 'recognition' proteins having high-affinity binding sites for particular stimulatory chemicals), or in genes coding for components associated with these proteins (Adler, 1975). Furthermore, the chemoreceptors simultaneously serve as the recognition site for chemotaxis and as the first element in a transport system that carries the chemotactically active compound across the cell membrane (Adler, 1975). However, transport of the compound is not a pre-requisite for the chemotactic response, since transport-specific mutations have been isolated that do not affect chemotaxis (Hazelbauer, 1975; Ordal and Adler, 1974).

While mutants in the receptors for galactose, maltose, ribose, glucose, mannose, mannitol, fructose, glucitol and galactitol have been isolated (Adler and Epstein, 1974; Aksamit and Koshland, 1974, Hazelbauer, 1975. Hazelbauer and Adler, 1971; Lengeler, 1975), chemoreceptor mutants for other stimulatory compounds have not been found. The reason for this is unclear, although it may be that such mutations are lethal, or that the compounds are detected by more than one chemoreceptor. In the latter case, a specifically non-chemotactic strain could only be produced by intro-ducing mutations simultaneously in all the chemoreceptors that detect the chemical, a situation which would occur rarely.

1.4.2 Multiply defective mutants

All members of this class are motile and tumble at relatively normal frequencies, but are defective in response to two or more structurally unrelated compounds. For example, mutants have been isolated that have all the known components of the galactose and ribose chemoreceptors, yet are unable to carry out chemotaxis towards any of the compounds detected by either of these chemoreceptors (Ordal and Adler, 1974). These strains are designated *trg*. Several different mutations are known that produce similar multiply defective phenotypes (Carl Ball, unpublished results). Since the mutants can respond normally to most stimuli they appear to be defective at a relatively early stage in the processing of chemotactic information, before a significant degree of convergence has occured.

Lesions in two additional genes, called *tar* and *tsr*, result in strains with more serious defects. These strains cannot respond properly to a large number of different stimuli, although their responses to some compounds are nearly normal (Mesibov and Adler, 1972; Silverman and Simon, 1977b; Springer *et al.*, 1977a; Tso and Adler, 1974). Hence, they are probably defective at later stages in the information-processing pathway. Taking this into account, it is not surprising that the functions of the *tar* and *tsr* genes appear to be closely related to the functions of the genes described in the next section (Section 1.4.3). This idea will be more fully developed throughout the remainder of the chapter.

1.4.3 Generally defective mutants

These strains either fail to respond or respond poorly to all stimuli. In addition, the generally defective mutants have highly aberrant patterns of motility. Lesions in 8 different genes result in such abnormalities and, as shown in Fig. 1.2, all but two of these genes are found in two closely linked operons (Parkinson, 1978a; Silverman and Simon, 1977a; Warrick *et al.*, 1977).

Although these mutants all show general defects in their ability to carry out chemotaxis, they do not all have the same phenotype. For example, *che A, che C, che D, che W* and *che Y* mutants fail to tumble in the absence of stimuli, and respond very poorly or not at all to attractants and repellents (Armstrong and Adler, 1969; Armstrong *et al.*, 1967; Parkinson, 1974, 1976, 1978a; Warrick *et al.*, 1977). Similarly, *che X* mutants also fail to tumble in the absence of stimuli (Parkinson, 1974, 1976, 1978a; Warrick *et al.*, 1977), but these strains can respond to the addition of repellents with an increase in tumbling, and this effect of repellents can be reversed by the subsequent addition of an attractant (Goy *et al.*, 1978; Parkinson, 1978b). However, the response of these strains is abnormal in several important respects (Goy *et al.*, 1978; Parkinson, 1978b; see below).

On the other hand, *che B* and *che Z* mutants tumble incessantly in the absence of stimuli (Parkinson, 1976, 1977, 1978a). Both *che B* and *che Z* strains can respond to the addition of attractants with a suppression of tumbling (Armstrong *et al.*, 1967; Parkinson, 1976, 1977, 1978a; Springer *et al.*, 1975) and this can be reversed by the subsequent addition of a repellent (Parkinson, 1978a). Thus, these strains can respond to temporal gradients of both attractants and repellents. However, their ability to respond to spatial gradients is seriously impaired due to the high frequency of spontaneous tumbling which prevents the cells from swimming far enough to detect the gradient. Moreover, they are generally less sensitive to temporal stimuli than are wild-type bacteria, showing higher thresholds and shorter response times (Parkinson, 1974, 1976; Springer *et al.*, 1975).

It should be pointed out that some uncertainty and confusion exists with regard to the relationship between the *tsr* and *che D* mutants. It has been proposed, on the basis of indirect evidence, that *che D* is a specific allele of the *tsr* gene (Parkinson, 1974), although the behavioral phenotypes of *che D* and *tsr* mutants are quite

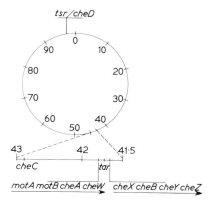

Fig. 1.2 Genetic map of *E. coli*, showing the location of some of the genes involved in chemotaxis.

Gene	Product molecular weight*	Product location†	Swimming pattern‡
che C	?	?	Fails to tumble
che A §	76 000 66 000	Mostly cytoplasm Cytoplasm	Fails to tumble
che W	12 000	Cytoplasm	Fails to tumble
tar	56 000–61 000	Cytoplasmic membrane	Normal
che X	28 000	Mostly cytoplasm	Fails to tumble
che B	38 000	Mostly cytoplasm	Tumbles incessantly
che Y	8 000	Cytoplasm	Fails to tumble
che Z	24 000	Mostly cytoplasm	Tumbles incessantly
tsr ¶	58 000–65 000	Cytoplasmic membrane	Normal
che D ¶	?	?	Fails to tumble

* Data from Silverman and Simon (1976) except those for *tar* and *tsr* which are from Springer *et al.* (1977a).
† Data from Ridgway *et al.* (1977) except those for *tar* and *tsr* which are from Kort *et al.* (1975).
‡ In the absence of stimuli. Data from Parkinson (1977).
§ Activity of the *che A* gene appears to be correlated with the production of two proteins; similarities between the two suggest that one may be derived from the other (Matsumura *et al.*, 1977).
¶ These two entries may represent alleles of the same gene. See text for details.

different. On the other hand, it has also been suggested that they may represent different genes (Springer *et al.,* 1977a). To further complicate the situation, *che D* has also been used to refer to mutants with the Tsr phenotype (Silverman and Simon, 1977b). Similarly, the *tar* gene has also been called *che M* (Silverman and Simon, 1977b). Hopefully, some common nomenclature will eventually be argreed upon.

1.4.4 Motility mutants

At first glance, this category appears to be of trivial importance. It seems obvious that if a cell cannot swim it will be unable to carry out chemotaxis. However, this obvious point should not obscure the possibility that these non-motile cells may also be defective in some component(s) of the chemotaxis machinery. Due to the intimate relationship between chemotaxis and motility it is not at all unlikely that some of the gene products involved in the functioning of the flagellum should also be involved in the processing of information.
involved in chemotaxis.

Several non-motile phenotypes have been identified. Two genes, *mot A* and *mot B,* control flagellar rotation. The *mot* mutants have flagella, but their flagella are paralyzed (Armstrong and Adler, 1967; Silverman and Simon, 1976). Another sixteen genes, collectively called *fla* genes, control the synthesis and assembly of the flagellar organelle (Silverman and Simon, 1977c), a subcellular structure that is anatomically very complex (de Pamphilis and Adler, 1971). All known *fla* mutants either totally fail to produce the organelle, or produce abnormal, incomplete flagellar structures (Silverman and Simon, 1977c; Suzuki, *et al.,* 1978).

1.5 IDENTIFICATION OF A PROTEIN METHYLATION REACTION INVOLVED IN CHEMOTAXIS

There is one further class of mutations that render cells unable to regulate tumbling behavior, although these mutations are not properly considered chemotaxis mutations since, in addition to abolishing chemotaxis, they have broad effects on cellular function. These are mutations which block the synthesis of the amino acid *L*-methionine In 1967, it was discovered that when a methionine auxotroph is deprived of methionine it loses the ability to tumble, although it can still swim, and thus it cannot carry out chemotaxis. However, normal behavior is readily restored simply by providing the cells with a fresh supply of methionine (Adler and Dahl, 1967). This requirement for a continual supply of methionine does not represent a need for protein synthesis, since cells show normal chemotaxis in the presence of inhibitors of protein synthesis, such as chloramphenicol (Armstrong, 1972a). On the contrary, a number of experiments provide evidence that the methionine requirement actually represents a requirement for *S*-adenosylmethionine (Armstrong, 1972a,b; Aswad and Koshland,

1974; Springer and Koshland, 1977), a compound derived from methionine which serves as a methyl donor in a variety of chemical reactions.

Since the addition of methionine to a methionine-starved cell rapidly restores its ability to carry out chemotaxis it seemed likely that supplying such cells with radioactively labelled methionine would result in a rapid incorporation of the isotope into *S*-adenosylmethionine, and subsequently into other chemotactically active compounds. In order to distinguish compounds that are involved in chemotaxis from those that are not, two criteria may be established: any metabolite (1) whose concentration or whose rate of turnover is affected by chemotactic stimuli, and/or (2) that is present in wild-type cells but missing in one or more mutant strains is likely to participate in some way in the biochemical reactions that underlie the chemotactic response.

Following this line of reasoning, Kort *et al.* (1975) were able to identify a reaction in which the methyl group of methionine is transferred to a protein in the cytoplasmic membrane, and were able to demonstrate that this reaction is involved in chemotaxis. The data that initially led to this conclusion are summarized in Fig. 1.3. In this experiment, radioactive methionine, isotopically labelled only in the methyl group, was supplied to the cells in the presence of a protein synthesis inhibitor. After incubating the cells with the radioactive methionine, all reactions were terminated by the addition of formaldehyde, a highly reactive fixative. Membranes were isolated and then solubilized with the detergent sodium dodecyl sulfate. Subsequently, the solubilized preparation was subjected to polyacrylamide gel electrophoresis, and the gel was exposed to film to produce a photographic image of the distribution of radioactivity. Each dark band in the figure represents a macromolecule that became radioactive due to incorporation of a methyl group from a radioactive methionine molecule. It is worth emphasizing that this radioactivity was not incorporated via protein synthesis, since a protein synthesis inhibitor was present, but rather was incorporated by a methylation reaction. The left-hand sample is from a wild-type strain. A number of radioactively labelled bands can be seen in a 15% polyacrylamide gel, as shown in Fig. 1.3. However, only two of these bands show any indication of involvement in chemotaxis, as judged by the criteria established above. When a mixture of attractants is added to the chemotactically wild-type strain, an increase in the amount of radioactivity incorporated in these bands is seen, while other bands show no change in degree of labelling. This satisfies the first of our criteria and suggests very strongly that the methylation reaction is involved in chemotaxis. In order to confirm this idea, mutants in each of the known chemotaxis genes were tested to see whether any of the mutations would affect the methylation of the two bands. Some of the mutants were dramatically altered in their methylation properties; the third and fourth samples in Fig. 1.3 are from a *che X* mutant, and demonstrate an almost complete lack of incorporation of label into these same two bands, although other methylated bands are not affected by the mutation. Furthermore, the addition of attractant to this strain has no effect on its methylation pattern. Thus, there appears to be a correlation between a methylation defect and a chemotaxis defect. In order to

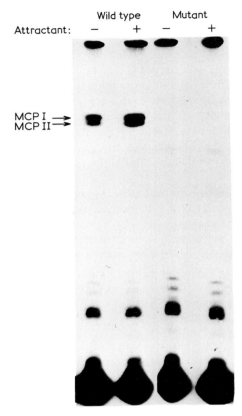

Fig. 1.3 SDS gel electrophoresis patterns of chemotactically wild-type *E. coli* and a *che X* mutant in the presence and absence of attractant. The cells were incubated with L-[methyl-^{3}H]-methionine in the presence of chloramphenicol (50 μg ml^{-1}). For the experiments shown in slots 2 and 4, L-aspartate and α-aminoisobutyrate were added 30 min after the addition of labelled methionine. All reactions were terminated at 60 min by the addition of formalin to 2.5%. Membrane were isolated, dissolved and boiled in sample buffer. Equal amounts of total protein were layered on a 15% polyacrylamide gel, a fluorographic image of which is shown in the figure. See Springer *et al.* (1977a) for procedural details.

show that the correlation is not spurious, due simply to the chance production of two independent mutations, one affecting chemotaxis and the other affecting methylation, a revertant was isolated that could carry out chemotaxis in the normal way. When this revertant was tested for its methylation properties it was found that the methylation defect had also reverted (Kort *et al.*, 1975), indicating that both phenomena are, indeed, a result of the same mutation.

The protein nature of the bands was established by the use of degradative enzymes. Treatment of isolated, labelled membranes with the proteases trypsin and pepsin resulted in the disappearance of the bands, while treatment with nucleases had little or no effect (Kort *et al.*, 1975). The bands were therefore called the methyl-accepting chemotaxis proteins (MCP). The methyl group is attached to one or more glutamic acid residues in these proteins by means of an ester linkage with the free carboxyl group of the amino acid (Kleene *et al.*, 1977; van der Werf and Koshland, 1977).

1.6 TWO COMPLEMENTARY PATHWAYS OF INFORMATION PROCESSING IN CHEMOTAXIS

When MCP is examined on 7% SDS polyacrylamide gels the two bands apparent on 15% gels are further resolved into a series of eight bands that range in molecular weight from 5.6×10^4 to 6.5×10^4 (Springer *et al.*, 1977a) (Fig. 1.4). A screening of the methylation patterns of the behavioral mutants produced the interesting observation that lesions in two genes, *tar* and *tsr*, caused the loss of some but not all of these bands. The *tar* mutants retain a subset of six bands, called MCP I, while the *tsr* mutants retain a subset of four bands, called MCP II (Fig. 1.4) (Springer *et al.*, 1977a). A specially constructed double mutant, carrying both *tsr* and *tar* defects, shows little or no methylation of any MCP bands (Silverman and Simon, 1977b; Springer *et al.*, 1977a).

In a series of deletion mapping experiments with specialized transducing phages carrying the *tar* and *tsr* regions of the *E. coli* chromosome, it has been shown that loss of these genes (as determined by complementation tests with *tsr* and *tar* mutants (Parkinson, 1977; Silverman and Simon, 1977b)) is correlated with a failure to synthesize a set of polypeptides with molecular weights very similar to those of the MCP bands (Silverman and Simon, 1977b). These results, taken together with the methylation defects noted above, suggest strongly that *tsr* and *tar* code for MCP I and MCP II respectively. However, it is not known whether all the bands in this region of the gel are coded for by only these two genes. It appears likely that they are, since the *tsr*–*tar* double mutant fails to methylate the entire set of bands. Alternatively, it may be that some of the methylated bands are not coded for by *tsr* and *tar*, but that these bands cannot be methylated in the double mutant due to the alteration of the *tsr* and *tar* gene products.

If all the bands are indeed coded for by the *tar* and *tsr* genes it is somewhat puzzling that only 8 bands are visible in the wild-type rather than the 10 expected from simple addition of the number of bands present in each of the mutants. This could be explained if some of the bands of MCP I and MCP II overlap, leading to a failure to distinguish them. Close scrutiny of Fig. 1.4 reveals that there are bands present in the *tsr* strain that have very nearly the same position on the gel as do bands in the *tar* strain. Furthermore, the bands that appear in the corresponding position in the wild-type strain are much darker than those observed in either of the

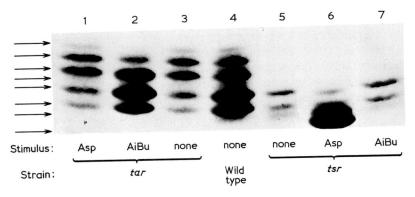

Fig. 1.4 Methylation patterns of the MCP's in wild-type, *tar*, and *tsr* mutants. Equal amounts of protein were layered in the sample wells of one 7% gel. The figure shows a fluorographic image of the region of the gel where proteins of molecular weights 56 000–65 000 are found. Arrows mark the positions of the 8 methylated bands referred to in the text. Note that the lowest band can only be seen clearly when it has been induced to incorporate extra methyl groups by the addition of the type II attractant aspartate (as in sample 6). (1) The *tar* mutant stimulated with 0.01 M L-aspartate. (2) The *tar* mutant stimulated with 0.05 M α-aminoisobutyrate. (3) The *tar* mutant (AW 539) unstimulated. (4) Wild-type unstimulated. (5) The *tsr* mutant unstimulated. (6) The *tsr* mutant stimulated with 0.01 M L-aspartate. (7) The *tsr* mutant (AW 518) stimulated with 0.05 M α-aminoisobutyrate. After Springer *et al.*, (1977a).

mutants, as though two less intense bands had overlapped to produce one of greater intensity.

Regardless of how many genes are ultimately shown to code for the methylated bands, it nevertheless seems clear that *tsr* is responsible for the synthesis of more than one of these bands, as is *tar*. It is not yet understood why a single gene gives rise to a product that migrates as several bands on an SDS gel. However, an analysis of the products of partial proteolytic digestion of the bands coded for by the *tar* gene shows that there is extensive sequence homology among them, which suggests that the *tar* bands may arise from post-translational modification of a single polypeptide (Matsumura *et al.*, 1977).

A combination of behavioral and biochemical experiments has led to the conclusion that there are two main pathways through which information is transmitted and processed in bacterial chemotaxis, one pathway relying on MCP I while the other relies on MCP II (see Fig. 1.5) (Silverman and Simon, 1977b; Springer *et al.*, 1977a). Receptors for one set of stimuli, called type II stimuli, appear to feed information through the pathway defined by MCP II. This is supported by three lines of evidence: (1) responses to type II stimuli are highly defective in *tar* strains, which

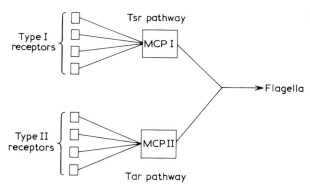

Fig. 1.5 Schematic representation of information flow in bacterial chemotaxis. After Springer *et al.* (1977a).

lack MCP II (Silverman and Simon, 1977b; Springer *et al.,* 1977a); (2) addition to type II stimuli to wild-type strains results in dramatic changes in methylation of MCP II (increases in methylation for type II attractants and decreases in methylation for type II repellents), but little or no change in methylation of MCP I* (Silverman and Simon, 1977b; Springer *et al.,* 1977a); see Fig. 1.4); (3) when several type II stimuli (attractants or repellents) are added simultaneously, the effects of these stimuli on both behavior and extent of methylation are integrated; thus two type II stimuli can make use of the pathway simultaneously (M.F. Goy and M.S. Springer, unpublished results).

In a similar way it has been shown that receptors for another set of stimuli, called type I stimuli, feed information primarily through the pathway defined by MCP I (see Fig. 1.5). However, under some conditions at least, type I receptors can also send information through the MCP II pathway, although the information has reversed its polarity (Muskavitch *et al.,* 1978). In *tsr* mutants, that have lost the MCP I pathway, type I repellents act as attractants and type I attractants may act as very weak repellents; this is apparently accomplished by feeding the information through MCP II in a reversed manner, since type I repellents cause an increase in methylation of MCP II and type I attractants cause a slight decrease in methylation of MCP II in these strains. The significance of this finding is not understood at present; it is not even known whether the phenomenon occurs in the wild-type strain, since overlap of MCP I and MCP II bands prevents the detection of any small 'reversed' changes of methylation in MCP II following type I stimulation.

There is a third set of stimuli that appear able to act through both MCP I and

* It is not possible to tell with complete certainty that there are no changes in methylation of MCP I, because MCP I and II bands overlap considerably. However, it appears unlikely that such changes occur, since when type II stimuli are given to a *tar* mutant, lacking MCP II, no changes in methylation of MCP I are observed (see Fig. 1.4).

Table 1.1 Effect of stimuli

	Receptor	Wild-type behavior	MCP	tar behavior	MCP	tsr behavior	MCP	tsr–tar behavior
Type I stimuli	serine, high affinity (AiBu)	att.	+	att.	+	rep?	slight –	none
	acetate	rep.	n.t.	rep.	n.t.	att.	n.t.	none
	benzoate	rep.	–	rep.	–	att.	+	none
	leucine	rep.	n.t.	rep.	n.t.	att.	n.t.	none
	indole	rep.	–	rep.	n.t.	att.	n.t.	none*
Type II stimuli	aspartate	att.	+	none	none	att.	+	none
	maltose	att.	+	none	none	att.	+	none
	serine, low affinity	att.	+	none	none	att.	+	none
	Ni, Co	rep.	–	none	none	rep.	–	none
Type III stimuli	galactose	att.	n.t.	att.	n.t.	att.	n.t.	none*
	ribose	att.	n.t.	att.	n.t.	att.	n.t.	none*

* In the wild-type strain, type I stimuli affect MCP I while type II stimuli affect MCP II. Only MCP I is present in the *tar* mutants and only MCP II is present in the *tsr* mutants. The *tsr–tar* double mutant lacks all of the methylated bands. Increases and decreases in methylation are indicated by + and – respectively; none means no change; n.t. means not tested. The behavior of the organism in response to stimuli is indicated by att. and rep. for attraction and repulsion respectively. None means no response. In some instances, marked with an asterisk, a stimulus had no effect in spatial assays but did produce some residual response in temporal assays. This may indicate either leakiness in the mutations or the existence of a third pathway (see text).

MCP II, since responses to these stimuli are not eliminated in either the *tsr* or the *tar* mutant, but *are* extremely defective in a *tsr−tar* double mutant (Mesibor and Adler, 1972; Silverman and Simon, 1977b; Springer *et al.,* 1977a). However, these compounds do have some residual effects on the behavior of *tsr−tar* strains (M.S. Springer and M.F. Goy, unpublished observations); thus, it may be that they act through an as-yet-unidentified third pathway that requires the presence of MCP I and MCP II in order to function properly. We call these type III stimuli. Table 1.1 presents a list of the various stimuli, classed by types, and indicates their effects on behavior and methylation.

1.7 METHYLATION PATTERN OF THE *fla, mot,* AND *che* MUTANTS

In addition to *tsr* and *tar,* mutations in a number of the *fla* and *che* genes have substantial effects on the methylation of MCP I and MCP II (Kort *et al.,* 1975; Silverman and Simon, 1977b; Springer *et al.,* 1977a, 1978). In all cases tested, mutations in any of the *fla* genes, which lead to an inability to synthesize normal flagella (Silverman and Simon, 1977c), also lead to an inability to incorporate label into MCP I and MCP II (Kort *et al.,* 1975; Springer *et al.,* 1978). This suggests that the MCP's are components of the flagellum, that they require the presence of an intact flagellum to function normally, or that their synthesis is co-regulated with the synthesis of the *fla* gene products. However, it is not necessary for the flagellum to be functional in order for methylation to occur, since *mot* mutants, which have paralyzed flagella, show normal methylation of the MCP's (Springer *et al.,* 1978).

When the *che* genes are tested, it is found that some of these genes are important in methylation but some are not (Kort *et al.,* 1975; Silverman and Simon, 1977b; Springer *et al.,* 1977a, 1978). Mutations in *che B, che D,* and *che X* produce strains that have both substantially decreased levels of incorporation and abnormal distributions of label in the MCP bands. Lesions in the other *che* genes have much less severe effects or none at all. It is interesting to note that those mutations which do substantially alter methylation affect bands in *both* MCP I and MCP II.

The products of some of these genes undoubtedly constitute the enzymes which methylate and demethylate the MCP's. In some way the methylating/de-methylating system must generate the specificity which allows the methylation of either MCP I or MCP II, but not both, to be altered in response to a given stimulus. The most straighforward mechanism by which this could be accomplished would be for the cell to employ separate methylating and demethylating enzymes for MCP I and MCP II. If this were the case, a methylase or demethylase-deficient mutant would be defective in chemotaxis either to the stimuli acting through MCP I or to the stimuli acting through MCP II, but not to both. Mutants defective in response to type I stimuli have the Tsr phenotype, and all the known mutants with this phenotype fall into one complementation group (Reader *et al.,* 1978), which defines the *tsr* gene.

As indicated above, this gene likely codes for MCP I. Similarly, all the known muta-tions blocking type II responses lie in the *tar* gene (Reader *et al.,* 1978), which probably codes for MCP II. No other Tsr- or Tar-type mutants exist to define an MCP I- or MCP II-specific methylase or demethylase. Furthermore, as mentioned above, all of the *che* mutations either do not affect methylation, or else they affect methylation of *both* MCP I and MCP II. Thus, no mutants have been isolated that show the properties required by a mechanism that employs separate methylating enzymes for the two MCP's, a result which implies that a single enzyme methylates both proteins.

Two other mechanisms can be envisioned for producing the required specificity. The first possibility is that the specificity does not lie in the methylating enzyme, but rather is vested in the MCP polypeptides themselves. Thus a particular stimulus might cause MCP I or MCP II to be altered in such a way that a change in its level of methylation takes place. The second, and equally likely, possibility is that specificity is achieved by regulating the activity of the methylating enzyme. For example, the relative ability to methylate MCP I or MCP II may be determined by regulatory sites on the enzyme which receive information from the chemoreceptors. In this regard, it is interesting to note that *che Z* mutants respond much better to aspartate (which acts through MCP II) than to serine (which acts largely through MCP I), whereas *che B* mutants respond much better to serine than to aspartate (Parkinson, 1974, 1977) When the methylation properties of these mutants are studied, it is found that *che Z* mutants, which show more or less normal methylation in the absence of stimuli, can alter their level of methylation in response to an aspartate stimulus somewhat more effectively than to a serine stimulus. Similarly, *che B* mutants, although relatively poor at methylating the MCP's to begin with, can nevertheless alter the level of methylation in response to stimuli, and do so more effectively to a serine stimulus than to an aspartate stimulus (Springer *et al.,* 1978). Thus, the *che Z* and *che B* gene products could serve as regulatory subunits which modulate the activity of the methylating enzyme, the *che B* gene product regulating methylation of MCP II in response to type II stimuli while the *che Z* gene product regulates methylation of MCP I in response to type I stimuli.

Although lesions in a number of genes affect the methylation of both MCP I and MCP II, the product of the *che X* gene is the most likely candidate for the catalytic function of the methylating and/or demethylating enzyme. A methylase mutant should be unable to methylate either of the MCP's; hence, it is expected to show very little incorporation of label into these bands. A demethylase mutant should be unable to demethylate the MCP's; hence, there should be no available sites for methylation when the radioactive methionine is added, and it is also expected to show very little incorporation of label. Mutations in *che X* produce strains which incorporate very few radioactive methyl groups into either MCP I or MCP II. Mutations in the other *che* genes have effects which are much less severe. In *Salmonella typhimurium* a species of bacteria related to *E. coli,* it has been suggested on the basis of this type of evidence that the *che R* gene, which corresponds genetically to the *che X* gene in

E. coli (Parkinson, 1978b), codes for the methylating enzyme (Springer and Koshland, 1977). Furthermore, *in vitro* methylation experiments with *Salmonella*, in which wild-type or mutant membranes containing acceptor proteins were mixed with wild-type or mutant cytoplasmic preparations containing the *che R* gene product, are consistent with this hypothesis: *che R* membranes could be methylated by the wild-type soluble fraction but wild-type membranes could not be methylated by the *che R* soluble fraction (Springer and Koshland, 1977).

The biochemical role of any of the *che, fla* and *mot* gene products, with the possible exception of *che X*, remains uncertain. Some of the genes may code for components involved in the control of methylation, and mutants with altered methylation properties are likely to represent genes of this type. Mutations in other genes have no apparent effect on methylation; these defects may occur at other stages of the chemotactic response, such as in the control of sensory excitation, or in the linkage between the methylation of the MCP's and the final control of the direction of flagellar rotation. Several genes are needed to code for the molecular gears that permit clockwise and counterclockwise rotation of the flagella, and for the molecular gearshift that permits the cell to change from one direction of rotation to the other. The products of the *fla, mot, che A, che C, che W* and *che Y* genes may function in these, or similar, capacities.

1.8 INVOLVEMENT OF THE METHYLATION REACTION IN SENSORY ADAPTATION

The data summarized in the preceding pages demonstrate that the methylation of MCP I and II is intimately involved in the mechanism that underlies bacterial chemotaxis. However these results do not indicate what the nature of that role might be. This question can be investigated directly by blocking the methylation reaction. If some particular aspect (or aspects) of the behavioral response is dependent on methylation, then a block of the methylation reaction will eliminate that part of the response. Two methods have been used to inhibit methylation, both of which have similar behavioral effects. The first procedure depends on depleting cells of the methyl donor by starving them of methionine. When a methionine auxotroph is washed free of methionine it still has a substantial internal pool of the amino acid, and a starvation period of some minutes is required to eliminate this pool. Thus these cells do not immediately lose the ability to tumble when methionine is removed, and they can be shown to respond to attractants during the starvation period. However, these responses have become abnormally prolonged (Aswad and Koshland, 1974; Springer *et al.*, 1975). If the cells are examined at longer and longer intervals after the removal of methionine, during which the residual intracellular pools of methionine presumably become further and further depleted, the time required to adapt to the stimulus grow steadily longer (Fig. 1.6) (Springer *et al.*, 1975). Thus adaptation appears to become more and more defective as the cells have less and

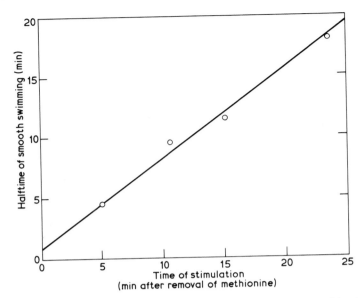

Fig. 1.6 Effect of methionine starvation on adaptation time. A methionine auxotroph of AW620, a tumbling mutant, was washed free of methionine at time 0. It was tested for response to the attractant L-serine $(1 \times 10^{-5}$ M) at the times indicated. Addition of methionine to cells starved for 25 min decreased the duration of the response to 60 s, which is the same as that found for unstarved cells. After Springer *et al.* (1975).

less methionine available. In order to test this idea more directly, several cultures of chemotactically wild-type bacteria were starved completely for methionine, and all but one were subjected to various attractant stimuli (Springer *et al.*, 1977b). The cells were subsequently incubated with the attractant, in the absence of methionine, for a long period of time in order to allow adaptation to occur, if indeed it could occur at all. Following this incubation period, methionine was added back to the cultures and the behavior of the cells was observed. In the control culture, which had never been exposed to attractant, normal swimming and tumbling resumed very shortly after the methionine was added. However, in every case where the cells had been stimulated with an attractant, an extended period of smooth swimming followed the addition of methionine. This period of smooth swimming represented the adaptation process, which had been arrested in the absence of methionine and could only occur when the amino acid was added back. The duration of the smooth swimming period was directly proportional to the length of the response that would have been observed had the attractant been given in the presence of methionine; however, for every attractant tested, this smooth-swimming interval was always 20% shorter than the normal adaptation time. This suggests that, although the bulk of the adaptation process is totally dependent on the presence of methionine, some part of the process is methionine-independent.

These findings indicate that the methylation reaction is involved in sensory adaptation, since in the absence of methionine neither adaptation nor methylation occurs. However, this does not prove the point, since starvation for methionine could have other effects on cellular metabolism, not related to methylation, that interfere with the adaptation process. Therefore, a second method of blocking the reaction was employed, since confirmation by an independent procedure would substantially strengthen the hypothesis.

The second procedure depends on the use of mutants that are unable to carry out the methylation reaction. For this purpose a *che X* mutant was chosen, since this strain still has the MCP polypeptides present in the membrane but lacks the ability to transfer methyl groups to them (Springer and Koshland, 1977; M.L. Toews and S. J. Kleene, unpublished results). When the *che X* mutant was subjected to attractant or repellent stimuli it initiated the appropriate changes in tumbling frequency. However, these responses were found to be unusually prolonged (Goy *et al.,* 1978; Parkinson, 1978b). For example, when 50 mM α-aminoisobutyrate (an attractant) was added to a culture of wild-type cells, the bacteria responded with a period of smooth swimming that lasted approximately five minutes, but when the same stimulus was added to the *che X* mutant, the cells showed no indication of adapting to the stimulus after more than 70 minutes (Goy *et al.,* 1978).

Thus, by a second, independent method we find that sensory adaptation cannot occur if the methylation reaction is blocked. Since the two approaches rely on different techniques to interfere with methylation they can, in some ways, serve as controls for one another. The only obvious property that *che X* mutants and methionine-starved, chemotactically wild-type cells have in common is an inability to carry out the methylation reaction, which suggests very strongly that it is, indeed, this defect that is the cause of the defect in adaptation.

The findings with the *che X* mutants in particular, bring up an important point. We have separated the chemotactic response into two processes, called excitation and adaptation, without really justifying this separation. The results obtained with the mutants allow us to state with some confidence that excitation and adaptation truly are two different processes, since excitation still occurs in these strains, although they have lost the ability to adapt due to the mutation.

1.9 INVOLVEMENT OF THE METHYLATED PROTEINS IN SENSORY EXCITATION

It is expected then that the *tsr, tar* and *tsr–tar* strains, which fail to carry out the methylation reaction due to a lack of functional acceptor protein, should also fail to carry out the adaptation process. However, when these mutants are tested with the appropriate stimuli it is found that they are defective in their ability to even *initiate* responses. The *tsr–tar* strain shows little or no change in tumbling frequency in response to any stimulus tested (Silverman and Simon, 1977b; Springer *et al,* 1977a).

Similarly the *tar* mutant, although it responds perfectly well to type I attractants and repellents, fails to initiate any response to type II stimuli. The *tsr* mutant does initiate responses to type I stimuli, but as described above, these responses are reversed in polarity, and appear in some way to be mediated by the MCP II pathway. Thus, even in *tsr*, the 'normal' process of excitation to type I stimuli is defective and has been replaced by an 'abnormal' process. These data suggest that the MCP molecules are essential not only in sensory adaptation, but in sensory excitation as well (Silverman and Simon, 1977b; Springer *et al.*, 1977a). However, it appears that some property of these polypeptides, other than their ability to be methylated, is responsible for this latter role, since *che X* strains, which have the MCP's but cannot methylate them, are capable of sensory excitation.

1.10 RELATIONSHIP OF THE PROPERTIES OF THE METHYLATION REACTION TO THE SENSORY ADAPTATION PROCESS

The data summarized in the preceding pages indicate convincingly that the methylation of MCP I and MCP II plays a role in sensory adaptation, since two independent methods of blocking methylation also result in a block of sensory adaptation. How could this chemical reaction function in adaptation? Following the delivery of a stimulus, two very different types of changes, both related to the adaptation process, must occur in the biochemical machinery that controls the chemotactic response. The first of these is a transient change in some parameter that regulates the direction of flagellar rotation. This parameter must change with a time course identical to the response itself, since it is in fact the biochemical analogue of the response. The second change, as described in detail earlier in this article, is a long-term alteration in the parameter that regulates the cell's sensitivity (or state of adaptation) to chemicals in the environment. A detailed study of the methylation reaction reveals that its characterisitics are consistent with the second role, but not the first (Goy *et al.*, 1977).

Fig. 1.7 illustrates some of the basic properties of the methylation of MCP I (identical data have been obtained for MCP II). Radioactive methionine is given at time zero, and is incorporated into MCP I until a stable plateau is reached. Apparently, the cells maintain a basal level of methylation in the absence of stimuli. If a type I attractant is given (at the arrow) the level of methylation of MCP I increases until a new plateau is reached. The methylation will remain at this new level indefinitely, as long as the attractant is present, and returns to the basal level only when the attractant is removed. Thus methylation has exactly the properties required of a parameter that regulates the cell's sensitivity to the stimulus. If so, this implies that the level of methylation at any point in time represents the state of adaptation of the cell at that time. Thus, (1) the level of methylation observed before the stimulus is added represents a state in which the cell is fully sensitive to the stimulus; (2) the increase in methylation that follows the attractant stimulus corresponds to the

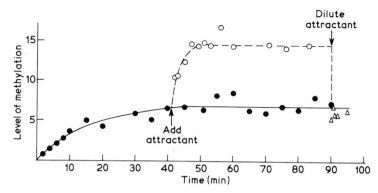

Fig. 1.7 Effects of the addition and removal of attractant on the methylation of MCP I. The 'level of methylation' of each sample is the amount of radioactivity in MCP I (as determined by densitometric scans of the MCP I bands) divided by the total protein concentration. This value is expressed in arbitrary units. Tritiated methionine was added at time zero. After 40 min of incubation the culture was divided in two. One group of cells (○) was stimulated by addition of the attractant α-aminoisobutyrate (50 mM final concentration), while the other group of cells (●) received no addition. The concentration of α-amino-isobutyrate was subsequently lowered by diluting the adapted cells 100-fold into medium containing no α-aminoisobutyrate (△) (Goy *et al.,* 1977). A 100-fold dilution of the adapted cells into medium containing α-amino-isobutyrate had no effect on the level of methylation (data not shown). Analogous data have been obtained for MCP II. From Goy *et al.* (1977), reproduced with permission of M. Goy, M. Springer, J. Adler, and the National Academy of Sciences, U.S.A.

process of adaptation itself; (3) the final steady-state level of methylation represents the state of complete adaptation to the stimulus, and maintenance of the level corresponds to the maintenance of the adapted state; and (4) demethylation, which results from removal of the attractant, represents the process of de-adaptation whereby sensitivitiy is re-established.

A considerable body of evidence supports these hypotheses (Goy *et al.,* 1977). First, the methylation and demethylation reactions show the same characteristic asymmetry as do the adaptation and de-adaptation processes. Specifically, methylation, like the process of adaptation which follows addition of an attractant, is slow, while demethylation, like the process of de-adaptation which follows removal of an attractant, is fast (see Fig. 1.7). Second, if the methylation reaction actually controls the adaptation process the cells should respond to the attractant only while the level of methylation is increasing. Data have been obtained which indicate that the time required for the increase in methylation is very similar to the time required for adaptation. In fact, when two stimuli are compared it is found that the ratio of the

Table 1.2 Correlation of behavioral properties with methylation of MCP

---

(1) If the methylation reaction is blocked adaptation does not occur.
(2) The attractant-induced increase in methylation and the half-time of this reaction are directly proportional to the adaptation time.
(3) Different stimuli presented simultaneously produce additive effects on the methylation reaction and the adaptation time.
(4) Attractants and repellents have opposite effects on both the methylation reaction and the behavior.
(5) Adaptation and methylation are slow.
(6) De-adaptation and demethylation are fast.
(7) Maintenance of the adapted state and maintenance of the attractant-induced level of methylation are both methionine-independent.
(8) De-adaptation and demethylation are both methionine-independent.

---

half-times of the responses to these two stimuli is equal to the ratio of the half-times of the methylation induced by the stimuli. Third, as discussed earlier, the parameter responsible for adaptation must undergo a long-term change that records the presence of the stimulus quantitatively as well as qualitatively. In agreement with this, it was found that the overall change in the steady-state level of methylation following an attractant stimulus is directly proportional to the change in the size of the stimulus, as detected by the chemoreceptors. Fourth, it has been found that, although adaptation is methionine-dependent, neither maintenance of the state of adaptation nor de-adaptation are dependent on the presence of the amino acid. In analogy with this, it was demonstrated that methylation requires the presence of methionine, but neither maintenance of an attractant-induced level of methylation nor demethylation when the attractant is removed require it. Several other correlations exist that provide additional evidence along these lines (see Table 1.2). Taken together, these observations are all consistent with the idea that the state of methylation of MCP I and MCP II regulates the state of adaptation of the bacterial cell as it encounters chemotactic stimuli in its environment. Table 1.2 provides a summary of all the data that support this idea.

1.11 THE TUMBLE REGULATOR

Regulation of the behavioral response must ultimately be manifested as control over the direction of flagellar rotation. Since the flagellum can rotate in either direction there appears to be a switching mechanism that allows the organelle to alternate between clockwise and counterclockwise rotation. Therefore, there should be some parameter that controls the state of the switch, and this parameter must be coupled to the excitation and adaptation processes. This parameter has been called the tumble regulator.

The tumble regulator directly controls the response by determining whether the cell swims or tumbles. For example, when an attractant is added the tumble regulator undergoes a transient change, first switching the cell exclusively into the smooth swimming mode, and subsequently returning the cell to the behavior that existed before the stimulus was given. This sort of transient phenomenon was alluded to earlier as one of two necessary changes which must occur in the chemotaxis machinery following a stimulus. It is an essential element of the chemotactic response and, hence, establishing the identity of the tumble regulator is central to understanding the molecular mechanisms that underlie the behavior.

In a species of chemotactic bacteria called *Bacillus subtilis,* recent evidence indicates that the intracellular concentration of calcium ions could play a role in tumble regulation (Ordal, 1977). By means of a calcium ionophore, Ordal was able to quantitatively control the intracellular levels of this ion. He showed that at very low levels an individual cell swims smoothly; at somewhat higher levels it shows mixed smooth swimming and tumbling; and at still higher levels it tumbles continuously. Normally, in bacteria the internal concentration of free calcium is fairly low, and is maintained at this level by an energy-driven efflux pump (Rosen and McClees, 1974; Silver *et al.,* 1975). If changes in intracellular calcium are important in chemotaxis, then some mechanism must exist to provide these changes, such as a process which selectively alters the permeability of the membrane to calcium. In this regard, there is evidence (Szmelcman and Adler, 1976), although it is not uncontested (Miller and Koshland, 1977), that membrane potential changes are associated with the chemotactic response. Thus, it is not unreasonable to imagine that the bacterial cell regulates its internal calcium ion concentration by a mechanism involving trans-membrane fluxes of the ion, and that the internal calcium concentration in turn controls the direction of flagellar rotation.

1.12 A MODEL FOR THE CHEMOTACTIC RESPONSE

In this section we would like to develop a *hypothetical* model which illustrates one possible scheme by which the methylation of the MCP molecules can be integrated into an overall mechanism that underlies bacterial chemotaxis. As described above, some parameter, called the tumble regulator, must directly control the rotation of the flagella. We assume for our model that this tumble regulator is the intracellular concentration of calcium ions. When the concentration of calcium is low the flagella rotate counterclockwise and the cell swims smoothly. When the concentration is high, rotation is clockwise and the cell tumbles. This internal concentration, which is lower than that of the surrounding medium, is controlled by a pump that regulates efflux and a gate, postulated to be the MCP molecules, that regulates influx. The operation of the pump is assumed to be unaffected by chemotactic stimuli. However, the relative permeability of the gate is *not* independent of the addition of stimuli. Rather, the net permeability at any time is determined by the interaction of two competing processes. One process, which we have called excitation, tends to close

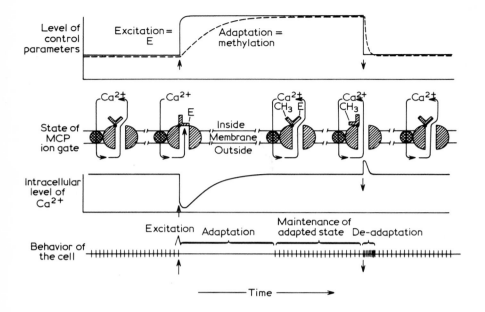

Fig. 1.8 A model for bacterial chemotaxis. Two control parameters, excitation and adaptation, regulate the operation of a gate (⬤◗) composed of MCP molecules, which in turn regulates the rate of influx of Ca^{2+} into the cell. The nature of the excitation parameter, designated as $-E$, is unknown. The adaptation parameter is the state of methylation of the MCP molecules, and is designated as $-CH_3$. Efflux of Ca^{2+} is controlled by a pump (⬤) which is assumed to be unaffected by chemotactic stimuli.

The levels of the control parameters are indicated at the top of the figure, as a function of time. Addition and removal of attractant occur at the first arrow (↑) and second arrow (↓) respectively. Immediately below this the state of the MCP ion gate is shown at various times: prior to the addition of attractant, immediately following addition, after the completion of adaptation, immediately following removal of attractant, and after completion of de-adaptation. The effects of the attractant on the intracellular level of Ca^{2+} and the behavior of the cell are also shown in the figure. See text for details.

For the sake of simplicity the gates have been shown in a continuum of states from fully open to fully closed. Biological precedent suggests that this type of gate typically has only two states: open and closed. In such a case the excitation and adaptation parameters would change the probability of whether a particular gate is open or closed, and thus would regulate the average number of gates in a population that are in a given state.

We have not specified the composition of the gates *vis-a-vis* MCP I and MCP II. The behavior of *tsr* and *tar* mutants, including a deletion mutant of *tar*, suggests that if the MCP molecules function as ion gates it is likely that an individual gate is composed exclusively of MCP I or exclusively of MCP II.

the gate to calcium, thereby decreasing the rate of entry of calcium into the cell. The other process, adaptation, has the opposite effect; it acts by methylating the gate molecules, which increases their permeability to calcium.

When the system is at rest, that is, when the cell is not responding to any stimulus, these two opposing processes are balanced so that the intracellular calcium is at a concentration that allows both smooth swimming and tumbling (see Fig. 1.8). Now an attractant is added. The chemoreceptors immediately produce a signal that results in a rapid increase in the activity of the excitatory process. This in turn leads to a decrease in the permeability of the gate, and the intracellular concentration of calcium falls. Tumbling is suppressed. At the same time, the receptor signal also causes a slower increase in the methylation of the MCP's. This tends to counteract the effects of the excitatory process. The permeability to calcium increases at the level of methylation increases, and thus the intracellular concentration of calcium begins to return to the resting level. Ultimately, when the new plateau level of methylation is reached, the two processes are again in balance, and the concentration of calcium is again at a level that allows both smooth swimming and tumbling. Thus the cell has adapted, and the response is terminated. When the attractant is removed, both the excitatory parameter and the level of methylation fall to their original value. However, the removal of methyl groups lags slightly behind the reversal of the effects of excitation. Hence there is a brief period during which the gate is more permeable than usual to calcium, resulting in a brief tumbling response. Once this is completed the cell has de-adapted and is ready to respond again.

At the heart of this model is the idea that there are two parameters, one excitational and the other adaptational, which change at different rates following a stimulus. This is a concept that has a long history in sensory biology (Delbruck and Reichardt, 1956), and has been proposed previously to explain some of the phenomena of bacterial chemotaxis (Berg and Tedesco, 1975; MacNab and Koshland, 1974). Whatever the merits of the scheme presented in the preceding paragraph, it appears that the processes of excitation and adaptation can be separated, as in the *che X* mutants, a finding which lends considerable support to two-process models in general.

1.13 CONCLUDING REMARKS

In summary, we know that in *E. coli* the sensory transduction process involves a methylation reaction in which two sets of proteins (MCP I and MCP II) serve as the methyl-accepting substrates. In addition, we know that the acceptor proteins play some role in the process of sensory excitation, and that the state of methylation of these proteins very likely regulates the process of sensory adaptation. Furthermore, some preliminary experiments indicate that excitation and adaptation may act to control the intracellular level of calcium ions. However, a large number of unanswered questions remain. First and formost, what is the actual function of the MCP molecules? Do they serve as an ion gate, as suggested above, or do they play some other role in the chemotactic response? In some way, the function of these molecules must be regulated by the addition or removal of methyl groups and, furthermore, their function must be affected by some as-yet-undefined excitational process. However, the exact mechanisms remain obscure. A second question concerns the nature of the linkage between the receptors and the MCP molecules, and between the MCP's and the flagella. In some way, information must be transferred from each of these locations to the next step in the sequence, but the way in which this is accomplished is unknown. Third, what is the explanation for the unusual multiplicity of bands derived from the MCP I and MCP II gene products? Does each band serve a unique function, or is the phenomenon simply an artifact? Fourth, what is the function of each of the *che, fla,* and *mot* gene products in chemotaxis and motility? Answers to these questions will likely provide a complete understanding of the sensory transduction process in *E. coli*.

One final question deserves special comment. This question concerns the relationship between the phenomena observed in *E. coli* and the cellular behaviors found in eukaryotic neurons or sensory receptor cells. In each case the cell acts as a signal transducer, and the analogies are striking. In support of the idea of universality of sensory transduction mechanisms, there is preliminary evidence in one eukaryotic system that the biochemistry which underlies the behavioral response includes a methylation reaction similar to that found in *E. coli*: O'Dea *et al.* (1978) have recently demonstrated that leukocyte chemotaxis involves changes in the activity of a methyltransferase system whose properties appear at first glance to be similar to those described for *E. coli*. However, the ability of *E. coli* to provide insights into the workings of eukaryotic systems will de determined in the long run by how conservative nature is in preserving the molecular mechanisms that underlie information transduction.

REFERENCES

Adler, J. (1975), Chemotaxis in Bacteria. *A. Rev. Biochem.,* **44**, 341–356.

Adler, J. and Dahl, M.M. (1967), A method for measuring the motility of bacteria and for comparing random and non-random motility. *J. gen. Microbiol.,***46**, 161–173.

Adler, J. and Epstein, W. (1974), Phosphotransferase-system enzymes as chemo-receptors for certain sugars in *Escherichia coli* chemotaxis. *Proc. natn. Acad. Sci. U.S.A.,* **71**, 2895–2899.

Adler, J., Hazelbauer, G.L. and Dahl, M.M. (1973), Chemotaxis towards sugar in *Escherichia coli. J. Bact.,* **115**, 824–847.

Aksamit, R.R. and Koshland, D.E., Jr. (1974), Identification of the ribose binding protein as the receptor for ribose chemotaxis in *Salmonella typhimurium. Biochemistry,* **13**, 473–478.

Armstrong, J.B. (1972a), Chemotaxis and methionine metabolism in *Escherichia coli. Can. J. Microbiol.,* **18**, 591–596.

Armstrong, J.B. (1972b), An *S*-adenosylmethionine requirement for chemotaxis in *Escherichia coli. Can. J. Microbiol.,* **18**, 1695–1701.

Armstrong, J.B. and Adler, J. (1967), Genetics of motility in *Escherichia coli*: complementation of paralyzed mutants. *Genetics,* **56**, 363—373.

Armstrong, J.B. and Adler, J. (1969), Complementation of non-chemotactic mutants of *Escherichia coli. Genetics,* **61**, 61—66.

Armstrong, J.B., Adler, J. and Dahl, M.M. (1967), Non-chemotactic mutants of *Escherichia coli. J. Bact.,* **93**, 390—398.

Aswad, D. and Koshland, D.E. Jr. (1974), Role of methionine in bacterial chemotaxis. *J. Bact.,* **118**, 640—645.

Berg, H.C. (1975), Bacterial behavior. *Nature,* **254**, 389—392.

Berg, H.C. and Anderson, R.A. (1973), Bacteria swim by rotating their flagellar filaments. *Nature,* **245**, 380—382.

Berg, H.C. and Brown, D.A. (1972), Chemotaxis in *Escherichia coli.* analysed by three-dimensional tracking. *Nature,* **239**, 500—504.

Berg, H.C. and Tedesco, P.M. (1975), Transient response to chemotactic stimuli in *Escherichia coli. Proc. natn. Acad. Sci. U.S.A.,* **72**, 3235—3239.

Boos, W., Gordon, A.S., Hall, R.E. and Price, H.D. (1972), Transport properties of the galactose-binding protein of *Escherichia coli:* substrate-induced conformational change. *J. biol. Chem.,* **247**, 917—924.

Brown, D.A. and Berg, H.C. (1974), Temporal stimulation of chemotaxis in *Escherichia coli. Proc. natn. Acad. Sci. U.S.A.,* **71**, 1388—1392.

Delbruck, M. and Reichardt, W. (1956), System analysis for the light growth reactions of phycomyces. In: *Cellular Mechanisms in Differentiation and Growth,* (Rudnick, D., ed), Princeton University Press, Princeton University, pp. 3—44.

De Pamphilis, M.L. and Adler, J. (1971), Fine structure and isolation of the hook-basal body complex of flagella from *Escherichia coli* and *Bacillus subtilis. J. Bact.,* **105**, 384—395.

Engelmann, T.W. (1883), *Bacterium photometricum.* Ein Beitrag zur vergleichenden Physiologie des Licht- und Farbensinnes. *Pfluegers Arch. Gesamte Physiol. Menschen Tiere.,* **30**, 95—124.

Goy, M.F., Springer, M.S. and Adler, J. (1977), Sensory transduction in *Escherichia coli:* role of a protein methylation reaction in sensory adaptation. *Proc. natn. Acad. Sci. U.S.A.,* **74**, 4964—4968.

Goy, M.F., Springer, M.S. and Adler, J. (1978), in preparation.

Hazelbauer, G.L. (1975), Maltose chemoreceptor of *Escherichia coli. J. Bact.,* **122**, 206—214.

Hazelbauer, G.L. and Adler, J. (1971), Role of the galactose binding protein in chemotaxis of *Escherichia coli.* toward galactose. *Nature New Biol.,* **230**, 101—104.

Hazelbauer, G.L. and Parkinson, J.S. (1977), Bacterial chemotaxis. In: *Microbial Interactions,* Receptors and Recognition Series B Vol. 3, (Reissig, J. ed), Chapman and Hall, London.

Kleene, S.J., Toews, M.L. and Adler, J. (1977), Isolation of glutamic acid methyl ester from an *Escherichia coli.* membrane protein involved in chemotaxis. *J. biol. Chem.,* **252**, 3214—3218.

Kort, E.N., Goy, M.F., Larsen, S.H. and Adler, J. (1975), Methylation of a membrane protein involved in bacterial chemotaxis. *Proc. natn. Acad. Sci. U.S.A.,* **72**, 3939—3943.

Koshland, D.E. Jr. (1976), Sensory Response in Bacteria. In: *Advances in Neuro-chemistry,* (Agranoff, B.W. and Aprison, M.H. eds.), Plenum Press, New York and London.

Koshland, D.E. Jr. (1977), A response regulator model in a simple sensory system. *Science,* **196,** 1055—1063.

Larsen, S.H., Reader, R.W., Kort, E.N., Tso, W.-W. and Adler, J. (1974), Change in direction of flagellar rotation is the basis of the chemotactic response in *Escherichia coli. Nature,* **249,** 74—77.

Leifson, E. (1960), *Atlas of Bacterial Flagellation.* Academic Press, New York.

Lengeler, J. (1975), Mutations affecting transport of the hexitols D-mannitol, D-glucitol, and galactitol in *Escherichia coli.* K12: isolation and mapping. *J. Bact.,* **124,** 26—38.

MacNab, R.M. (1977), Bacterial flagella rotating in bundles: a study in helical geometry. *Proc. natn. Acad. Sci. U.S.A.,* **74,** 221—225.

MacNab, R.M. and Koshland, D.E. Jr. (1972), The gradient-sensing mechanism in bacterial chemotaxis. *Proc. natn. Acad. Sci. U.S.A.,* **69,** 2509—2512.

MacNab, R. and Koshland, D.E. Jr. (1974), Bacterial motility and chemotaxis: Light-induced tumbling response and visualization of individual flagella. *J. mol. Biol.,* **84,** 399—406.

Matsumura, P., Silverman, M. and Simon, M. (1977), Synthesis of *mot* and *che* gene products of *Escherichia coli.* programmed by hybrid Col E1 plasmids in minicells. *J. Bact.,* **132,** 996—1002.

Mesibov, R. and Adler, J. (1972), Chemotaxis towards amino acids in *Escherichia coli. J. Bact.,* **112,** 315—326.

Miller, J.B. and Koshland, D.E. Jr. (1977), Sensory electrophysiology of bacteria: relationship of the membrane potential to motility and chemotaxis in *Bacillus subtilis. Proc. natn. Acad. Sci. U.S.A.,* **74,** 4752—4756.

Muskavitch, M.M., Kort, E.N., Springer, M.S., Goy, M.F. and Adler, J. (1978), Attraction by repellents: an error in sensory information processing by bacterial mutants. *Science,* in press.

O'Dea, R.F., Viveros, O.H., Aswanikumar, S., Schiffman, E., Corcoran, B.A. and Axelrod, J. (1978), Rapid stimulation of protein carboxymethylation in leukocytes by a chemotactic peptide. *Nature,* in press.

Ordal, G.W. (1977), Calcium ion regulates chemotactic behavior in bacteria. *Nature,* **270,** 66—67.

Ordal, G.W. and Adler, J. (1974), Isolation and complementation of mutants in galactose taxis and transport. *J. Bact.,* **117,** 509—516.

Parkinson, J.S. (1974), Chemotaxis in *Escherichia coli:* Data processing by the chemotaxis machinery of *Escherichia coli. Nature,* **252,** 317—319.

Parkinson, J.S. (1976), *che A, che B,* and *che C* genes of *Escherichia coli* and their role in chemotaxis. *J. Bact.,* **126,** 758—770.

Parkinson, J.S. (1977), Behavioral genetics in bacteria. *A. Rev. Genet.,* **11,** 397—414.

Parkinson, J.S. (1978a), Complementation analysis and deletion mapping of *Escherichia coli* mutants defective in chemotaxis. *J. Bact.,* in press.

Parkinson, J.S. (1978b), in preparation.

Pfeffer, W. (1883), Locomotorische Richtungsbewegungen durch chemische Reize. *Berichte der Deutschen Botanischen Gesellschaft,* **1,** 524—533.

Reader, R.W., Tso, W.-W., Goy, M.F., Springer, M.S. and Adler, J. (1978), in preparation.

Ridgeway, H.F., Silverman, M. and Simon, M.I. (1977), Localization of proteins controlling motility and chemotaxis in *Escherichia coli. J. Bact.,* **132,** 657–665.

Rosen, B.P. and McClees, J.S. (1974), Active transport of calcium in inverted vesicles of *Escherichia coli. Proc. natn. Acad. Sci. U.S.A.,* **71,** 5042–5046.

Schenk, S.L. (1893), Die Thermotaxis der Mikroorganismen und ihre Bezeihung zur Erkaltung. *Zentr. Bakteriol. Parasitenk.,* **14,** 33–43.

Silver, S., Toth, K. and Scribner, H. (1975), Facilitated transport of calcium by cells and subcellular membranes of *Bacillus subtilis* and *Escherichia coli. J. Bact.,* **122,** 880–885.

Silverman, M. and Simon, M. (1974), Flagellar rotation and the mechanism of bacterial motility. *Nature,* **249,** 73–74.

Silverman, M. and Simon, M. (1976), Genes controlling motility and chemotaxis in *Escherichia coli:* the mocha operon. *Nature,* **264,** 577–580.

Silverman, M. and Simon, M. (1977a), Identification of polypeptides necessary for chemotaxis in *Escherichia coli. J. Bact.,* **130,** 1317–1325.

Silverman, M. and Simon, M. (1977b), Chemotaxis in *Escherichia coli:* methylation of *che* gene products. *Proc. natn. Acad. Sci. U.S.A.,* **74,** 3317–3321.

Silverman, M. and Simon, M. (1977c), Bacterial flagella. *A. Rev. Microbiol.,* **31,** 397–419.

Springer, M.S., Goy, M.F. and Adler, J. (1977a), Sensory transduction in *Escherichia coli:* two complementary pathways of information processing that involve methylated proteins. *Proc. natn. Acad. Sci. U.S.A.,* **74,** 3312–3316.

Springer, M.S., Goy, M.F. and Adler, J. (1977b), Sensory transduction in *Escherichia coli:* requirement for methionine in sensory adaptation. *Proc. natn. Acad. Sci. U.S.A.,* **74,** 173–177.

Springer, M.S., Goy, M.F. and Adler, J. (1978), Effects on a chemotaxis-related methylation reaction of mutations in the *che, mot,* and *fla* genes of *Escherichia coli,* in preparation.

Springer, M.S., Kort, E.N., Larsen, S.H., Ordal, G.W., Reader, R.W. and Adler, J. (1975), Role of methionine in bacterial chemotaxis: requirement for tumbling and involvement in information processing. *Proc. natn. Acad. Sci. U.S.A.,* **72,** 4640–4644.

Springer, W.R. and Koshland, D.E. Jr. (1977), Identification of a protein methyltransferase as the *che R* gene product in the bacterial sensing system. *Proc. natn. Acad. Sci. U.S.A.,* **74,** 533–577.

Spudich, J.L. and Koshland, D.E. Jr. (1975), Quantitation of sensory response in bacterial chemotaxis. *Proc. natn. Acad. Sci. U.S.A.,* **72,** 710–713.

Strange, P.D. and Koshland, D.E. Jr. (1975), Receptor interactions in a signalling system: competition between ribose receptor and galactose receptor in the chemotaxis response. *Proc. natn. Acad. Sci. U.S.A.,* **73,** 4387–4391.

Suzuki, T., Iino, T., Horiguchi, T. and Yamaguchi, S. (1978), Incomplete flagellar structures in nonflagellate mutants of *Salmonella typhimurium. J. Bact.,* **33,** 904–915.

Szmelcman, S. and Adler, J. (1976), Change in membrane potential during bacterial chemotaxis. *Proc. natn. Acad. Sci. U.S.A.,* **73**, 4387–4391.

Tsang, N., MacNab, R. and Koshland, D.E. Jr. (1973), Common mechanism for repellents and attractants in bacterial chemotaxis. *Science,* **181**, 60–63.

Tso, W.-W., and Adler, J. (1974), Negative chemotaxis in *Escherichia coli. J. Bact.,* **118**, 560–576.

van der Werf, P. and Koshland, D.E. Jr. (1977), Identification of a γ-glutamyl methyl ester in a bacterial membrane protein involved in chemotaxis. *J. biol. Chem.,* **252**, 2793–2795.

Warrick, H.M., Taylor, B.L. and Koshland, D.E. Jr. (1977), Chemotactic mechanism of *Salmonella typhimurium*: preliminary mapping and characterization of mutants. *J. Bact.,* **130**, 223–231.

Zukin, R.S., Hartig, P.R. and Koshland, D.E. Jr. (1977), Use of a distant reporter group as evidence for a conformational change in a sensory receptor. *Proc. natn. Acad. Sci. U.S.A.,* **74**, 1932–1936.

2 Bacterial Phototaxis

EILO HILDEBRAND

Acknowledgements

Most of the experiments on *Halobacterium halobium* reported here have been done by Norbert Dencher and Edita Janković. I would like to thank both for their kind permission to cite unpublished results. Valuable suggestions provided by the Editor which improved the manuscript are gratefully acknowledged. I am also indebted to Drs F. Lenci and G. Colombetti, who made their review on photobehaviour of micro-organisms available before publication, and to Helga Gaube and Edith Brentgens for their help in preparing the manuscript. The work on *Halobacterium* was supported by the Deutsche Forschungsgemeinschaft, SFB 160.

2.1 INTRODUCTION

Light is one of the most important pre-requisites of life. Most plants including blue-green algae and some bacteria contain photopigments which enable these organisms to utilize luminous energy for their cellular metabolism. When the *energy* of an absorbed photon is converted and utilized to drive metabolic processes, the photopigment functions in *photocoupling* (Oesterhelt and Stoeckenius, 1973). For example, chlorophyll converts light into chemical energy which is finally stored by means of carbohydrate synthesis.

Another important photobiological phenomenon is reaction to light by distinct movements, resulting in orientation with respect to the environment. The majority of animals and many motile micro-organisms can utilize light for that purpose. Photobehaviour is commonly mediated by a mechanism in which light triggers a chain of reactions which are driven by metabolic energy previously stored in the cell. In this case the organism uses the *information* carried by light rather than its energy, and the function of the photoreceptor pigment is signal transduction or *photosensing.* The most complicated photosensory organs are the eyes of vertebrates and insects. More primitive light-sensitive structures can be found in less evolved animals and in some unicellular organisms, e.g. in the flagellate *Euglena.* Although blue-green algae and bacteria do not contain specialized photosensory organelles some of them show distinct photoresponses.

Light-dependent behaviour in bacteria was first studied by Engelmann (1883, 1888). Since that time the photobehaviour of unicellular organisms has been investigated by several authors using different species of bacteria and other micro-organisms. It is not the aim of this article to give an encyclopedic survey of all these studies. The interested reader is referred to some excellent reviews which have appeared in recent years (see for instance Clayton, 1964; Feinleib and Curry, 1974; Haupt, 1966; Lenci and Colombetti, 1978; Nultsch, 1975). Bacterial photobehaviour has been quantitatively studied by Clayton (1953a,b,c, 1958) with *Rhodospirillum rubrum,* and most of our fundamental knowledge in this field comes from his excellent work. (For review of the older literature see Clayton, 1959.)

Sensory and neural systems have elicited growing interest and bacteria are considered particularly suitable model systems for the study of elementary mechanisms by which stimulus and response are coupled. Unlike higher developed systems, unicellular organisms have integrated receptor and effector sites in one cell. This has the great experimental advantage that the system acts independently of other cells. However, it sometimes makes it difficult to separate the mechanisms associated with receptor and effector function.

A remarkable progress in understanding the chemosensory mechanisms of bacteria

37

has been made during the last decade (see Chapter 1 in this volume and recent reviews by Adler, 1975; Berg, 1975b; Hazelbauer and Parkinson, 1977; Koshland, 1977). The mechanism of receptor—effector coupling in chemobehaviour is still obscure, but many ideas developed in this field can be adopted for bacterial photobehaviour.

This article will describe fundamental mechanisms of photobehaviour as they are presently understood or as one might expect they might function. Therefore it seems reasonable to concentrate on a few examples which are well characterized or are being studied on a molecular level. Other systems will be considered only in so far as they seem suitable for such an approach and might help to elucidate the problems — not for the sake of comparison. We are far from understanding the molecular mechanisms of photobehaviour, thus many of the considerations will be hypothetical or even speculative.

Recently, light-induced motor responses have been discovered in *Halobacterium halobium*, an extreme halophilic organism which is of particular current interest with respect to molecular aspects of photoreception and membrane-bound processes. We will therefore focus primarily on this system as representative of the problems of bacterial photobehaviour.

2.2 GENERAL CHARACTERISTICS OF PHOTOBEHAVIOUR IN MICRO-ORGANISMS

Several species of micro-organisms, mainly flagellates, blue-green algae and some bacteria show light-dependent alterations of their motor activity which cause certain changes of movement or orientation. Since such photoresponses, although often different in nature, usually result in a net movement with respect to the light source, the phenomenon is frequently called *phototaxis*. Properly the term phototaxis should, however, be restricted to the orientation of a single organism towards the light (positive phototaxis) or away from it (negative phototaxis) (Diehn *et al.*, 1977). There is so far no evidence for phototaxis in this sense in bacteria.

2.2.1 Types of photoresponses

Two types of light-controlled motor responses can be distinguished. In *photokinesis* a change in light intensity causes an alteration in linear velocity, the photokinetic response. Photokinetic activity is normally maintained as long as the light intensity remains constant, i.e. adaptation does not occur. The action spectra of photokinesis correspond quite closely to the absorption spectra of chlorophyll or to the *in vivo* absorption spectra of the organisms, respectively. Thus photokinesis appears to be linked directly to the photocoupling function and lacks most of the properties of a sensory process. It will be considered only marginally here.

A *phobic response* consists of a sudden disturbance of normal movement followed by a resumption of the original behaviour, whereby the direction of movement is changed. The first step may be either a cessation of movement (stop response) or a transient tumbling or reversal.

Photophobic responses are the common reactions in all light-sensitive procaryotes (bacteria and blue-green algae) and the elementary motor response in eucaryotes, e.g. flagellates, diatoms, several swarmspores and gametes (for review see Nultsch, 1975) and in desmids (Häder and Wenderoth, 1977). Photophobic responses are rather varied but each species exhibits a characteristic pattern dependent on the morphology of the organism and the action of its motor organelles. Under normal conditions the response is all-or-none.

The photophobic response is determined by a temporal change in light intensity, dI/dt, (step-up or step-down) rather than by the absolute magnitude of the stimulus. Another striking feature of photophobic behaviour is that the organism normally adapts if the stimulus is sustained or frequently repeated. This means that the sensitivity of the system can change under certain light conditions.

Photophobic responses have been observed in the photosynthetic purple bacteria and recently also in *Halobacterium*. While halobacteria show both a step-up response (evoked by an increase of light intensity) and a step-down response (evoked by a decrease of light), which differ with respect to their spectral sensitivity (Hildebrand and Dencher, 1975), only the latter has been reported for purple bacteria (Clayton, 1959).

Light pulses of high intensity induce tumbling reactions in *Salmonella typhimurium* and *Escherichia coli* (Macnab and Koshland, 1974; Taylor and Koshland, 1975) and backward swimming of *Pseudomonas citronellolis* (Taylor and Koshland, 1974). These can also be regarded as step-up photophobic responses. Blue light is most efficient and a flavin is postulated to be the photoreceptor. As prolonged exposure to light leads to paralysis of the organisms, the responses are thought to be unimportant in the normal physiology of the bacteria (Taylor and Koshland, 1975). Recently a light-dependent behaviour which does not depend on photosynthesis was observed in aerobically cultivated *Rhodospirillum rubrum* (Harayama and Iino, 1976). After a sudden reduction of strong light phobic responses occurred more frequently than under steady illumination or after an abrupt increase of the light intensity. Further experiments (Harayama and Iino, 1977a) strongly suggest that the response is mediated by the photoreduction of ferric ions in the medium, so that the effect seems to be a chemoresponse rather than a true photoresponse.

The purple bacteria *Chromatium* and *Rhodospirillum* exhibit quite different photobehaviour (Fig. 2.1). The former has an ellipsoid shape and bears flagella only on one pole (the rear), the latter is elongated and bipolarly flagellated. Both normally swim parallel to their long axis. *Chromatium okenii*, pushed by its flagellar bundle, shows a well-defined polarity, whereas *Rhodospirillum* swims equally well in either direction always keeping its bundles in a 'head-tail' position. If *Chromatium* swims from an illuminated area into the dark, which is equivalent to a sudden decrease in light intensity, the organism rapidly moves backward, bundle-first, several body lengths and thereafter resumes its original forward movement, but in a direction

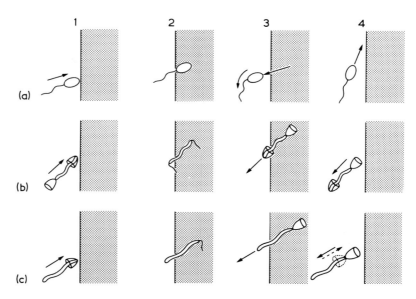

Fig. 2.1 Step-down photophobic responses of photosynthetic bacteria *Chromatium* (a), *Rhodospirillum* (b), and *Thiospirillum* (c). For further description see text. (After Buder, 1915 and Metzner, 1920; adapted from Clayton, 1971.)

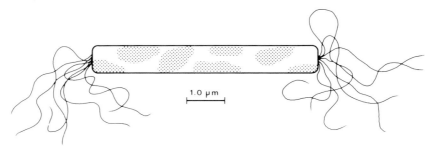

Fig. 2.2 Scheme of *Halobacterium halobium* showing patches of purple membrane and bipolar flagellation (from Hildebrand, 1977).

randomly deviating from the previous one (Engelmann, 1883; Buder, 1915, 1919). In contrast, *Rhodospirillum rubrum* simply reverses its swimming direction and continues to swim in a new direction until the next response occurs which can be either spontaneous or stimulus-induced (Buder, 1915). The same kind of response is exhibited by *Halobacterium,* a rod-shaped bacterium which also carries flagellar bundles on both poles (Fig. 2.2). *Halobacterium halobium* swims in a more or less straight course with a rate of about 2.5 μm s^{-1} (at 24°C). Upon an appropriate stimulus the organism stops moving after a latent period of at least 0.5 s and thereafter starts again in nearly the opposite direction. The unipolarly flagellated purple bacterium *Thiospirillum jenense* represents an intermediate type (Fig. 2.1). It can swim in both directions, either pushed or pulled by the flagellar bundle. The bacterium responds quickly with a single reversal like *Rhodospirillum* or *Halobacterium.* Under less optimal conditions, however, the movement in one direction is preferred and the photophobic response looks more like in *Chromatium* (Buder, 1915; Pfennig, 1964).

2.2.2 Biological significance

Most micro-organisms which show light-induced motor reactions utilize light energy for their cellular metabolism. *Halobacterium* can use light energy for ATP synthesis by means of bacteriorhodopsin which acts as a light-driven proton pump (Oesterhelt and Stoeckenius, 1973). A close relation between the photosensing and the photo-coupling function has been demonstrated in bacteria, blue-green algae and in some eucaryotes. In these cases the action spectra for the step-down photophobic response coincide quite well with the absorption spectra of the photocoupling pigment, i.e. of chlorophyll or bacteriorhodopsin, respectively (see also Section 2.4.1), which indicates that the motor response is mediated in some way by this pigment. As the response results in an accumulation of organisms in the illuminated area, the biological relevance seems evident: The photosensing system enables the organisms to find optimal conditions for their energy supply. For instance it can be observed under the microscope that halobacteria accumulate in a spot of yellow-green or white light within some minutes. The mechanism by which this is accomplished is sketched in Fig. 2.3a.

At the first glance it looks as if a decrease in the energy-yielding process is associated with the phobic response of these organisms and one could argue that the reaction results from a sudden decrease in the energy available through metabolism. This view has been stressed by Links (1955) who proposed that the changed amount of energy-supplying substance for the motor apparatus, probably ATP, is responsible for photoaccumulation. This hypothesis is certainly an oversimplification, as will be discussed later (see Section 2.5.1). It may be the primary steps of photocoupling that are involved in the sensory trigger mechanism rather than the high-energy end products.

In other motile cells such as flagellates and gametes of higher plants the photo-phobic response is not functionally related to photosynthesis. Photosensory systems independent of the energy-converting apparatus have been developed in these organisms.

It is beyond the scope of this article to describe all the kinds of behavioural mechanisms by which micro-organisms can adapt to the environment, but it is amazing how many different strategies organisms have developed to search for favourable light conditions and to survive.

Halobacterium shows a distinct photophobic response upon an increase of light

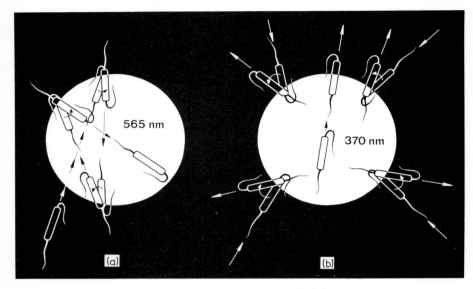

Fig. 2.3 'Phototactic' behaviour of *Halobacterium halobium* as a consequence of photophobic responses. (a) Accumulation of bacteria in a light spot of yellow-green (565 nm) resulting from step-down (light-off) photophobic responses carried out at the border to the dark. (b) Avoiding of UV light (370 nm) as a result of step-up (light-on) photophobic responses at the border to the light (from Hildebrand, 1977).

intensity in the blue and ultraviolet (step-up response). However, it seems questionable whether this photosystem is of biological significance. As the response results in an avoidance of blue and UV light (Fig. 2.3b) one could argue that this photosystem either protects the bacterium from irradiation which would damage its DNA or, considering the spectral transmittance of water, helps the organism to stay at a certain depth. This response might represent an evolutionary remnant, formerly important in avoidance of intense UV irradiation, or it might be only a by-product of bacteriorhodopsin synthesis and have no biological relevance.

Photokinesis of micro-organisms capable of photosynthesis is obviously not significant with respect to utilization of light energy. Positive photokinetic activity results in a statistical preference for the dark areas; it can therefore not serve as a mechanism to find optimal light conditions for the photocoupling mechanism.

2.2.3 Analogy to excitation

The intimate relation between photobehaviour and photosynthesis in *Rhodospirillum rubrum* led Manten (1948) to the hypothesis that the motor response is associated with a decrease in the rate of photosynthesis, and Links (1955) proposed that the photoresponse may be simply associated with the amount of energy available for the organism's locomotor apparatus. Clayton (1958) criticized Links' hypothesis and postulated a mechanism closely related to the excitation process in sensory cells (e.g. visual cells) and neurons. Examining the photobehaviour of bacteria for the most important criteria of sensory activity and excitation one can indeed find that most of them are fulfilled.

(1) *Light perception* Changes in light energy flow are detected by the organism. Stimulus perception is mediated by the interaction of light with specific receptor substances which have been identified in most cases (see also Section 2.4.1).

(2) *Sensory transduction* The kind of energy carrying sensory information is changed, most probably in a process closely related to stimulus perception. This transduction mechanism is entirely unknown, but it must be assumed that the light stimulus is converted in some way into a chemical or electrical signal which is propagated to and can be detected by the motor organelles.

(3) *Amplification* It is an important property of sensory cells that the energy change of the stimulus is small compared to the energy flow controlled by it at the cellular level. The sensory mechanism acts as a switch and can be considered as an amplifier. This principle is most evident in the visual cells of animals where absorption of a single photon leads to a measurable displacement of electrical charge across the cell membrane. On the other hand, Clayton (1958) calculated that the single quantum at a wavelength of 890 nm has much more energy than is expended by the motor organelles during the photophobic response of *Rhodospirillum rubrum.* The same seems to be true for *Halobacterium.* Hence it may become senseless to claim amplification as an essential criterion for the bacterial sensory system. Generally, the sensitivity of bacterial photosensory systems is considerably lower than that of visual cells.

(4) *All-or-none response* A classical property of nervous excitation is the all-or-none nature of the response, the action potential. At a first glance the photophobic response of bacteria seems to meet this criterion, but the all-or-none nature of the response has not been tested carefully enough. Some observations with *Halobacterium* indicate that upon weak stimulation, incomplete responses can occur. This would be in agreement with the graded action potential and the incomplete ciliary reversal which can be elicited in *Paramecium* by weak mechanical stimulation (Naitoh and Eckert, 1969; Machemer, 1974).

(5) *Strength-duration relation* Nerve cells obey the Bunsen–Roscoe Law which means that the response remains constant if the product ($I \times t$) of strength (intensity, I) and duration (t) of the stimulus is kept constant. This is also true for sensory cells as long as the stimulus duration is short as compared to the latent period. Strength-duration curves measured with *Rhodospirillum rubrum* (Clayton, 1953c) correspond fairly well with theoretical curves. The step-up photophobic response (photosystem 370) of *Halobacterium halobium* obeys the strength–duration criterion over the range examined (Fig. 2.4). In contrast, the step-down response (PS 565) does not adhere to this rule, probably because of the relatively weak and accordingly long-duration stimuli applied.

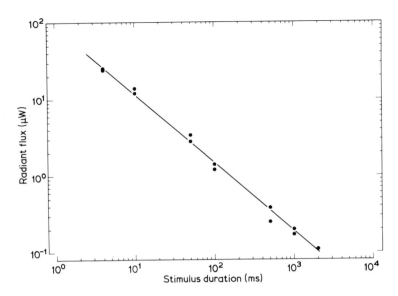

Fig. 2.4 Stimulus strength–duration relation of the step-up photophobic response (PS 370) of *Halobacterium halobium*. Linear regression coefficient of a double logarithmic plot of the data is $\beta = -0.93$). (After Dencher, 1974).

(6) *Weber Law* Sensory systems commonly obey Weber's Law which predicts that the response will be constant over a certain range, if the relative change of the stimulus energy ($\Delta I/I_0$) is kept constant. Adherence to this law could be demonstrated with *Rhodospirillum rubrum* by Schrammeck (1934) and to a far less extent by Clayton (1953a). The relationship does not hold for the step-down response of *Halobacterium* (Dencher, 1974), but has not been systematically tested in the step-up response. (For further details see Section 2.4.6). It should be emphasized that adherence to Weber's Law differs widely in various sensory systems.

(7) *Accommodation* An abrupt change of the stimulus energy is more effective than a gradual one. This phenomenon, intensively investigated in nerve cells, was also found in *Rhodospirillum rubrum* (Clayton, 1953c). Accommodation has not been tested in *Halobacterium halobium.*

(8) *Refractoriness* For a certain duration after excitation of a nerve fiber it is impossible to evoke another response. This temporary loss of excitability is called *absolute* refractoriness. In the subsequent *relative* refractory period excitability is reduced. That means a larger stimulus has to be applied to evoke a standard response. Clayton (1953c) found an absolute refractory period of about 0.25 s and a recovery phase of about 3 s in *Rhodospirillum rubrum.* The absolute refractoriness for both photophobic responses of *Halobacterium* (light-on and light-off) is less than 0.3 s, the relative refractory period lasts about 1.5 s, but may be superimposed by an

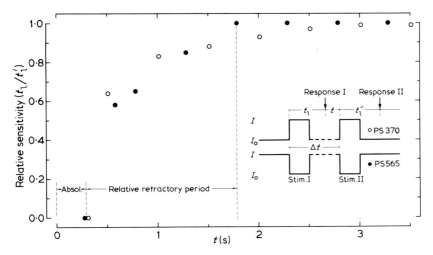

Fig. 2.5 Refractoriness of step-up (○) and step-down (●) photophobic response of *Halobacterium halobium*.

adaptation effect (see below) in the case of the light-on response (Fig. 2.5).

(9) *Rhythmicity* Under sustained stimulation nerve fibers show repeated response (rhythmicity). This phenomenon is closely related to refractoriness and has been reported for *Rhodospirillum rubrum*, but has not been established with certainty in *Halobacterium*. Rhythmicity can also be induced by temperature changes (Metzner, 1920) and through application of certain drugs (Clayton, 1953c).

(10) *Adaptation* The stimulus strength necessary to elicit a constant response varies depending on the preceding activation (light adaptation) or recovery (dark adaptation). Adaptation can be easily demonstrated with visual cells of invertebrates and vertebrates. In bacteria, however, it is difficult to distinguish from refractoriness. In the case of *Halobacterium* which contains two different sensory photosystems the phenomena can be separated experimentally to a certain extent, because only the light-on system (PS 370) adapts whereas the light-off system (PS 565) does not (Hildebrand and Dencher, 1975; Hildebrand and Janković, unpublished results). Probable mechanisms of adaptation will be discussed in Sections 2.4.6 and 2.5.4.

On the basis of these criteria the photophobic activity of bacteria can be regarded as an excitatory phenomenon (Clayton, 1958) comparable to the excitation of nerve cells. Bacterial behaviour has a great similarity to both sensory activation and nervous excitation. However, the time scale is in the order of seconds rather than milliseconds, and, for the most part, bacterial behaviour corresponds more closely to that of ciliate protozoa, e.g. *Paramecium*, than to nerve cells. The similarity between bacterial behaviour and the activity of higher developed excitable cells suggests that some fundamental mechanisms are universal for all sensory systems.

2.2.4 Steps in the causal chain

Sensory function in aneural organisms requires the following steps in a causal chain connecting stimulus to response:

(1) *Stimulus perception* Changes in light intensity to which the organism responds must be detected by a photoreceptor organelle or a photosensitive substance acting as a receptor.

(2) *Sensory transduction* The photoreceptor molecule must function as a signal transducer converting information carried by the light stimulus into a qualitatively different form, probably electrochemical, which can be detected or transmitted by certain cellular constituents. In other words: The temporal stimulus pattern has to be translated into a language which is understood by the cell.

(3) *Signal transmission* The converted signal must be transmitted to and detected by the effector organelles. Theoretically more than one step may be involved in this process.

(4) *Motor response* The signal finally controls the activity of the effector organelle which in turn brings about the observable motor response of the organism. Activation of the locomotor apparatus may be considered another transduction process by which the chemical or electrical signal is converted into a mechanical force.

The mechanisms of light perception are partially understood in those cases where the photoreceptor pigment has been isolated or identified. During recent years we have obtained important insight into the functioning of bacterial flagella, but the nature of the intermediate steps is rather obscure at present, and it appears to be difficult to analyse directly the mechanisms involved in sensory transduction and signal transmission. Because of the small size of bacteria it seems impossible to insert a micro-electrode for intracellular voltage recording, so that the application of this classical electrophysiological method is out of the question. From the standpoint of systems analysis we have to consider the bacterium mainly as a black box. The most promising method for obtaining information about the mechanisms involved in the stimulus-response sequence seems the adoption of certain working hypotheses from other excitable systems and the study of input—output relations under conditions which have been examined in those systems.

2.3 HOW BACTERIA SWIM

All species in which photophobic responses have been observed bear flagella which enable them to swim. Bacterial flagella may be either randomly distributed over the entire surface or concentrated at one or both poles of the cell. In normally swimming bacteria the flagella form bundles which act as a unit. Such a bundle may occur at one or both ends of the bacterium. Among photosensitive bacteria both unipolarly and bipolarly flagellated species are known. The diameter of a single flagellum is far below the resolution of the light microscope, but individual flagella could be visualized in

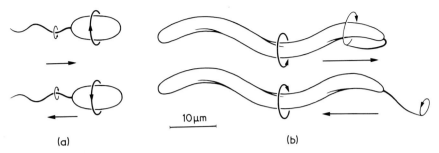

Fig. 2.6 Reversal of motion and flagellar orientation in the photosynthetic bacteria *Chromatium okenii* (a) and *Thiospirillum jenense* (b) (after Buder, 1915).

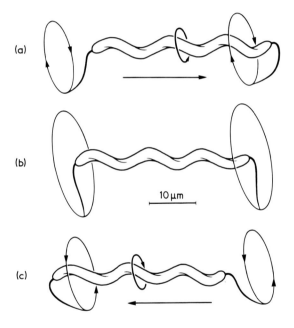

Fig. 2.7 Reversal of motion and flagellar orientation in *Spirillum volutans* (after Krieg *et al.,* 1967, and Metzner, 1920).

living bacteria by means of dark-field microscopy using very bright light (Macnab and Ornston, 1977). The actual position and form of flagellar bundles in living bacteria can also be seen by the application of the dark-field technique. Using this method, Buder (1915) observed that in *Chromatium* the helical-shaped flagellar bundle rotates in one direction whereas the cell body rotates in the opposite (Fig. 2.6a). In bipolarly

flagellated species such as *Spirillum volutans* or *Rhodospirillum rubrum* one bundle
is normally in the 'head' position while the other is in the 'tail' position (Fig. 2.7). We
have not been able to visualize flagella of live *Halobacterium halobium,* but we know
from electron micrographs of negatively stained preparations that this species has
flagellar bundles on both poles (Hildebrand and Dencher, 1975), consisting of 5—10
single flagella (Houwink, 1956). Their orientation during the normal movement and
during the photophobic response is unknown, and at the present time we are dependent on analogy with other bipolarly flagellated forms, e.g. *Spirillum volutans.*

2.3.1 The bacterial flagellum

Unlike cilia and flagella of eucaryotic organisms, the bacterial flagellum represents a
thin filamentous structure which measures some microns in length and 12—14 nm in
diameter. The whole filament consists of a polymeric protein, flagellin, which shows
no enzymatic activity and cannot actively bend (for review see Berg, 1975a). Intensive
electronmicroscopic studies carried out by DePamphilis and Adler (1971a) on isolated
flagella of *Escherichia coli* and *Bacillus subtilis* revealed that each flagellum consists
of a helical filament, a short intercalated segment, the hook, and a basal apparatus
with wheel-like structures. The latter is embedded in the cytoplasmic membrane and

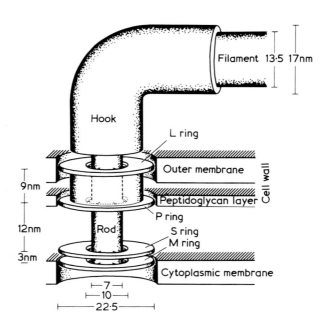

Fig. 2.8 Model of the basal part of a flagellum from a Gram-negative bacterium
(after DePamphilis and Adler, 1971a,b).

the cell wall (DePamphilis and Adler, 1971b). A model of the proximal part of the flagellum of a Gram-negative bacterium is shown in Fig. 2.8.

2.3.2 Movement and motor response

Excellent experiments performed by Berg and Anderson (1973), Silverman and Simon (1974) and others provided evidence that flagella rotate and that the sense of rotation can be altered. This occurs when the bacterium changes its swimming direction or enters a tumbling phase (Silverman and Simon, 1974; Larsen *et al.*, 1974b). The flagellar filaments rotate about 50 revolutions per second while the cell body rotates more slowly in the opposite direction (Berg, 1975a).

Rotation of flagella implies that in the bundle filaments rotate side by side. Macnab (1977) could demonstrate with a working model that in fact a co-ordinated helical bundle is formed if a set of semi-rigid helices, which rotate separately, interact with each other. If the sense of rotation is changed the filaments come apart and this causes the tumbling response which is the characteristic motor response in peritrichously flagellated bacteria, e.g. *Escherichia coli* and *Salmonella typhimurium.*

In polarly flagellated bacteria such as *Chromatium, Rhodospirillum* or *Halobacterium* a change of the direction of rotation has less dramatic effects. When these species are subjected to a light stimulation they simply reverse their swimming direction approximately 180°. In *Rhodospirillum* and in the non-photosensitive *Spirillum volutans* one can observe that both flagellar bundles simultaneously snap over, like an umbrella, from the 'tail' position to the 'head' position and *vice versa* (Fig. 2.7). This behaviour must be caused by a simultaneous change of the sense of rotation of all flagella. It seems typical for bipolarly flagellated bacteria and we believe the same mechanism is valid in the case of *Halobacterium*. From the photobehaviour of *Chromatium* (= *Bacterium photometricum*) described by Engelmann (1883) and Buder (1915) we must conclude that the stimulus-induced reversal of the direction of rotation is transient and the original direction is spontaneously resumed after some time following the response. *Thiospirillum,* the other unipolarly flagellated type of photosensitive bacteria (Fig. 2.6b), can behave either like *Rhodospirillum* or like *Chromatium* (see Section 2.2.1). Its photoresponses be explained in an analogous way.

2.3.3 The problem of the motive force

Berg (1974) suggested that the M-ring is rigidly mounted on the rod, whereas the S-ring is attached to the cell wall, and that the torque is generated between the rings. The M-ring is assumed to rotate freely in the cytoplasmic membrane and the more distally located pair of rings, found only in Gram-negative bacteria is thought to function as bushing for the rod.

The energy source for the motor is most probably not ATP, rather an intermediate of oxidative phosphorylation (Larsen *et al.*, 1974a). This is reminiscent of a mechanism for powering active transport, and one could argue that the motor may be driven by translocation of certain ions through the M-ring which interact with fixed charges on the surface of the S-ring (Berg, 1975a). Recent experimental results (Manson *et al.,* 1977; Matsuura *et al.,* 1977) and theoretical considerations (Läuger, 1977) indicate that the bacterial flagellum is driven by a proton motive force. This is consistent with the chemiosmotic theory of Mitchell (1966) which states that the intermediate of oxidative phosphorylation is an electrochemical potential gradient of protons across the membrane. An alternative mechanism for flagellar rotation has been proposed by Adam (1977), namely that a directed streaming of the cytoplasmic membrane drives the M-ring. Both ideas involve a conformational transition of spoke-like subunits of the M-ring, which were observed by DePamphilis and Adler (1971a), as the basis for reversal of rotational direction.

2.3.4 Co-ordination of flagellar activity

According to the working model presented by Macnab (1977), the combined action of several filaments in a bundle requires an identical sense of rotation of all flagellar motors. Consequently one has to assume that reversal occurs simultaneously in all flagella of the bundle. Moreover, bipolarly flagellated bacteria, e.g. *Spirillum volutans,* show a co-ordinated reversal of both bundles (Metzner, 1920). These properties point to a central co-ordinating mechanism controlling the activity of all flagella. Since the bundles at each pole change their rotational direction within about 10 ms or less (Krieg *et al.,* 1967) the co-ordinating signal must spread rapidly over the entire cell. The nature of this signal is unknown. An electrochemical mechanism, connected with certain properties of the cytoplasmic membrane, similar to that of ciliate protozoa (Eckert and Naitoh, 1970) seems to be the most likely candidate.

2.4 THE DETECTION OF LIGHT

For both photosensing and photocoupling, light quanta must be absorbed by specific receptor molecules. Among micro-organisms various types of photopigments are used to accomplish this function. In some cases the same pigment serves as photoreceptor for both photocoupling and photosensing, for instance in blue-green algae and purple bacteria, where chlorophyll *a* or bacteriochlorophyll, respectively, act as receptor molecules. The same is true for the step-down photophobic response and photo-coupling of *Halobacterium* which are both mediated by bacteriorhodopsin. In other organisms the two systems are functionally separated and specific photosensory receptor pigments other than chlorophyll are found. This is true for *Euglena,* where a flavoprotein has been identified as the sensory pigment (Diehn, 1969; Benedetti and Lenci, 1977 and references therein) and in other flagellates in which carotenoids probably act as sensory photoreceptors (e.g. Forward, 1973; Schletz, 1975). *Halobacterium* represents a unique example in so far as it possesses a second sensory photosystem, which mediates the step-up response independently of bacteriorhodopsin

Sensory photopigments can be either concentrated in special photoreceptor organelles (e.g. the paraflagellar body of *Euglena*) or distributed over the entire cell surface. No differentiated light-sensitive parts of the cell have been found in purple bacteria. Photophobic responses can be elicited in *Thiospirillum jenense* when only one end of the cell is stimulated (Pfennig, 1964), which suggests that the receptor pigment is equally distributed. *Halobacterium* also shows a response if it experiences a stimulus (light-on or light-off) at only one pole. It has not yet been established whether the middle part of the bacterium is sensitive as well.

Sensory photopigments may be present only in extremely small amounts which cannot be isolated or spectroscopically detected. The method most frequently used to identify receptor pigments is to obtain action spectra of the organism's photoresponse.

2.4.1 Photoreceptor pigments

The receptor chromophores responsible for light-dependent motor responses in micro-organisms can be roughly divided into five groups, namely: chlorophylls, flavins, carotenoids, retinals, and phycobilins. All these substances are characterized by a system of conjugated double bonds making them suitable for absorption in the visible and near UV part of the spectrum.

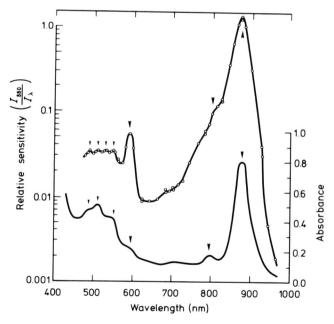

Fig. 2.9 Action spectrum of step-down photophobic response (upper curve) and *in vivo* absorption (lower curve) of *Rhodospirillum rubrum*. Large arrowheads indicate bacteriochlorophyll maxima, small arrowheads indicate carotenoid maxima. (After Clayton, 1953a and from Haupt, 1966).

Phycobilins seem to be restricted to certain blue-green and red algae (Nultsch, 1975) and will not be considered further. A flavin-like pigment has been identified in *Euglena*, and may also be responsible for the step-up responses to high-intensity blue light observed in *Salmonella typhimurium* and *Escherichia coli* (see Section 2.2.1). Bacteriochlorophyll is the receptor pigment for the step-down response of *Rhodospirillum rubrum* (Fig. 2.9) and most probably all purple bacteria. The photochemistry of chlorophylls has been intensively studied and is reviewed elsewhere. Carotenoids are widespread and seem to be involved in the photobehaviour of many micro-organisms, including bacteria (see Sections 2.4.2 and 2.4.4), at least as accessory or shielding pigments. Although retinals are related to carotenoids they should be considered as a separate group since retinal is normally complexed with a protein by a Schiff base linkage thereby shifting its absorption spectrum to the red and making it spectroscopically different from carotenoids. Retinal–protein complexes (rhodopsins) are the common photoreceptor pigments in the eyes of animals. Among micro-organisms, halobacteria are the only group in which retinal–protein complexes have been found. The sensory photosystems based on this class of receptor pigments will be described in detail in Sections 2.4.3 and 2.4.4.

2.4.2 Accessory pigments

Substances other than the effective receptor pigment may participate in quantum capture. Especially carotenoids are thought to act as so-called accessory pigments. Accessory pigments alone are inactive and act only together with the effective receptor substance. An important requirement for an accessory action is that the absorption spectra of the two substances are near each other, the fluorescence spectrum of the accessory pigment overlapping the absorption spectrum of the effective pigment so that radiationless energy transfer from the former to the latter becomes possible. The accessory action results in a composite action spectrum, and theoretically the band caused by the accessory pigment may be larger than that of the effective pigment. The action spectra obtained by Clayton (1953a) for photosynthetic activity and photobehaviour of *Rhodospirillum rubrum* indicate that in both mechanisms a carotenoid, spirilloxanthin, acts as an accessory pigment to bacteriochlorophyll (Fig. 2.9). An accessory action of carotenoids could also be demonstrated in the step-up photophobic response (PS 370) of *Halobacterium halobium* (see Section 2.4.4).

2.4.3 Bacteriorhodopsin, photosystem 565

Some years ago Oesterhelt and Stoeckenius (1971) discovered a retinal–protein complex in the extremely halophilic bacterium *Halobacterium halobium*. They called this – in analogy to the visual pigment – bacteriorhodopsin (BR). BR acts as a light-driven proton pump converting light into electrochemical energy which can be utilized by the cell to synthesize ATP (Oesterhelt and Stoeckenius, 1973).

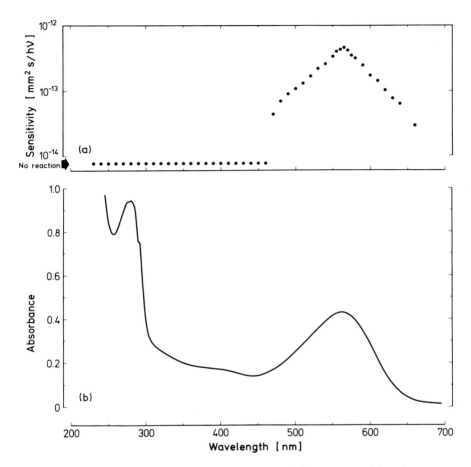

Fig. 2.10 Action spectrum of step-down photophobic response (a) and absorption of isolated purple membrane bacteriorhodopsin (b) of *Halobacterium halobium* (after Hildebrand and Dencher, 1975).

Halobacteria also exhibit light-dependent motor responses which have been studied more recently by Hildebrand and Dencher (1975). Photophobic responses in *Halobacterium* can be evoked either by an increase ('step-up' or 'light on' response) or by a decrease of the light intensity ('step-down' or 'light-off' response). The motor response is identical in both cases, but the spectral sensitivity differs, indicating the existence of two different sensory photosystems. The light-on response has a maximum sensitivity in the blue and UV, and we called it photosystem 370 (PS 370). The light-off response is maximally sensitive in the yellow-green part of the spectrum and is therefore called PS 565. The action spectrum of PS 565 corresponds

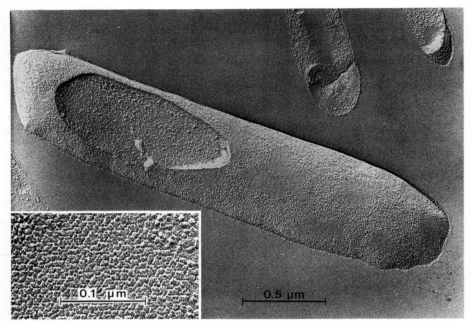

Fig. 2.11 Freeze-etched preparation of *Halobacterium halobium* showing purple membrane patches (smooth surface structure). Inset: Purple membrane structure at higher magnification. (Courtesy of Dr W. Schröder.)

to the absorption spectrum of BR in the visible region (Fig. 2.10), and the receptor pigment is therefore thought to be this substance.

Bacteriorhodopsin is located in distinct patches, the so-called purple membrane, within the cell membrane (Figs. 2.2 and 2.11). The molecule consists of a retinal chromophore, and a polypeptide of about 25 000 daltons (Oesterhelt and Stoeckenius, 1971; Reynolds and Stoeckenius, 1977). The chromophore is linked to the protein *via* a Schiff-base formed by the aldehyde group of retinal and the ε-amino-group of a lysine. It is assumed there are additional polar interactions between the two components which account for the absorption shift to longer wavelength. An excellent article by Henderson (1977) is available, which reviews the structure and function of the purple membrane.

Bacteriorhodopsin, the only protein of the purple membrane, makes up about 75% of the total mass and forms a rigid two-dimensional crystal of hexagonally arranged molecules (Blaurock and Stoeckenius, 1971). Each molecule consists of seven α-helices (Henderson, 1975; Henderson and Unwin, 1975) which are oriented perpendicular to the membrane (Fig. 2.12). The overall dimensions of the molecule are about 2.5 x 3.5 x 4.5 nm. The protein molecules always form clusters of three leaving a space of about 2 nm between them. The interspaces are occupied by lipids

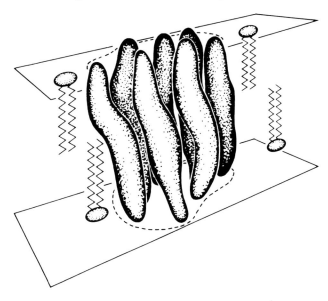

Fig. 2.12 Three-dimensional model of bacteriorhodopsin molecule consisting of seven α-helices embedded in bilipid membrane (after Henderson and Unwin, 1975 and Henderson, 1977).

which are arranged in a bilayer. Electron density profiles show that BR is asymmetrically oriented in the purple membrane (Blaurock and King, 1977). The exact position of the chromophore is not yet known, but the amino acid sequence of the protein chain is presently under study (e.g. Ovchinnikov *et al.,* 1977).

The crystalline nature of bacteriorhodopsin favours interaction between neighbouring molecules. Consistent with this an electron coupling effect has been deduced from circular dicroism measurements (Bauer *et al.,* 1976; Becher and Ebrey, 1976). It may be interesting to note that a paracrystalline structure has been found also in the paraflagellar body of *Euglena* which serves as the sensory photoreceptor organelle, containing a flavoprotein as the receptor pigment.

The retinal in BR can exist either in the 13-*cis* form or in the *trans* configuration (Fig. 2.13). BR kept in the dark for several hours contains equal amounts of 13-*cis* and *trans* retinal (Dencher *et al.,* 1976). Illumination shifts the equilibrium completely towards the *trans* isomer. After absorption of a photon, *trans*-BR undergoes a rapid reaction cycle (Fig. 2.14) during which protons are released and subsequently taken up (Oesterhelt and Stoeckenius, 1973; Oesterhelt and Hess, 1973). At 20°C the whole cycling is completed in less than 10 ms (Stoeckenius and Lozier, 1974; Dencher and Wilms, 1975; Lozier *et al.,* 1975), hence in contrast to rhodopsin no noticeable bleaching occurs in BR at room temperature. It is believed that the release and uptake of protons by the BR molecule is the basis for the net translocation of

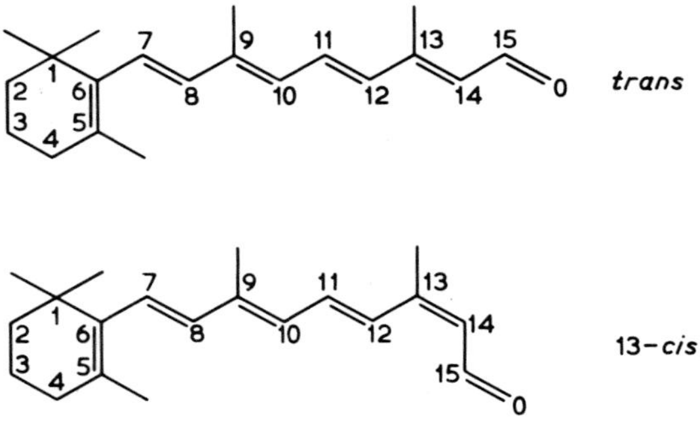

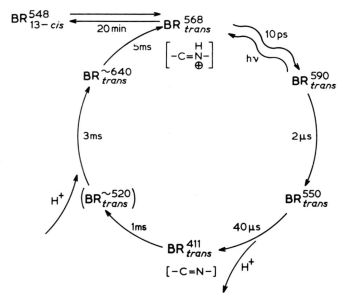

Fig. 2.13 Isomeric conformations of retinal chromophore in bacteriorhodopsin (from Sperling *et al.*, 1977).

Fig. 2.14 Photochemical cycle of bacteriorhodopsin (after Dencher and Wilms, 1975; Lozier *et al.*, 1975 and other authors).

protons across the bacterial cell membrane (Oesterhelt and Stoeckenius, 1973).

13-*cis* BR is also subjected to photochemical and subsequent dark reactions which have been studied recently (Dencher *et al.*, 1976). These reactions, however, may not have any biological function since under the conditions required for the photo-coupling as well as for the photosensing mechanism (e.g. in the light) only the *trans* configuration exists.

It is not known how BR may act as the sensory receptor. Since the effective stimulus consists of a temporal decrease in light intensity we can assume that the photochemical cycle is interrupted and the proton translocation rate will be transiently decreased. The possibility that a sudden decrease in light intensity may act *via* a *trans-cis* isomerization seems improbable because of the considerably long half-time of about 20 min for the isomerization (Oesterhelt *et al.*, 1973).

The sensitivity of the BR-photosystem is rather low. A decrease of light intensity of at least 2×10^{11} quanta mm^{-2} s^{-1} at a wavelength of 565 nm was required to elicit a phobic response of the bacterium (Hildebrand and Dencher, 1975). The sensitivity of the step-down response of *Rhodospirillum rubrum* is about 100 times higher (Clayton, 1953a). One may ask why the 280 nm band is absent in the spectral sensitivity curve of the light-off response of *Halobacterium* (Fig. 2.10). But as long as the UV part of the action spectrum for ATP synthesis is not known this question is difficult to answer. Probably the energy transfer from the protein part to the reactive center of the molecule is limited as has been found also in frog rhodopsin (Kropf, 1967).

2.4.4 The UV receptor of *Halobacterium*, photosystem 370

The step-up photophobic response of *Halobacterium* shows an action spectrum (Fig. 2.15) which is quite different from that of the step-down response. The curve exhibits two distinct maxima at 280 nm and 370 nm, the former being typical for aromatic amino acids of a protein. Smaller secondary peaks occur towards longer wavelengths, but light stimuli at wavelengths beyond 530 nm are ineffective. It was impossible to identify unequivocably the effective receptor pigment on the basis of this action spectrum. The receptor could be either a flavoprotein or a retinylidene protein, a retinal-protein complex, which can be obtained *in vitro* by CTAB* treatment of the purple membrane at alkaline pH (Oesterhelt and Stoeckenius, 1971; Peters *et al.*, 1976). In both cases α-bacterioruberine, a carotenoid, which has been found in large amounts in *Halobacterium* (Kelly *et al.*, 1970) was thought to participate, either as a shielding substance or as an accessory pigment.

In order to answer this question N. Dencher cultured halobacteria, mutant strain $R_1 L_3$, lacking most of the carotenoid content, in the presence of 1 mM nicotine, which inhibits the cyclization of lycopene to β-carotene (Howes and Batra, 1970) and hence blocks the synthesis of retinal. Bacteria grown under these conditions failed to respond both to light-off and light-on stimuli. After addition of *trans*-retinal to nicotine cells the light-on response reappeared first (Fig. 2.16) and the light-off response appeared after a delay of about 60 min. Since both photosystems can be regenerated by *trans*-retinal in the presence of nicotine an inhibitory effect of nicotine on another step of the sensory process seems to be ruled out. Addition of riboflavin or carotenoids instead of retinal did not reconstitute the photosystems.

* Cetyltrimethyl ammonium bromide, a detergent.

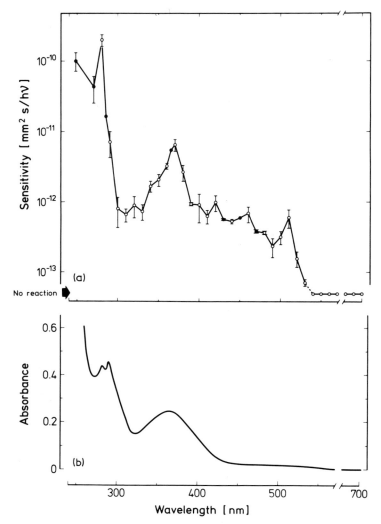

Fig. 2.15 Action spectrum of step-up photophobic response of *Halobacterium halobium*, strain R_1 (a) and absorption of retinylidene protein obtained after treatment of purple membrane with CTAB at pH $\geq$ 8.5 (b). (After Hildebrand and Dencher, 1975).

We conclude that the receptor pigment responsible for the light-on response is a retinal–protein complex, although obviously different from BR with respect to its spectroscopic and hence chemical properties. The spectral sensitivity of the regenerated light-on system is similar to the PS 370 except that regenerated cells fail to

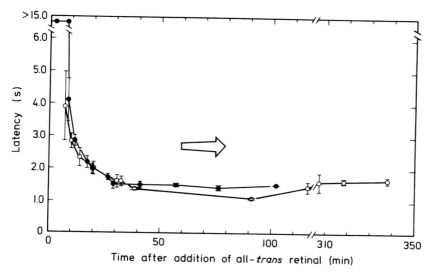

Fig. 2.16 Regeneration of PS 370 (step-up photophobic response) of *Halobacterium halobium* after addition of *trans*-retinal to a suspension of bacteria whose retinal synthesis was inhibited by nicotine. Decreasing latency means increasing sensitivity. Data points (○, ●) represent experiments from different cultures. Arrow indicates reappearance of PS 565 (step-down photophobic response).

respond to light of wavelengths longer than 450 nm (Fig. 2.17). It may be argued that loss of sensitivity in this region is due to the absence of bacterioruberine in the strain, $R_1 L_3$, used for these experiments and, indeed, addition of carotenoids extracted from strain R_1 to the regenerated cells reinstated the sensitivity around 500 nm (Fig. 2.17).

We were unable to isolate or to detect spectroscopically the effective blue receptor. The characteristic peak at 370 nm in the action spectrum indicates a retinal Schiff base, and we assume a complex in which the retinal is less intimately embedded in the protein moiety than bacteriorhodopsin. This complex may be either a precursor of BR or a side-product of its biosynthesis since in a growing culture as well as in regenerated cells the light-on system always preceeds the light-off system. In any case PS 370 seems to be located in areas of the cell membrane adjacent to the purple membrane, most probably in the 'brown membrane' which is believed to be the site of BR synthesis (Sumper *et al.*, 1976).

The reconstitution experiments clearly demonstrate that protein as well as carotenoids act as accessory pigments in PS 370. However, it remains unclear how energy is transferred from the carotenoids to the reactive site of the retinal. One possibility is that excited triplet states are involved.

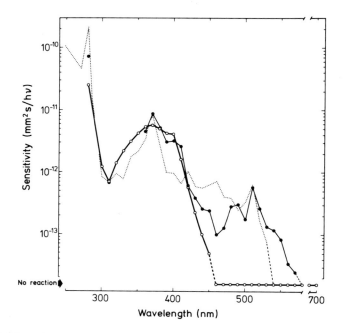

Fig. 2.17 Action spectrum of step-up photophobic response of *Halobacterium halobium,* strain $R_1 L_3$, after regeneration of PS 370 by addition of *trans*-retinal (○) and after addition of carotenoids extracted from strain R_1 to regenerated cells (●). For comparison action spectrum of strain R_1 (dotted curve) as in Fig. 2.15a.

The sensitivity of the light-on response at 370 nm is about 10 times that of the light-off response at 565 nm.

2.4.5 Primary events in photoreception

The *cis-trans* isomerization of 11-*cis* retinal in rhodopsin was proposed as the primary event in visual photoreception several years ago (Hubbard and Kropf, 1959; Wald, 1968). However, the photochemical reactions of bacteriorhodopsin begin with *trans*-BR and isomerization has not been detected with certainty in the reaction cycle. Both *trans*-BR and 11-*cis* rhodopsin exhibit similar absorption changes after excitation: the spectrum shifts to the red in about 10 ps and subsequently back towards the blue (for references see Hildebrand, 1977). This parallelism indicates that the primary reactions may be identical in both rhodopsins. Deprotonation of the Schiff base found in both BR and rhodopsin (Lewis *et al.,* 1974; Lewis, 1976) could well be an early reaction in all retinal–protein complexes, including PS 370, and may lead finally to more extensive conformational changes of the receptor molecule initiating the transduction process.

2.4.6 Pigment adaptation

It is a common feature of sensory systems that they can change sensitivity depending on the stimulus conditions. Visual cells of vertebrates and invertebrates show a considerable change in sensitivity which depends on background light intensity and on preceding activation. This adaptation phenomenon is partially due to rhodopsin bleaching or regeneration, and partially to transient changes of membrane properties. For the sake of simplicity the former may be called *pigment adaptation*, the latter *membrane adaptation.*

A sensitivity change dependent on background light has been found in *Rhodospirillum rubrum* (Clayton, 1953a, see Section 2.2.3 of this chapter) and in PS 370 of *Halobacterium halobium* but is absent in PS 565 (Hildebrand and Dencher, 1975). The adaptation of PS 370 may account for the slightly slower recovery of sensitivity in the double stimulus experiments shown in Fig. 2.5. The absence of an adaptation effect in the BR system (PS 565) is of particular interest. It indicates that the absolute decrease in light energy flow is detected by the receptor and that there is no noticeable 'bleaching', i.e. decomposition, of receptor pigment. This result is quite consistent with the rapid cycling of bacteriorhodopsin.

In contrast, the sensitivity of PS 370 gradually decreases with increasing background light. With blue background illumination ($\lambda = 420-490$ nm) the threshold intensity was about 50 times that with red background light ($\lambda > 645$ nm) which does not excite PS 370. The decreased sensitivity of both photosystems, persisting about 1.8 s after a phobic response can be attributed to transient refractoriness of the signalling system or the effector organelles. If we assume that both photosystems induce an identical kind of excitation, which seems most reasonable, the adaptation of PS 370 must be an inherent property of the receptor. In addition to the possibility that the pigment is partially decomposed by light and hence the dark adaptation (sensitivity increase) depends on its regeneration we have to consider another mechanism, namely that the amount of unknown intermediates may control the sensitivity of the system.

Sensory adaptation has been also found in the behavioural responses of bacteria towards chemicals (Macnab and Koshland, 1972; Tsang *et al.*, 1973). Adaptation in *Escherichia coli* requires methionine (Springer *et al.*, 1977), and a methylation of cytoplasmic membrane proteins is thought to control the state of adaptation (Goy *et al.*, 1977). The role of methionine in sensory adaptation of *Halobacterium* has not been examined. Given the properties of PS 565, one may argue that any methylation of proteins would be connected with the transducer function of certain receptors rather than with the excitation process or the effector activity.

2.5 RECEPTOR–EFFECTOR COUPLING

The functional pathway which links motor organelle to receptor can be divided into three main steps listed in Section 2.2.4 (1) sensory transduction, (2) signal transmission, and (3) motility transduction. Mechanisms of receptor—effector coupling seem to be the basis for other important properties of a sensory system, for instance amplification, data processing, 'memory' (i.e. adaptation and refractoriness), and response regulation.

2.5.1 Sensory transduction

Although the molecular mechanism of sensory transduction is obscure even in the intensively studied photoreceptor cells of animals, it is well established that the receptor membrane undergoes a permeability change for Na^+ ions (and to some extent for Ca^{2+}) and that the signal created by transduction is an electrochemical one, i.e. a transient change of the membrane potential. There is also an agreement on the assumption that the permeability change is brought about by certain conformational alterations of membrane proteins which in turn are linked in some way to the excited state of the rhodopsin molecule (for review see Stieve, 1974). A similar mechanism holds for the mechanosensitivity of *Paramecium* except that it is the calcium permeability which is increased, thereby causing the receptor potential (Eckert *et al.*, 1972).

In photosensitive bacteria it could be considered that the flagella simply sense the cellular ATP level. However, this is improbable for the following reasons:

(1) ATP is not the energy source for the flagella.

(2) Bipolarly flagellated bacteria show a co-ordinated flagellar reversal on both poles and the stimulation of one end of *Halobacterium* is sufficient to cause the cell to back up. The diffusion rate of ATP in the cytoplasm is certainly too low to manage the co-ordination within about 10 ms, a time which was calculated from filmed *Spirillum volutans* (Krieg *et al.*, 1967).

(3) The light-on photoresponse as well as chemoresponses of other bacteria are not related to ATP synthesis of the cell. The second point argues against any transmitter substances of a size comparable to that of ATP. A direct coupling *via* the proton gradient has been suggested (Larsen *et al.*, 1974a). This mechanism would be consistent with proton translocation mediated by BR, and a change in proton motive force could be easily detected by the flagella. In the blue-green alga *Phormidium uncinatum*, a sudden interruption of the photosynthetic electron flow has been proposed as the event leading to the step-down photophobic response (Häder, 1974, 1976). The same may be true in the case of purple bacteria, but it is questionable whether this signal can be directly detected by the flagella.

Hence, the nature of the cellular signal generated by the bacterial transduction process remains obscure. Since receptor molecules are inherent constituents of the cell membrane, membrane properties may be involved. Some arguments, discussed below, favour the assumption that the stimulus is transduced into an electrochemical signal, most likely a change of membrane potential, which would resemble the receptor potential of ciliate protozoa and other sensory systems.

2.5.2 Signal transmission and processing

Three possibilities for the signal transmission other than ATP level can be considered:
(1) Release and diffusion of a low molecular weight transmitter, e.g. a cation,
(2) alteration of the proton gradient across the cytoplasmic membrane, and (3) fluctuation of the membrane potential. The third could be either a result of the second or independent of proton distribution. In order to decide between these possibilities it becomes particularly interesting to know whether bacteria can integrate signals generated by different receptors. In the chemosensory function chemicals interacting with different receptor sites act additively if applied simultaneously (Tsang *et al.,* 1973; Adler and Tso, 1974). Thus, signals generated by different receptors are most probably of the same nature and signals caused by attractants and repellents are different in sign. Light-on and light-off stimuli of proper wavelengths applied simultaneously to *Halobacterium* also act additively (Hildebrand and Janković, unpublished results) indicating an identical mechanism of signal transduction. Halobacteria seem to be attracted by certain chemicals and it would be interesting to test whether chemically and light-induced 'excitation' compensate.

The capability of bacteria to balance internally the effects of antagonistically acting stimuli is difficult to explain by a transmitter substance and favours rather an electrochemical mechanism. Moreover, the diffusion of a substance of low molecular weight would be too slow to account for the signalling over a distance of 50 μm (Berg, 1975b) which must occur for flagellar co-ordination (see next section). Diffusion of a common cation discussed in the case of *Volvox* (Schletz, 1975) can be ruled out for bacteria.

2.5.3 Response regulation and co-ordination

Bacteria moving in a gradient of perceptible chemicals show motor responses (tumbling) less frequently if their swimming direction is towards a higher concentration of attractant or lower concentration of repellent (Berg and Brown, 1972. Macnab and Koshland, 1972; Tsang *et al.,* 1973). This response regulation, which is the basis of 'chemotaxis', has been explained on the assumption of an internal 'twiddle generator' (Berg and Brown, 1972) whose frequency is modulated by stimuli. The nature of the response regulator is presently unknown.

A response generator also seems reasonable for bacterial photobehaviour. Purple bacteria as well as halobacteria exhibit spontaneous reversal responses in the absense of stimuli. Hence, a stimulus might simply increase the frequency of signals from the response generator. Fluctuations of the proton gradient across the membrane or of the membrane potential itself could well serve as the response generator. The all-or-none nature of the response suggests a threshold behaviour of either the output control mechanism (response regulator) or the effector mechanism itself. An electrochemical mechanism would be best suited to fulfill these requirements.

We have to assume that all flagella in a bundle reverse the direction of rotation simultaneously and, moreover, the activity of both flagellar bundles of bipolarly flagellated bacteria has to be synchronized (see Section 2.3.4). Recently, Lee and Fitzsimons (1976) reported that filamentous forms of *Rhodospirillum rubrum* up to 60 μm long respond to a decrease of light in the same way as normal forms of 2 μm length. This makes a chemical transmitter improbable and strongly favours the assumption of a central co-ordinating mechanism of a quasi-nervous nature, i.e. a membrane-controlled ionic mechanism.

However, bacterial flagella may show relative autonomy under certain conditions. Metzner (1920) reported a lack of synchronization of the two flagellar bundles in spirilla, only one carrying out reversal upon stimulation, resulting in an antagonistic action of the bundles so that the cell became motionless. Several agents have been tested by Caraway and Krieg (1972) for their uncoordinating action in *Spirillum volutans*. Nearly all those effective act on the cell membrane. The K^+ ionophores valinomycin and gramicidin as well as tetrodotoxin (TTX), an inhibitor of the Na^+ conductance in nerve fibers, failed to affect the co-ordinated reversal, and the authors concluded that action potentials along a polarized membrane are not a factor in flagellar co-ordination. It must be emphasized that these results do not rule out an excitation mechanism which depends on cations different from those involved in nervous conduction.

2.5.4 The membrane concept

The foregoing considerations point strongly to a quasi-nervous mechanism for receptor-effector coupling in bacteria similar to that found in *Paramecium* and other ciliates (Naitoh and Eckert, 1974). The great advantage of such an electrochemica mechanism would be its general applicability to qualitatively different sensory functions of bacteria such as chemo- and photoreception. Before presenting a model for the functioning of this coupling in bacteria, the excitation mechanism of *Paramecium* will be briefly reviewed (for details see Chapter 3 in this volume).

Paramecium swims by means of cilia whose effective stroke is normally oriented to the rear of the organism. If the cell experiences a stimulus at its front the ciliary beat is transiently reversed causing a short phase of backward movement, thereafter the normal behaviour is restored. In the non-excited state the internal K^+ concentration is maintained at a high level relative to the environment, whereas the internal Ca^{2+}-concentration is kept low at about 10^{-8} to 10^{-7}M, both by active transport processes. This cation distribution together with a relatively high permeability of the membrane for K^+ and a comparatively low one for Ca^{2+} causes the cytoplasmic membrane to be polarized to about 25 mV, inside negative. Upon a stimulation of the frontal receptor sites the cell becomes locally depolarized, probably as a result of an increased Ca^{2+} permeability. This signal, the receptor potential, spreads passively and triggers the opening of voltage-sensitive Ca^{2+} channels in the membrane of the cilia, allowing Ca^{2+} to flow in down its electrochemical gradient and to cause, in a way which is not yet understood, the ciliary reversal. The calcium mechanism implies that ciliary reversal can occur only as long as the Ca^{2+} gradient is sufficient to allow a Ca^{2+} influx, and in fact it can be demonstrated that the organisms fail to respond if the external Ca^{2+} concentration is below 10^{-8} M (Hildebrand and Dryl, results to be published). A similar dependence upon the external Ca^{2+} concentration exists for the flagellar response of *Chlamydomonas* (Schmidt and Eckert, 1976).

The validity of the calcium influx mechanism has been recently tested in *Escherichia coli* (Ordal, 1977) and in *Halobacterium halobium* (Hildebrand and Janković, unpublished results). Both species failed to show phobic responses, i.e. tumbling or directional changes, respectively, if the external Ca^{2+} concentration was lowered to 10^{-8} M or less. This indicates a further analogy to ciliates although important dissimilarities with respect to sensory transduction and motility transduction may exist.

What would be a reasonable electrochemical mechanism connecting photoreceptor function to effector activity in bacteria? We know that *Halobacterium* is capable of actively extruding protons either by the photocoupling activity of bacteriorhodopsin or by respiration (Oesterhelt and Stoeckenius, 1973). Also that the photosynthetic electron flow of purple bacteria is converted into a proton gradient across the membrane. The H^+ extrusion is always electrogenic and therefore accompanied by an electrical polarization of the cell membrane, making the interior at least 100 mV negative with respect to the outside (for review see Harold, 1977). Hence, H^+ gradient, electron flow and membrane potential are in a way interconvertible.

Light-induced electrogenesis has been demonstrated after the incorporation of BR into proteoliposomes (Kayushin and Skulachev, 1974; Drachev *et al.*, 1974) and bilayer lipid membranes (Dancsházy and Karvaly, 1976). The membrane potential or proton gradient drive the transport of ions across the bacterial membrane. *Halobacterium,* for example, will accumulate K^+ to about 4 M (e.g. Garty and Caplan, 1977) and extrude Na^+ (e.g. Eisenbach *et al.,* 1977). A proton/calcium antiport which keeps the internal Ca^{2+} concentration at a low level has been found in *E. coli* (Tsuchiya and Rosen, 1976). The membrane potential depends on the distribution of all ions and on the membrane permeability for them. Its actual value may therefore be smaller than determined by the H^+-gradient.

The hypothesis presented here (Fig. 2.18) says that random fluctuations of membrane potential of a depolarizing nature lead to spontaneous reversal responses of bacterial flagella, as they do in *Paramecium*, and may represent the 'response generator'. Any effective stimulus applied to the bacterium would modulate the membrane potential. The way in which this happens may be different. Light-on and light-off stimuli in photosensitive bacteria, an increasing repellent or decreasing attractant concentration would cause a depolarization whereas a decrease in repellent or an increase in attractant would cause a hyperpolarization. In photosensory systems the depolarization may be brought about in different ways, for purple bacteria, like *Rhodospirillum*, by a sudden drop of photosynthetic electron flow, for PS 565 of *Halobacterium* by a sudden decrease in proton extrusion, and in PS 370 of *Halobacterium* by an increase of the passive membrane permeability for protons (and/or other cations).

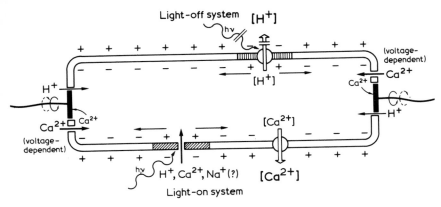

Fig. 2.18 Scheme illustrating a hypothetical mechanism of photosensory function in bacteria. For further explanation see text.

The electrical signal mediated by the receptor, the receptor potential, might be passively transmitted with decrement to the effector site, or a Ca^{2+}-dependent electrical excitation may be interposed. Since the distance between receptor site and effector is short a generally excitable membrane is not necessarily required. However, voltage-sensitive Ca^{2+} gates would have to exist in the neighbourhood of the flagella. An influx of Ca^{2+} ions triggered by the depolarizing signal would cause the flagella to reverse their rotation. It seems quite possible that Ca^{2+} causes the conformational changes of the substructure of the M-ring postulated by Adam (1977) and Läuger (1977).

An alteration of the membrane potential as the trigger impulse for behavioural responses of bacteria has been already suggested by Doetsch (1972) and several attempts have been made to test this hypothesis. Electrical stimulation of *Spirillum volutans* by an extracellularly applied voltage, which can be interpreted as a perturbation of the membrane potential, caused the bacteria to reverse their swimming direction (Caraway and Krieg, 1972). Szmelcman and Adler (1976) measured membrane potential changes in *E. coli* using the uptake of triphenylmethylphosphonium ($TPMP^+$) and found that both attractants and repellents produce a hyperpolarizing wave which the authors attribute to the chemosensory activity. This result is surprising. It would indicate that the membrane potential does not determine the tumbling frequency. Different ions are thought to be responsible for the hyperpolarization caused by opposing stimuli. It must be noted, however, that the temporal resolution of the $TPMP^+$-method is rather low as compared to the behavioural response, so that rapid changes of membrane potential might not have been detected.

Using a fluorescent dye, Miller and Koshland (1977) were able to show with *Bacillus subtilis* that a hyperpolarization of the membrane causes a supression of tumbling whereas a depolarization leads to a period of transient tumbling followed by a return to the normal behaviour. However, attractants which alter the swimming behaviour failed to cause a change in the membrane potential. It appears that a temporal change in the membrane potential (dV_m/dt) and not its absolute level determines the response frequency. But, although experimentally induced alterations of the membrane potential led to the expected behaviour, a change in the overall membrane potential accompanied by the action of chemoeffectors could not be demonstrated by these experiments.

Recently, Harayama and Iino (1977b) measured a change in membrane potential as an absorbance change of carotenoids in *Rhodospirillum rubrum.* Both the motor response and the change in membrane potential could be prevented by antimycin, an inhibitor of the photosynthetic electron transfer, and by valinomycin plus potassium. The experiments confirm the hypothesis that the photophobic response of purple bacteria is induced by a transient disturbance of the photosynthetic electron transfer (Throm, 1968) and that the membrane potential plays an important role in the signalling process.

An interruption of the electron transport chain caused by a disturbance of the flavin system may also be the event which leads to the motor responses of *Salmonella typhimurium* and *E. coli* when subjected to high intensity blue light (Taylor and Koshland, 1975).

The membrane concept for the photosensory function of bacteria presented above remains speculative and requires further experimental support. Clear evidence for the role of membrane potential in signal transmission is necessary. One approach would be to measure stimulus-dependent changes in membrane potential by means of fluorescent indicators, another to apply an external electrical field and determine whether the sensory process is disturbed under these conditions. Neither approach has yet been applied to photosensitive bacteria.

2.6 CONCLUDING REMARKS

A membrane-bound electrochemical mechanism, similar to that of ciliate protozoa, can best account for the various properties of bacterial photosensory systems. It guarantees rapid signal transmission and flagellar co-ordination, permits data processing and can probably explain membrane adaptation, refractoriness and rhythmicity. Not least, it could well represent the response generator. This concept has the great advantage of explaining both the photosensory and the chemosensory function on a common basis. Moreover, it appears that procaryotes and eucaryotes may use similar principles in their sensory function. In particular, the role of Ca^{2+} ions in controlling sudden changes of the activity of motor organelles seems to be an universal phenomenon of motility.

Sensory physiology is one of the most fascinating fields of biology and great progress has been made during the last decade in understanding the mechanisms of sensory activation. Micro-organisms, and particularly bacteria, are well suited for the study of sensory processes on the molecular level.

Nevertheless, more questions have been raised in this chapter than can be answered at present, and the conclusions drawn should be considered primarily as working hypotheses and guidelines for further experiments. The discovery of two sensory photosystems in *Halobacterium* has re-awakened interest in bacterial photobehaviour. Further study of these systems, including the characterization of mutants defective in steps of the photosensory process should contribute to our understanding of sensory mechanisms.

REFERENCES

Adam, G. (1977), Rotation of bacterial flagella as driven by cytomembrane streaming. *J. theor. Biol.*, **65**, 713−726.

Adler, J. (1975), Chemotaxis in bacteria. *A. Rev. Biochem.*, **44**, 341−356.

Adler, J. and Tso, W.W. (1974), 'Decision'-making in bacteria: Chemotactic response of *Escherichia coli* to conflicting stimuli. *Science*, **184**, 1292−1294.

Bauer, P.-J., Dencher, N.A. and Heyn, M.P. (1976), Evidence for chromophore−chromophore interactions in the purple membrane from reconstitution experiments of the chromophore-free membrane. *Biophys. Struct. Mech.*, **2**, 79−92.

Becher, B. and Ebrey, T.G. (1976), Evidence of chromophore−chromophore (exciton) interaction in the purple membrane of *Halobacterium halobium*. *Biochem. biophys. Res. Comm.*, **69**, 1−6.

Benedetti, P.A. and Lenci, F. (1977), *In vivo* microspectrofluorometry of photo-receptor pigments in *Euglena gracilis*. *Photochem. Photobiol.*, **26**, 315−318.

Berg, H.C. (1974), Dynamic properties of bacterial flagellar motors. *Nature,* **249**, 77−79.

Berg, H.C. (1975a), Bacterial behaviour. *Nature*, **254**, 389−392.

Berg, H.C. (1975b), Chemotaxis in bacteria. *A. Rev. Biophys. Bioeng.*, **4**, 119−136.

Berg, H.C. and Anderson, R.A. (1973), Bacteria swim by rotating their flagellar filaments. *Nature*, **245**, 380−382.

Berg, H.C. and Brown, D.A. (1972), Chemotaxis in *Escherichia coli* analysed by three-dimensional tracking. *Nature*, **239**, 500−504.

Blaurock, A.E. and King, G.I. (1977), Asymmetric structure of the purple membrane. *Science*, **196**, 1101−1104.

Blaurock, A.E. and Stoeckenius, W. (1971), Structure of the purple membrane. *Nature New Biol.*, **233**, 152−154.

Buder, J. (1915), Zur Kenntnis des *Thiospirillum jenense* und seiner Reaktionen auf Lichtreize. *Jahrb. wiss. Bot.*, **56**, 529−584.

Buder, J. (1919), Zur Biologie des Bakteriopurpurins und der Purpurbakterien. *Jahrb. wiss. Bot.*, **58**, 525−628.

Caraway, B.H. and Krieg, N.R. (1972), Uncoordination and recoordination in *Spirillum volutans. Can. J. Microbiol.*, **18**, 1749−1759.

Clayton, R.K. (1953a), Studies in the phototaxis of *Rhodospirillum rubrum*. I. Action spectrum, growth in green light, and Weber law adherence. *Arch. Mikrobiol.*, **19**, 107−124.

Clayton, R.K. (1953b), Studies in the phototaxis of *Rhodospirillum rubrum*. II. The relation between phototaxis and photosynthesis. *Arch. Mikrobiol.*, **19**, 125–140.

Clayton, R.K. (1953c), Studies in the phototaxis of *Rhodospirillum rubrum*. III. Quantitative relations between stimulus and response. *Arch. Mikrobiol.*, **19**, 141–165.

Clayton, R.K. (1958), On the interplay of environmental factors affecting taxis and motility in *Rhodospirillum rubrum*. *Arch. Mikrobiol.*, **29**, 189–212.

Clayton, R.K. (1959), Phototaxis of purple bacteria. In: *Encyclopedia of plant physiology*, (Ruhland, W., ed.), **17**, 1, pp. 371–387, Springer-Verlag, Berlin.

Clayton, R.K. (1964), Phototaxis in microorganisms. In: *Photophysiology*, (Giese, A.C., ed.), **2**, pp. 51–77, Academic Press, New York.

Clayton, R.K. (1971), *Light and living matter. A guide to the study of photobiology*. Vol. II: The biological part. MacGraw-Hill, New York.

Dancsházy, Z. and Karvaly, B. (1976), Incorporation of bacteriorhodopsin into a bilayer lipid membrane: A photoelectric-spectroscopic study. *FEBS Letters*, **72**, 136–138.

Dencher, N. (1974), Photophobische Reaktion von *Halobacterium halobium* R_1 und ihre Beziehung zur Purpurmembran. Diplomarbeit, Aaachen, Jülich.

Dencher, N.A., Rafferty, Ch. N. and Sperling, W. (1976), 13-*cis* and *trans* bacteriorhodopsin: Photochemistry and dark equilibrium. *Ber. KFA Jülich* Nr. 1374.

Dencher, N. and Wilms, M. (1975), Flash photometric experiments on the photochemical cycle of bacteriorhodopsin. *Biophys. Struct. Mech.*, **1**, 259–271.

DePamphilis, M.L. and Adler, J. (1971a), Fine structure and isolation of the hook-basal body complex of flagella from *Escherichia coli* and *Bacillus subtilis*. *J. Bact.*, **105**, 384–395.

DePamphilis, M.L. and Adler, J. (1971b), Attachment of flagellar basal bodies to the cell envelope: Specific attachment to the outer, lipopolysaccharide membrane and the cytoplasmic membranes. *J. Bact.*, **105**, 396–407.

Diehn, B. (1969), Action spectra of the phototactic responses in *Euglena*. *Biochim. Biophys. Acta*, **177**, 136–143.

Diehn, B., Feinleib, M., Haupt, W., Hildebrand, E., Lenci, F. and Nultsch, W. (1977), Terminology of behavioral responses of motile microorganisms. *Photochem. Photobiol.*, **26**, 559–560.

Doetsch, R.N. (1972), A unified theory of bacterial motile behavior. *J. theor. Biol.*, **35**, 55–66.

Drachev, L.A., Kaulen, A.D., Ostroumov, S.A. and Skulachev, V.P. (1974), Electrogenesis by bacteriorhodopsin incorporated in a planar phospholipid membrane. *FEBS Letters*, **39**, 43–45.

Eckert, R. and Naitoh, Y. (1970), Passive electrical properties of *Paramecium* and problems of ciliary coordination. *J. gen. Physiol.*, **55**, 467–489.

Eckert, R., Naitoh, Y. and Friedman, K. (1972), Sensory mechanism in *Paramecium*. I. Two components of the electric response to mechanical stimulation of the anterior surface. *J. exp. Biol.*, **56**, 683–694.

Eisenbach, M., Cooper, S., Garty, H., Johnstone, R.M., Rottenberg, H. and Caplan, S.R. (1977), Light-driven sodium transport in sub-bacterial particles of *Halobacterium halobium*. *Biochim. Biophys. Acta*, **465**, 599–613.

Engelmann, T.W. (1883), *Bacterium photometricum*. Ein Beitrag zur vergleichenden Physiologie des Light- und Farbensinnes. *Arch. ges. Physiol.*, **30**, 95–124.

Engelmann, T.W. (1888), Die Purpurbacterien und ihre Beziehung zum Licht. *Bot. Z.*, **46**, 661–670; 677–690; 693–701; 709–720.

Feinleib, M.E. and Curry, G.M. (1974), The nature of the photoreceptor in phototaxis. In: *Handbook of Sensory Physiology*, (Loewenstein, W.R., ed.), **1**, pp. 366–395. Springer-Verlag, Berlin, Heidelberg, New York.

Forward, R.B., Jr. (1973), Phototaxis in a dinoflagellate: Action spectra as evidence for a two-pigment system. *Planta*, **111**, 167–178.

Garty, H. and Caplan, S.R. (1977), Light-dependent rubidium transport in intact *Halobacterium halobium* cells. *Biochim. Biophys. Acta*, **459**, 532–545.

Goy, M.F., Springer, M.S. and Adler, J. (1977), Sensory transduction in *Escherichia coli*: Role of a protein methylation reaction in sensory adaptation. *Proc. natn. Acad. Sci. U.S.A.*, **74**, 4964–4968.

Häder, D.-P. (1974), Participation of two photosystems in the photo-phobotaxis of *Phormidium uncinatum*. *Arch. Mikrobiol*, **96**, 255–266.

Häder, D.-P. (1976), Further evidence for the electron pool hypothesis *Arch. Mikrobiol.* **110**, 301–303.

Häder, D.-P. and Wenderoth, K. (1977), Role of three basic light reactions in photo-movement of desmids. *Planta*, **137**, 207–214.

Harayama, S. and Iino, T. (1976), Phototactic response of aerobically cultivated *Rhodospirillum rubrum*. *J. gen Mikrobiol.*, **94**, 173–179.

Harayama, S. and Iino, T. (1977a), Ferric ion as photoreceptor of photophobotaxis in non-pigmented *Rhodospirillum rubrum*. *Photochem. Photobiol.*, **25**, 571–578.

Harayama, S. and Iino, T. (1977b), Phototaxis and membrane potential in the photosynthetic bacterium *Rhodospirillum rubrum*. *J. Bact.*, **131**, 34–41.

Harold, F.M. (1977), Ion currents and physiological functions in microorganisms. *A. Rev. Microbiol.*, **31**, 181–203.

Haupt, W. (1966), Phototaxis in plants. *Int. Rev. Cytol.*, **19**, 267–299.

Hazelbauer, G.L. and Parkinson, J.S. (1977), Bacterial chemotaxis. In: *Microbial Interactions*, Receptors and Recognition, Series B, Volume 3, (Reissig, J.L., ed.), pp. 61–98, Chapman and Hall, London.

Henderson, R. (1975), The structure of the purple membrane from *Halobacterium halobium*: Analysis of the X-ray diffraction pattern. *J. mol. Biol.*, **93**, 123–138.

Henderson, R. (1977), The purple membrane from *Halobacterium halobium*. *A. Rev. Biophys. Bioeng.*, **6**, 87–109.

Henderson, R. and Unwin, P.N.T. (1975), Three-dimensional model of purple membrane obtained by electron microscopy. *Nature*, **257**, 28–32.

Hildebrand, E. (1977), What does *Halobacterium* tell us about photoreception? *Biophys. Struct. Mech.*, **3**, 69–77.

Hildebrand, E. and Dencher, N. (1975), Two photosystems controlling behavioural responses of *Halobacterium halobium*. *Nature*, **257**, 46–48.

Houwink, A.L. (1956), Flagella, gas vacuoles and cell-wall structure in *Halobacterium halobium*; an electron microscope study. *J. gen. Microbiol.*, **15**, 146–150.

Howes, C.D. and Batra, P.P. (1970), Accumulation of lycopene and inhibition of cyclic carotenoids in *Mycobacterium* in the presence of nicotine. *Biochim. Biophys. Acta*, **222**, 174–179.

Hubbard, R. and Kropf, A. (1959), Molecular aspects of visual excitation. *Ann. N.Y. Acad. Sci.*, **81**, 388–398.

Kayushin, L.P. and Skulachev, V.P. (1974), Bacteriorhodopsin as an electrogenic proton pump: Reconstitution of bacteriorhodopsin proteoliposomes generating $\Delta\psi$ and Δ pH. *FEBS Letters*, **39**, 39–42.

Kelly, M., Norgard, S. and Liaaen-Jensen, S. (1970), Bacterial carotenoids. XXXI. C_{50}-carotenoids 5. carotenoids of *Halobacterium salinarium*. *Acta chem. scand.*, **24**, 2169–2182.

Koshland, D.E., Jr. (1977), A response regulator model in a simple sensory system. *Science*, **196**, 1055–1063.

Krieg, N.R., Tomelty, J.P. and Wels, J.S. (1967), Inhibition of flagellar coordination in *Spirillum volutans*. *J. Bact.*, **94**, 1431–1436.

Kropf, A. (1967), Intramolecular energy transfer in rhodopsin. *Vision Res.*, **7**, 811–818.

Larsen, S.H., Adler, J., Gargus, J.J. and Hogg, R.W. (1974a), Chemomechanical coupling without ATP: The source of energy for motility and chemotaxis in bacteria. *Proc. natn. Acad. Sci. U.S.A.*, **71**, 1239–1243.

Larsen, S.H., Reader, R.W., Kort, E.N., Tso, W.-W. and Adler, J. (1974b), Change in direction of flagellar rotation is the basis of the chemotactic response in *Escherichia coli*. *Nature*, **249**, 74–77.

Läuger, P. (1977), Ion transport and rotation of bacterial flagella. *Nature*, **268**, 360–362.

Lee, A.G. and Fitzsimons, J.T.R. (1976), Motility in normal and filamentous forms of *Rhodospirillum rubrum*. *J. gen. Microbiol.*, **93**, 346–354.

Lenci, F. and Colombetti, G. (1978), Photobehaviors of microorganisms. A biophysical approach. *A. Rev. Biophys. Bioeng.*, **7**, (in press).

Lewis, A. (1976), Tunable laser resonance Raman spectroscopic investigations of the transduction process in vertebrate rod cells. *Fedn. Proc. fedn. Am. Socs. exp. Biol.*, **35**, 51–53.

Lewis, A., Spoonhover, J., Bogomolni, R.A., Lozier, R.H. and Stoeckenius, W. (1974), Tunable laser resonance Raman spectroscopy of bacteriorhodopsin. *Proc. natn. Acad. Sci. U.S.A.*, **71**, 4462–4466.

Links, J. (1955), An hypothesis for the mechanism of (phobo-) chemotaxis. II. The carotenoids, steroids, and fatty acids of *Polytoma uvella.*, Ph. D. Thesis, Leiden.

Lozier, R.H., Bogomolni, R.A. and Stoeckenius, W. (1975), Bacteriorhodopsin: A light-driven proton pump in *Halobacterium halobium*. *Biophys. J.*, **15**, 955–962.

Machemer, H. (1974), Frequency and directional responses of cilia to membrane potential changes in *Paramecium*. *J. comp. Physiol.*, **92**, 293–316.

Macnab, R.M. (1977), Bacterial flagella rotating in bundles: A study in helical geometry. *Proc. natn. Acad. Sci. U.S.A.*, **74**, 221–225.

Macnab, R.M. and Koshland, D.E. Jr. (1972), The gradient-sensing mechanism in bacterial chemotaxis. *Proc. natn. Acad. Sci. U.S.A.*, **69**, 2509–2512.

Macnab, R. and Koshland, D.E. Jr. (1974), Bacterial motility and chemotaxis: Light-induced tumbling response and visualization of individual flagella. *J. mol. Biol.*, **84**, 399–406.

Macnab, R.M. and Ornston, M.K. (1977), Normal-to-curly flagellar transitions and their role in bacterial tumbling. Stabilization of an alternative quaternary structure by mechanical force. *J. mol. Biol.,* **112**, 1–30.

Manson, M.D., Tedesco, P., Berg, H.C., Harold, F.M. and van der Drift, C. (1977), A protonmotive force drives bacterial flagella. *Proc. natn. Acad. Sci. U.S.A.,* **74**, 3060–3064.

Manten, A. (1948), Phototaxis in the purple bacterium *Rhodospirillum rubrum,* and the relation between phototaxis and photosynthesis. *Leeuwenhoek nederl. Tijdschr.,* **14**, 65–86.

Matsuura, S., Shioi, J. and Imae, Y. (1977), Motility in *Bacillus subtilis* driven by an artificial protonmotive force. *FEBS Letters,* **82**, 187–190.

Metzner, P. (1920), Die Bewegung und Reizbeantwortung der bipolar begeisselten Spirillen. *Jahrb. wiss. Bot.,* **59**, 325–412.

Miller, J.B. and Koshland, D.E. Jr. (1977), Sensory electrophysiology of bacteria: Relationship of the membrane potential to motility and chemotaxis in *Bacillus subtilis. Proc. natn. Acad. Sci. U.S.A.,* **74**, 4752–4756.

Mitchell, P. (1966), Chemiosmotic coupling in oxidative and photosynthetic phosphorylation. *Biol. Rev.,* **41**, 445–502.

Naitoh, Y. and Eckert, R. (1969), Ionic mechanisms controlling behavioral responses of *Paramecium* to mechanical stimulation. *Science,* **164**, 963–965.

Naitoh, Y. and Eckert, R. (1974), The control of ciliary activity in Protozoa. In: *Cilia and Flagella,* (Sleigh, M.A., ed.), pp. 305–352, Academic Press, London, New Yorl

Nultsch, W. (1975), Phototaxis and photokinesis. In: *Primitive Sensory and Communication Systems,* (Carlile, M.J., ed.), pp. 29–90, Academic Press, New York, London, San Francisco.

Oesterhelt, D. and Hess, B. (1973), Reversible photolysis of the purple complex in the purple membrane of *Halobacterium halobium. Eur. J. Biochem.,* **37**, 316–326.

Oesterhelt, D., Meentzen, M. and Schumann, L. (1973), Reversible dissociation of the purple complex in bacteriorhodopsin and identification of 13-*cis* and all-*trans*-retinal as its chromophores. *Eur. J. Biochem.,* **40**, 453–463.

Oesterhelt, D. and Stoeckenius, W. (1971), Rhodopsin-like protein from the purple membrane of *Halobacterium halobium. Nature New Biol.,* **233**, 149–152.

Oesterhelt, D. and Stoeckenius, W. (1973), Functions of a new photoreceptor membrane. *Proc. natn. Acad. Sci. U.S.A.,* **70**, 2853–2857.

Ordal, G.W. (1977), Calcium ion regulates chemotactic behavior in bacteria. *Nature,* **270**, 66–67.

Ovchinnikov, Yu.A., Abdulaev, N.G., Feigina, M.Yu., Kiselev, A.V. and Lobanov, N.A. (1977), Recent findings in the structure-functional characteristics of bacterio-rhodopsin. *FEBS Letters,* **84**, 1–4.

Peters, J., Peters, R. and Stoeckenius, W. (1976), A photosensitive product of sodium borohydride reduction of bacteriorhodopsin. *FEBS Letters,* **61**, 128–134.

Pfennig, N. (1964), *Thiospirillum jenense* (Thiorhodaceae) – Lokomotion und phototaktisches Verhalten. Film No. E 678, Inst. wiss. Film, Göttingen.

Reynolds, J.A. and Stoeckenius, W. (1977), Molecular weight of bacteriorhodopsin solubilized in Triton X-100. *Proc. natn. Acad. Sci. U.S.A.,* **74**, 2803–2804.

Schletz, K. (1976), Phototaxis in *Volvox*. Pigments involved in the perception of light direction, *Z. Pflanzenphysiol.*, **77**, 189–211.

Schmidt, J.A. and Eckert, R. (1976), Calcium couples flagellar reversal to photo-stimulation in *Chlamydomonas reinhardtii. Nature,* **262**, 713–714.

Schrammeck, J. (1934), Untersuchungen über die Phototaxis der Purpurbakterien. *Beitr. Biol. Pflanz.,* **22**, 315–379.

Silverman, M.R. and Simon, M. (1974), Flagellar rotation and the mechanism of bacterial motility. *Nature,* **249**, 73–74.

Sperling, W., Carl, P., Rafferty, Ch. N. and Dencher, N.A. (1977), Photochemistry and dark equilibrium of retinal isomers and bacteriorhodopsin isomers. *Biophys. Struct. Mech.,* **3**, 79–94.

Springer, M.S., Goy, M.F. and Adler, J. (1977), Sensory transduction in *Escherichia coli*: A requirement for methionine in sensory adaptation. *Proc. natn. Acad. Sci. U.S.A.,* **74**, 183–187.

Stieve, H. (1974), On the ionic mechanisms responsible for the generation of the electrical response of light sensitive cells. In: *Biochemistry of Sensory Functions*, (Jaenicke, L., ed.), pp. 79–105. Springer-Verlag, Berlin, Heidelberg, New York.

Stoeckenius, W. and Lozier, R.H. (1974), Light energy conversion in *Halobacterium halobium. J. Supramol. Struct.,* **2**, 769–774.

Sumper, M., Reitmeier, H. and Oesterhelt, D. (1976), Biosynthesis of the purple membrane of halobacteria. *Angew. Chem. Int.* Ed. Engl. **15**, 187–194.

Szmelcman, S. and Adler, J. (1976), Change in membrane potential during bacterial chemotaxis. *Proc. natn. Acad. Sci. U.S.A.,* **73**, 4387–4391.

Taylor, B.L. and Koshland, D.E. Jr. (1974), Reversal of flagellar rotation in mono-trichous and peritrichous bacteria. Generation of changes in direction. *J. Bact.,* **119**, 640–642.

Taylor, B.L. and Koshland, D.E. Jr. (1975), Intrinsic and extrinsic light responses of *Salmonella typhimurium* and *Escherichia coli. J. Bact.,* **123**, 557–569.

Throm, G. (1968), Untersuchungen zum Reaktionsmechanismus von Phototaxis und Kinesis an *Rhodospirillum rubrum. Arch. Protistenk.,* **110**, 313–371.

Tsang, N., Macnab, R. and Koshland, D.E. Jr. (1973), Common mechanism for repellents and attractants in bacterial chemotaxis. *Science,* **181**, 60–63.

Tsuchiya, T. and Rosen, B.P. (1976), Calcium transport driven by a proton gradient in inverted membrane vesicles of *Escherichia coli. J. biol. Chem.,* **251**, 962–967.

Wald, G. (1968), The molecular basis of visual excitation. *Nature,* **219**, 800–807.

3 Behavior of Paramecium: Chemical, Physiological and Genetic Studies

DAVID L. NELSON and CHING KUNG

Acknowledgement

We thank the following for providing manuscripts in advance of publication:
P. Brehm, S. Dryl, K. Dunlap, R. Eckert, A. Grebecki, H. Hansma, F. Harold,
M. Levandowsky, H. Machemer, M. Takahashi and J. Van Houten.

Research done in the author's laboratories was supported by NSF grant #
BNS 75-10433 (C.K.), NIH Grant # GM 2271403 (C.K.), NSF grant # BNS 76-11490
(D.L.N.), NIH grant # 00085 (D.L.N.), Dreyfus Foundation Teacher-Scholar Award
(D.L.N.), Steenbock Career Advancement Award (D.L.N.), and grants from the
Graduate School of the University of Wisconsin (C.K. and D.L.N.).

Taxis and Behavior
(*Receptors and Recognition,* Series B. Volume 5)
Edited by G.L. Hazelbauer
Published 1978 by Chapman and Hall, 11 New Fetter Lane, London EC4P 4EE
© Chapman and Hall

3.1 INTRODUCTION

Jennings, in his classic monograph of 1906, described in detail the variety of swimming behavior seen in *Paramecium* in response to several types of stimuli. Recent years have seen a renewal of interest in the behavior of *Paramecium*, which appears to be well-suited for studies of sensory transduction, membrane excitation, and the regulation of behavior in eucaryotes. *Paramecium* is a free-living freshwater protozoan with an excitable surface membrane that governs the organism's swimming behavior by coupling the receptors for various stimuli to the cilia that cover its surface (Fig. 3.1).

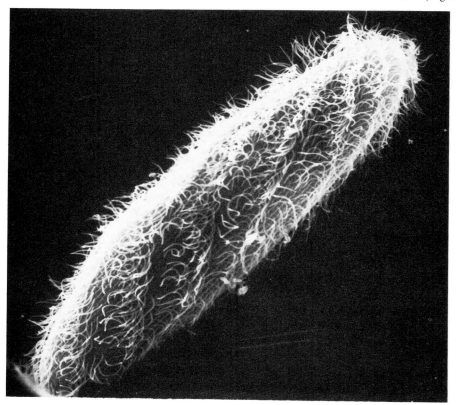

Fig. 3.1 Scanning electron micrograph of a wild-type *Paramecium tetraurelia* fixed during forward swimming. Note that the cell is covered with cilia. The cell is asymmetric. Dorsal left surface showing; upper end anterior; cell 114 μm in length. (Courtesy S.L. Tamm.)

Paramecium swims forward through its medium in a left-handed helical path, propelled by the co-ordinated beating of its several thousand cilia. There is only a low rate of spontaneous change of direction in the normal medium. When a cell collides with an obstacle or enters the zone of a certain chemical repellent, it backs away momentarily, then resumes forward swimming in a new direction. The result of a series of such avoiding reactions is net movement away from the obstacle or repellent.

3.2 AVOIDING REACTION AND ITS IONIC BASIS

3.2.1 Ciliary reversal: the basis of the avoiding reaction

The reversal in swimming direction is a result of the alteration of the direction of the power stroke of each cilium, which occurs in all of the cilia during a fraction of a second after the obstacle is encountered. The ionic basis of ciliary reversal has been worked out by studies of the ionic requirements of the process and the electrophysiological events that accompany the change in swimming behavior.

3.2.2 Ionic basis of ciliary reversal

Paramecium is a large enough cell (e.g. 30 x 120 μm for *P. tetraurelia*) to allow the insertion of one or more microelectrodes. Kinosita, Naitoh, Eckert, Machemer, Kung, Schein, and their collaborators have made extensive electrophysiological studies of *Paramecium,* which have been reviewed (Eckert, 1972; Naitoh and Eckert, 1974; Naitoh, 1974; Eckert *et al.,* 1976; Machemer and de Peyer, 1977) and can be briefly summarized thus:

The surface membrane of *Paramecium* is normally polarized (V_m inside negative at -10 to -40 mV, depending on the external ionic species and strength). When cells are mechanically stimulated by a stylus on their anterior end or electrically stimulated by injection of an outward current through an intracellular microelectrode (Naitoh and Eckert, 1968, 1969), a sudden membrane depolarization may occur, during which V_m becomes less negative. The rise occurs in a few milliseconds and is followed by a slower decrease to the prestimulation V_m (Fig. 3.2). This depolarization is regenerative, as in squid axon and frog muscle. However, unlike the all-or-none action potentials in those membranes, but similar to crustacean muscle, the regenerative depolarization is graded in *Paramecium*; stronger stimuli produce greater depolarizations (Fig. 3.2). Such graded action potentials change the direction of the power strokes of the cilia. Thus, the swimming behavior of the organism, which is easily observed with a dissecting microscope, is the visual correlate of the electrical activity of the cell membrane.

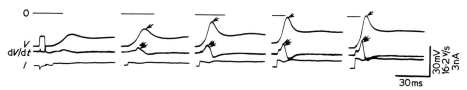

Fig. 3.2 Membrane responses evoked by injected currents in a wild-type
P. tetraurelia. Panels from left to right show responses to increasing strength
of injected current. Outward current (*I*) delivered through one electrode
causes the membrane potential (*V*, recorded with a second electrode) to become
less negative (reference level, 0). Action potentials (arrows) are triggered by
stronger currents. Note that the amplitude of the action potentials is graded to
the strength of injected currents. The maximal rate of rise of the action
potential (double arrows on d*V*/d*t* traces) also increases according to the
current strength. The injected currents are 2, 3, 5, 7, and 10×10^{-10} A from
left. The square pulse on the *V* trace in the first panel is a 10 mV, 5 ms
calibration. The paramecium is bathed in a solution of 4 mM KCl, 1 mM
$Ca(OH)_2$, 1 mM citrate, 1.3 mM Tris, pH 7.2. (Courtesy Y. Satow.)

3.2.3 Ca^{2+} carries both the depolarizing current and the message

The electrical events described above clearly involve ion fluxes across the cell membrane. Electrophysiological studies (see Naitoh and Eckert, 1974) provide strong
evidence that the inward current (the upstroke of the action potential) is carried by
Ca^{2+} and indicate that the membrane conductance to Ca^{2+} increases in a regenerative
manner upon suprathreshold stimulation. The downstroke of the action potential is
due to a delayed K^+ efflux.

Does Ca^{2+} entry trigger ciliary reversal? Naitoh and Kaneko (1972) prepared
permeable models of *Paramecium* by treating mildly with a detergent, and showed
that these ghosts could be made to swim quite normally by the addition of MgATP
to the medium. The *direction* of swimming by such ghosts was determined by the
Ca^{2+} concentration in the medium; at low Ca^{2+} (10^{-7}M), cells moved forward, but
at higher Ca^{2+} ($> 10^{-6}$ M) ciliary reversal occurred, and swimming was exclusively
backwards. These experiments established that Ca^{2+} carries not only the current, but
also the *message* : swim backwards; reverse the direction of the ciliary power stroke.

3.2.4 A model for the avoiding reaction

A simple model for the mechanism of coupling between membrane depolarization
and ciliary reversal has been proposed (Eckert, 1972; Naitoh and Eckert, 1974;
Naitoh and Kaneko, 1972; Eckert *et al.*, 1976). Normally, the internal concentration
of Ca^{2+} is maintained at a low level by an efficient, active extrusion of Ca^{2+}. Stimulation triggers an increase in Ca^{2+} conductance and the resultant Ca^{2+} influx raises

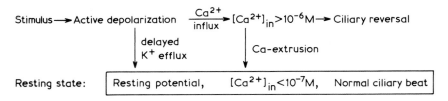

Fig. 3.3 Ca^{2+} control of ciliary beat direction in *Paramecium.* See text for detail.

the internal Ca^{2+} concentration enough to activate a 'muscle'* which reorients the ciliary beat. The ciliary reversal is transient; Ca^{2+} extrusion and/or sequestration reduces the internal level of Ca^{2+}; below the 'muscle's' threshold, the direction of ciliary beat returns to normal, and forward swimming resumes. This model predicts the existence of *at least* four biochemical components:

1. A receptor that receives the stimulus;
2. A Ca^{2+} channel through the membrane, with a voltage-sensitive gate;
3. A Ca^{2+}-activated 'muscle' which reorients ciliary beat; and
4. An active Ca^{2+} extrusion pump.

Other electrophysiological and genetic evidence reviewed later also shows, as in other excitable membranes, the existence of:

5. A gated K^+ channel through the membrane which is responsible for the down-stroke of the action potential.

Biochemical evidence for the existence of some of these components is described later. The model for the avoiding reaction is summarized in Fig. 3.3. The nature of the 'muscle' and how Ca^{2+} acts on it are not known.

3.2.5 Membrane potential controls rate as well as direction of ciliary beat

By combining electrophysiological measurements with high-speed microcinematography Machemer and Eckert (1973) have shown that the rate of both forward and reverse ciliary beating varies with membrane potential. These studies show clearly that both rate and direction vary in a graded fashion; they are not all-or-none phenomena. Fraenkel and Gunn (1961) have pointed out that a free-swimming organism such as *Paramecium* can seek or avoid a certain region either by varying the speed of swimming in response to some stimulus (orthokinesis) or by altering the frequency of direction changes (klinokinesis). In *Paramecium,* both types of behavior are

---

* The word 'muscle' refers to the as yet unidentified mechanism which receives the Ca^{2+} and causes the change in beat direction of the cilium. There is no evidence that the mechanism involves actomyosin.

apparently regulated by the membrane potential. In studies of chemotaxis, thermo-taxis etc., by this organism, it is therefore important to determine which of the mechanisms is involved.

<h3 style="text-align:center">3.3 DIRECT MEASUREMENT OF ION FLUXES IN
PARAMECIUM</h3>

Browning and Nelson (1976) and Browning *et al.* (1976) have obtained evidence in support of the Ca hypothesis by measuring directly the influx and efflux of ^{45}Ca across the membranes of intact *Paramecium.* Normally, the extrusion of Ca^{2+} is so efficient that only immeasurably small accumulations of radiocalcium could be expected. However, by assaying Ca influx at low temperature, where the efflux mechanism is inhibited, accumulation of Ca was demonstrated. The influx of Ca^{2+} was stimulated by the same conditions that cause membrane depolarization and ciliary reversal. For example, the addition of Na^+ or K^+ (which stimulate ciliary reversal) resulted in a 10-fold increase in the rate of Ca^{2+} influx (Fig. 3.4). Mutants which have electrophysiological properties indicating a defect in the Ca gate (Pawns, see below) were defective in this stimulated Ca influx (Fig. 3.4). Ca influx into *Paramecium* had the properties of a passive process, and was saturable at relatively low Ca^{2+} (c. 10^{-5} M). Ca^{2+} efflux from cells previously loaded with ^{45}Ca at low temperature took place rapidly at room temperature, and was an active process, occurring against a concentration gradient. These studies therefore document the existence of the gated Ca channel and the Ca pump predicted by the model. This assay must be done at an unphysiological (low) temperature, but Ling and Kung (in preparation) have used $^{133}Ba^{2+}$ as an analog of Ca, and with it have measured Ba^{2+} fluxes through the Ca channel at physiological temperatures. Andrivon (1970) has measured the influx of Ni^{2+} into *Paramecium,* and although Ni^{2+} is potentially an analog of Ca^{2+}, the fact that Ni^{2+} uptake is energy-dependent indicates that Ni^{2+} does not enter via the Ca(Ba) channel.

Browning (1976) has also measured the fluxes of monovalent cations across the *Paramecium* membrane, using radioisotopes and flame photometry. Cells actively accumulated K^+ (and its analog Rb^+) from a medium containing that ion at 100 μM. Since the internal concentration of K^+ is about 100 times greater than this, transport was clearly uphill. K^+ influx was rapid at $25°C$ but was strongly inhibited at $0°C$ or by energy poisons. The apparent K_m for external K was about 30 μM, although we obtained evidence suggesting that there may be a second system with lower affinity. In contrast to K^+ influx, the efflux of K^+ was a passive process, only slightly inhibited at $0°C$ or by energy poisons. Both influx and efflux of Na^+ were about 10 times slower than the corresponding movement of K^+. Hansma and Kung (1976) have characterized the Na^+ uptake system in some detail and have detected differences between the Na^+ uptake of wild-type cells and certain behavioural mutants (see below) which also showed abnormal K^+ permeabilities.

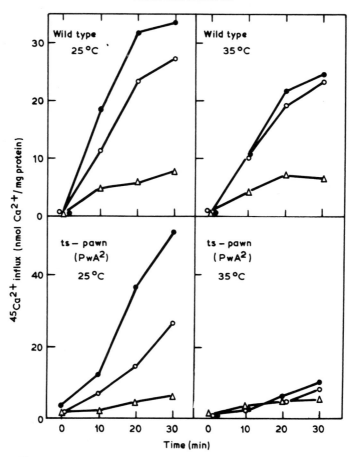

Fig. 3.4 ^{45}Ca influx into wild type and a behavioral mutant. Cells of the wild type or a temperature-sensitive Pawn (which behaves normally when grown at 25°C but is defective when grown at 35°C) were grown either at 25°C or 35°C, and Ca influx was assayed with 15 mM KCl (●) or 15 mM NaCl (○) as stimuli or with no addition (△). (a) wild type, 25°C; (b) wild type, 35°C; (c) ts-pawn, 25°C; (d) ts-pawn, 35°C. (From Browning *et al.,* 1976.)

3.4 CILIA: STRUCTURE, FUNCTION AND COMPOSITION

3.4.1 Cilia: the motor elements

The cilia of *Paramecium* closely resemble those of other eucaryotic cells. A central motile apparatus, the axoneme, contains the classical 9 + 2 arrangement of microtubules (Fig. 3.5a). The proteins of the *Paramecium* axoneme have not been well characterized, but those of the related ciliate *Tetrahymena*, and the flagellate *Chlamydomonas,* have been extensively studied. Associated with the tubulin of the microtubules are a group of high-molecular-weight proteins, dyneins, with Mg-dependent ATPase activity. The sliding of the microtubules relative to one another, in which dynein plays a critical role and for which Mg-ATP hydrolysis supplies energy (Warner, 1976), is presumably the driving force of the ciliary beat. The details of ciliary motion are outside the scope of this review but have been reviewed elsewhere (e.g., Sleigh, 1974). It is not known how a bend is formed in the cilium or what goes on within the cilium during reversal or beat acceleration.

3.4.2 The ciliary membrane: a highly differentiated structure

Enclosing the length of the axoneme and continuous with the cell's surface membrane is the ciliary membrane (Fig. 3.5a,b). Electron microscopic examination of freeze-fractured cilia reveals two ordered sets of structures within this membrane (Fig. 3.5c). Two rows of 8 nm particles, called the necklace, encircle the cilium near its base (Plattner, 1975). Distal to the necklace are 9 discrete arrays, called plaques, each consisting of 10 nm particles in a 3 x 5 rectangular arrangement. Each plaque is opposite and connected to one of the 9 outer doublets of the axoneme (Fig. 3.5d). The plaque region corresponds to a region of negative charges capable of binding polycationic ferritin (Dute and Kung, 1977) (Fig. 3.5e). Dense deposits are seen immediately beneath the plaques in cells fixed in solutions containing large amounts of calcium (Plattner, 1975; Fisher *et al.,* Tsuchiya and Takahashi, 1976) (Fig. 3.5f). Electron microprobe analysis has demonstrated these deposits to consist of calcium and phosphorus (Plattner and Fuchs, 1975; Tsuchiya, 1976). Comparison of *Tetrahymena* strains with and without plaques suggests that the plaques correlate with a Ca-activated ATPase (Baugh *et al.,* 1976). Byrne and Byrne (1978) found that many plaques are deranged in a strain of 'paranoiac' mutants (below).

3.4.3 Deciliation: evidence for functional differentiation in *Paramecium* surface membranes

When intact ciliates are exposed to combinations of Ca^{2+} and ethanol (Gibbons, 1965) or local anesthetics (Thompson, Baugh and Walker, 1974), virtually all cilia are lost without destruction of the cell bodies (for review, see Nozawa, 1975). The zone between necklace and plaques is where cilia break when cells are deciliated. Deciliated cells can regenerate cilia over a period of hours under appropriate conditions (Satir *et al.,* 1976). Deciliated cells (*P. caudatum*) have the same resting membrane potential as intact cells, but lose their ability to generate the action potential (Ogura and Takahashi, 1976; Dunlap, 1977). When cells are allowed to regenerate cilia, they recover excitability. The deciliated cells retain a K-mediated hyperpolarization to mechanical stimulation at the posterior end, indicating that at least one kind of K^+ channel is retained in deciliated cells. These findings strongly suggest that the

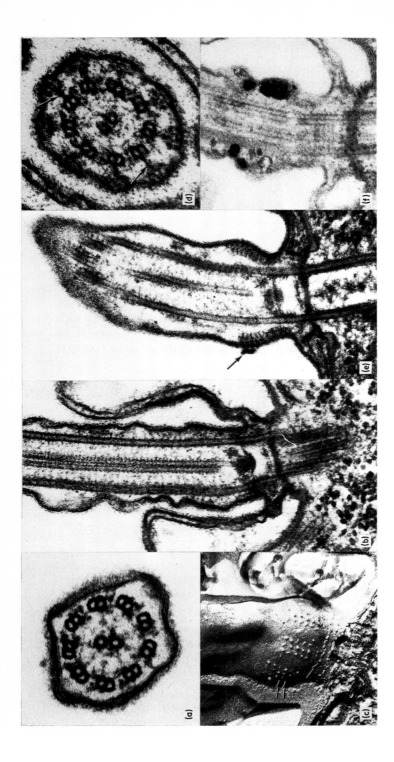

Fig. 3.5 Structures of cilia in *P. tetraurelia*. (a) Cross-section of the shaft of a cilium, showing the 9 + 2 microtubular arrangement and the surrounding membrane (x 140 000). (b) Longitudinal section of a cilium near the base (x 69 000). (c) Freeze-fractured electron micrograph of the base of a cilium showing the necklace (arrow) and the plaques (double arrows) (x 68 000). (d) Cross-section of a cilium at the level of the plaques (x 124 000). Note the connections between the membrane plaque particles and the microtubules (arrows). (e) Thin section of a cilium from a cell incubated with polycationic ferritin before fixation. Note polycationic-binding sites correspond to the positions of the plaques (arrow) (x 71 000). (f) A cilium from a cell fixed in the presence of Ca^{2+}. Note the large, dense deposits beneath the membrane at the plaque region (x 81 000). (Courtesy of R. Dute.)

voltage-sensitive Ca channels that regulate ciliary motion are themselves localized in the ciliary membrane, and are not generally distributed over the entire surface of the cell. The ciliary membrane is *functionally differentiated* for excitability.

3.4.4 Proteins of the cilium and ciliary membrane

The surface antigens of *Paramecium* have been studied extensively. The principal antigen (immobilization or i-antigen) is one of the largest known single polypeptides (mol. wt. about 300 000) (Hansma, 1975). It is released as a soluble protein when intact cells are washed with a salt-ethanol solution (Preer, 1959). An immunologically related protein is tightly bound to the membrane, and differs slightly in molecular weight (Hansma and Kung, 1976); this peptide may be a precursor of the i-antigen. These two proteins are major components of the *Paramecium* surface; the i-antigen may represent 1% of the cell's dry mass, and the membrane-bound form constitutes 75% of the total membrane protein. The peripheral (non-integral) nature of the i-antigen and the paramecium's ability to synthesize over 12 different kinds of such proteins one at a time (see Preer, 1969), make it unlikely that such proteins play a direct role in membrane excitation.

Hansma (1974) has used polyacrylamide gel electrophoresis in SDS to resolve a number of minor protein species in the ciliary membrane of *Paramecium* and several workers in our laboratories have used two-dimensional gel electrophoresis to resolve about 100 protein species in cilia. It is possible that among the species seen on such gels are proteins involved in ion gating or pumping, and we hope that a careful comparison of mutant and wild-type cells by this technique will allow us to recognize such proteins.

At least ten of the proteins of the cilium are phosphoproteins (Lewis and Nelson, unpublished), and in view of the emerging role of membrane protein phosphorylation in excitable membranes, it will be of interest to see whether behavioral mutants show altered patterns of protein phosphorylation. Protein kinase activity has not been demonstrated in *Paramecium* but, in the related ciliate *Tetrahymena,* protein kinases dependent upon either cAMP or cGMP, as well as adenyl cyclase, are present in cilia (Dickinson *et al.,* 1976; Morofushi, 1973; Morofushi, 1974).

Doughty and Dodd (in press) have used low concentrations of glutaraldehyde to cross-link surface membrane proteins of *Paramecium.* Glutaraldehyde-treated cells are altered in their response to certain metal ions, and the authors conclude that some critical protein(s) in the excitable membrane have been altered.

Riddle and Nelson (in preparation) have characterized a Ca-activated ATPase released from *Paramecium* upon deciliation. This soluble enzyme is distinctly different from dynein, another ATPase activity that, in conjunction with tubulin, is responsible for the beating action of the cilia. Doughty (personal communication) has identified several forms of dynein in *Paramecium* cilia, and has also purified a Ca-ATPase released from cilia by mild treatment with detergent (Doughty, in press). The roles of these non-dynein ATPases have not been established, but it is possible that they are involved either in active extrusion of Ca, or are part of the Ca-activated reversal mechanism described above.

3.4.5 Lipid composition: evidence of chemical differentiation in ciliary membranes of *Paramecium* and *Tetrahymena*

The phospholipid, sterol, and fatty acid composition of several membrane fractions from *Tetrahymena,* including cilia, pellicle and microsomes, have been compared (Holtz and Conner, 1973), and ciliary membranes were found to contain similar kinds, but different amounts, of these lipids. For example, isolated cilia of *Tetrahymena* were richer in ethanolamine phosphonolipids than other membrane fractions, and correspondingly less rich in ethanolamine glycerophosphatides. Lipid composition, distribution, biosynthesis and turnover has been thoroughly studied in *Tetrahymena,* and these studies have been reviewed recently by Thompson and Nozawa (1977). *Paramecium* lipids are far less well studied. Andrews and Nelson (1977) and Rhoads *et al.* (1977) have found similar enrichments of phosphonolipids in the isolated cilia of *Paramecium* (Table 3.1). We have also shown (Andrews, 1977) that six sphingolipids

Table 3.1 Phospholipids of *Paramecium**

	Whole cells	Cilia	Deciliated bodies
Cardiolipin	4†	—	4
Glyceryl-aminoethylphosphonate	16	30	13
Phosphatidyl ethanolamine	41	37	37
1-alkyl-phosphatidylcholine	30	11	30
Ceramide aminoethylphosphonate	3	15	1
Phosphatidylinositol	3	2	3
Sphinolipids	1	2	0

* from Andrews (1977)
† % of total

are readily detected in cilia but undetectable in other membrane fractions. *Paramecium* phospholipid composition changes very little with growth stage, and six behavioral mutants in three different classes (Pawn, Paranoiac and Fast, see below) have phospholipid compositions indistinguishable from that of wild type. We (Andrews and Nelson, 1977) and Kaneshiro's group (Kaneshiro *et al.,* 1977) have noted significant differences between the fatty acid composition of ciliary and other membranes of *Paramecium.*

3.5 STIMULI TO WHICH *PARAMECIUM* RESPONDS

Jennings (1906) cataloged the impressive behavioral repertoire of *Paramecium*, and several more recent reviews (Jahn and Bovee, 1967; Dryl, 1973, 1974; Levandowsky and Hauser, 1978; Machemer and de Peyer, 1978) provide useful discussions of the variety of stimuli to which *Paramecium* and related organisms respond. The response may be a change of swimming velocity (orthokinesis) or a change in the frequency of avoiding reactions (klinokinesis). The result in either case is net movement of the cell toward an attractant or away from a repellent, by a process of biased trial-and-error. When a stimulus alters the orientation of the body axis with respect to the source of the stimulus, the response is *taxis*. Both taxis and kinesis have been observed in *Paramecium.*

Negative geotaxis (the tendency to swim upward) is very pronounced in *Paramecium* and provides the basis for several selection procedures in isolating behavioral mutants (below). The orientation induced by weak electical potential gradient (galvanotaxis) has been extensively documented, and the tendency to swim upstream (rheotaxis) has also been described (Dryl, 1974; Jennings, 1906).

Mechanical stimulation may elicit any of several responses, depending upon the part of the cell that is touched and other factors that are not well understood. The tendency to stop swimming when a physical obstacle is encountered, called thigmotaxis by Jennings, sometimes dominates a cell's response. Under other circumstances a physical stimulus at the anterior end elicits the classical avoiding reaction, and the same stimulus delivered at the posterior end causes faster swimming.

There is no evidence of a response by *Paramecium* to visible light, but high and low temperature are sensed, as are certain inorganic ions and simple organic compounds in the medium. Strictly speaking these responses are kineses, not taxes, but to keep our teminology consistent with that used in the previous literature on *Paramecium* and bacteria, we have used the terms thermotaxis and chemotaxis in the following discussions.

3.5.1 Chemotaxis

Jennings (1906) directly observed the responses of individual paramecia to drops of salt or acid solutions and bubbles of gases. He noted that paramecia collect in drops or disperse from drops or bubbles by avoiding reactions at the boundary. He also cataloged a large number of chemicals that cause avoiding reactions in *Paramecium* and dissociated the stimulation from the osmotic or general toxic effects of the chemicals. More recently, a dark-field photographic technique has been adopted to study the locomotion of paramecia. Using this technique Dryl (1973, 1974) has studied and reviewed paramecium's chemotaxis in different pH, cation solutions, quinine, and lower alcohol solutions.

Chemotaxis has been re-examined in large populations of paramecia responding to chemical gradients. Two methods have been employed (Van Houten *et al.,* 1975).

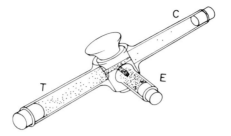

Fig. 3.6 T-maze for assaying chemotaxis. Paramecia are placed in the 'entry arm', E; test solution in the 'test arm', T; control solution in the 'control arm', C, and the stopcock in the center. The relative number of paramecia found in T after 30 min measures chemotaxis. (From Van Houten *et al.*, 1975.)

A counter-current flow method originally devised for the study of chemotaxis of nematodes (Dusenbery, 1973) has been adopted for paramecium work. A simpler method is the 'T-maze' (Fig. 3.6). The maze is essentially a three-way stopcock. Paramecia entering from one arm must 'choose' between one arm with the test solution and one with the control solution. The fraction of paramecia that arrive at the test arm is taken as the index of chemotaxis (I_{che}). Thus, I_{che} approaches unity when attraction is strong; zero when repulsion is strong; 0.5 when there is no chemotaxis. Using the 'T-maze', Van Houten (1977) has surveyed paramecium's chemotaxis to sugars, fermentation by-products, amino acids, and other organic compounds as well as inorganic ions known or suspected to affect membrane or behavior. She found that, among other chemicals, acetate and lactate are attractants; quinidine-HCl and tetraethylammonium are repellents. To see if the avoiding reaction is required for these attractions and repulsions, the I_{che}'s of wild types are compared with those of pawns, the mutants that lack avoiding reactions but swim forward normally (Pawn B, see below). While the I_{che}'s of wild types show clear chemotaxis, those of pawns hover around 0.5 (Table 3.2). Thus, the avoiding reaction is a necessary condition for chemotaxis to these chemicals. Van Houten (1977) also discovered a form of repulsion (e.g. by OH^-) in *Paramecium* which results from the increase in swimming speed. Pawns can be repelled by this means. A unifying hypothesis on the physiological basis of chemotaxis has been proposed by her (Van Houten, in press). It states that ordinarily there is a ground rate of action potential, hence a basal frequency of avoiding reactions. Repellents like quinidine-HCl depolarize the membrane, causing a higher frequency of action potential. The resultant increase in the frequency of avoiding reactions leads to klinokinetic repulsion. Attractants like acetate slightly hyperpolarize the membrane, causing a lower frequency of action potential. The resultant decrease in the frequency of avoiding reaction leads to klinokinetic attraction. Repellents like OH^- strongly hyperpolarize the membrane, abolish all action potentials and avoiding reactions and increase the swimming speed. The speeding leads to orthokinetic repulsion. Preliminary results from

Table 3.2 Indices of chemotaxis in *P. tetraurelia* *

	Wild type	Pawn
Attractants:		
5 mM acetate†	0.84	0.55
5 mM lactate†	0.83	0.46
Repellents: I:		
0.1 mM quinidine-HCl‡	0.08	0.44
5 mM tetraethylammonium§	0.08	0.58

* Using the T-maze (Fig. 3.6) tested for 30 min. For the counter ions and other
details see Van Houten (1978).
† Control: 5 mM Cl^-.
‡ A modified T-maze with a two-way plug used. The I_{che}'s are calculated in the
same manner. Control 0.1 mM KCl.
§ Control: 5 mM Na^+.

intracellular recording support this hypothesis (Satow and Van Houten, personal
communication).

3.5.2 Geotaxis and Galvanotaxis

Forward-swimming paramecia tend to orient their anterior end upward, and the
resulting upward movement (negative geotaxis) leads to their accumulation at the top
of the vessel. The mechanism of geotaxis has been reviewed recently (Dryl, 1974;
Machemer and de Peyer, 1978). The simplest explanation of geotaxis is that of Winet
and Jahn (1974). Winet and Jahn propose that orientation is upward because the
center of propulsion (sum of the driving forces of all cilia) is anterior to the center of
gravity. Grebecki and Nowakowska (1978) and Nowakowska and Grebecki (1978)
have recently elaborated on this idea. In any case, reorientation of the body axis
through avoiding reactions is not the mechanism since pawn mutants (see below) can
perform negative geotaxis perfectly. The avoiding reaction, in fact, interferes with the
geotaxis (Kung, 1971a).

When an electrical current is flowing through the medium, paramecia migrate
toward the cathode. Dryl (1974), Naitoh and Eckert (1974) and Machemer and de Pey
(1977) have reviewed the extensive literature on this subject and favor the explanation
that ciliary reversal, due to depolarization at the cathodal end, and ciliary augmentatio
due to hyperpolarization at the anodal half of the cell, cause the cell to turn to face
the cathode. Pawn is capable of galvanotaxis (Kung, 1971a) although the galvanotaxis
has not been quantified. It is not known whether ciliary augmentation alone is
enough for orientation, or whether pawn shows ciliary reversal under this condition.

3.5.3 Responses to thermal stimuli

Early work by Jennings (1906) and by Mendelssohn (1902a,b,c) established that *Paramecium* avoided regions of extreme temperature and tended to aggregate in a region of intermediate temperature, the 'optimal temperature' zone, which for cells grown at 25°C was 24—28°C. Such thermal avoidance could in principle be accomplished by regulation either of swimming velocity (orthokinesis) or swimming direction (klinokinesis). Jennings showed that near the optimal temperature, orthokinesis was primarily responsible for responses to thermal stimuli, but that very warm or very cool regions were avoided by klinokinesis; cells encountering extremes of temperature gave classical avoidance responses.

Glaser (1924) and Yapp (1941) studied the swimming velocity of *Paramecium* as a function of temperature, and both reported that velocity increased with temperature. Yapp noted that as the temperature exceeded 30°C, the frequency of avoiding reactions increased dramatically, so that forward motion practically ceased.

More recently, Tawada and Oosawa (1972) and Tawada and Miyamota (1973) have documented the occurrence of orthokinesis in *Paramecium* subjected to thermal stimuli near the optimal temperature. Cells shifted toward the temperature optimum temporarily swam faster, then returned to a 'steady velocity' within a few minutes. This 'steady velocity' was greatest at growth temperature and decreased markedly at either higher or lower temperatures. In a spatial gradient of temperature, cells swam faster when moving toward the temperature optimum than when swimming away from it. This difference of velocity, combined with spontaneous avoiding reactions that occurred regardless of the direction of swimming, resulted in the accumulation of cells at the temperature optimum. However, Nakaoko and Oosawa (1977) have recently shown that the rate of discontinuous directional change is the basis of accumulation at temperature optimum. The transient decrease or increase of this rate when the paramecia approach or leave the optimum (i.e., klinokinesis) appear to be the crucial mechanism. The disagreement in the results and interpretations is puzzling.

Hildebrand and Dryl (personal communication) studied thermal avoidance by klinokinesis in *Paramecium*. They observed the behavior of cells as they approach a heated wire, and found that vigorous avoiding reactions occurred as cells entered a zone where the temperature was between 35° and 40°C. Hennessey and Nelson (in preparation) have adapted the apparatus used by Van Houten *et al.* (1975) for quantitative studies of thermal avoidance. A T-shaped devise of glass tubing, in which each of the three arms is connected through a stopcock (Fig. 3.7), is arranged so that when cells are introduced into a lower arm (E in diagram) their negative geotaxis will lead them to swim upward, where they can either enter a control arm (C) at the same temperature or a test arm (T) containing warmer medium. Thermistors placed as shown in the diagram allow one to monitor the temperatures at the exit of E and the entry of T. After introducing about 5000 cells into the entry arm E, one waits 5 minutes, then count cells in the control and test arms to determine the 'index of thermotaxis', I_T:

$$I_T = \frac{\text{cells in T}}{\text{cells in C + cells in T}}$$

When I_T is near unity, little thermal avoidance has occurred; with effective thermal avoidance, the value of I_T approaches zero. To control for variations in motility, the fraction of cells that escape the entry arm is measured, and expressed as I_M:

$$I_M = \frac{\text{cells in T + cells in C}}{\text{total cells (T+C+E)}}$$

When the temperature at the entry to T is 40°C, good thermal avoidance is observed. Thermal avoidance is stimulated by a monovalent cation, and does not occur in Pawn mutants (Pawn B, see below), which are incapable of the avoidance response (Table 3.3).

Table 3.3 Indices of thermotaxis in *P. tetraurelia*

Temperature in T-arm (°C)	Additions	Index of thermotaxis (I_T)	
		Wild type	Pawn
25	none	0.95 ± 0.03	—
25	1 mM Na$^+$	0.95	0.95 ± 0.02
40	none	0.41	—
40	0.5 mM Na$^+$	0.22	—
40	1.0 mM Na$^+$	0.12	0.95
40	2.0 mM Na$^+$	0.06	—
40	0.5 mM K$^+$	0.37	—
40	0.5 mM Rb$^+$	0.18	—
40	0.5 mM Li$^+$	0.14	—

Results with Pawn confirm the observations of Jennings and of Tawada and Miyamoto, that the avoidance of regions of high temperatures is accomplished primarily by klinokinesis, not orthokinesis.

3.6 'ADAPTATION'

Paramecium can 'adapt'. Dryl (1959) and, more recently, Hildebrand and Dryl (1976) showed that *P. caudatum* fail to show ciliary reversal to various stimuli after prolonged incubation in a K$^+$-enriched (15.8 mM) medium. This process is reversible; upon returning the cells to K$^+$-deficient medium the avoiding reactions return with a half time of about 10 min. Hildebrand and Dryl postulated that the Ca channel is being regulated during 'adaptation'. They propose that the amount of Ca^{2+} or K$^+$ bound to the outer or inner face of the membrane controls conductance. Ca^{2+} bound to the inside would determine sensitivity.

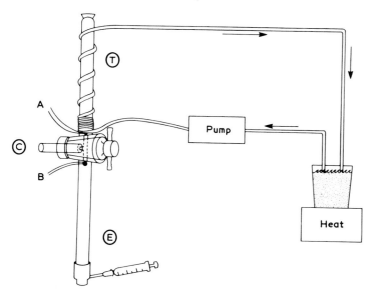

Fig. 3.7 Apparatus for assay of thermotaxis. Cells injected into the entry arm (E) swim upward by negative geotaxis, entering either arm C (same temperature as E) or T (heated by a tube carrying hot water.)

Although the kinetics are different, *P. tetraurelia* also shows similar 'adaptation'. Intracellular recording showed that the 'adapted' paramecia often fail to generate action potentials (Satow, Shusterman and Kung, unpublished). These paramecia also fail to accumulate ^{133}Ba above a background level (Ling and Kung, unpublished). Thus, the failure in ciliary reversal after adaptation is indeed due to a modification of the excitable membrane and not a modification of the ciliary axoneme. However, the membrane modification may not be on the Ca channel. For example, prolonged incubation in K^+-enriched medium might increase non-specific leakage or open a K^+-specific channel. In either case, the short-circuiting effect of cation efflux could render excitation impossible, even though the Ca channel had not been modified by 'adaptation'. Whether 'adaptation' is correlated with the closure of the Ca channel, the opening of an efflux channel or with the changes in internal ion concentrations is now being tested.

A group of mutants have been isolated that 'adapt' poorly, if at all (Shusterman, Thiede and Kung, in preparation). These mutants were originally selected for their ability to survive K^+ at a concentration ($\simeq 35$ mM) lethal to wild type (see below). Leaky mutants which have intermediate resistance to K^+ also show weak 'adaptation'. The strict correlation of K^+-resistance with lack of 'adaptation' in over 30 lines of independent mutants shows that 'adaptation' at $\simeq 15$ mM K^+ and killing by $\simeq 35$ mM K^+ share a common mechanism. Finding the basis of the K^+-resistance in the mutants may lead us to this mechanism. Note that 'adaptation' in *Paramecium* differs from sensory adaptation in animals in that the former is a general loss of excitability and the latter is a loss of response to a specific stimulus.

3.7 BEHAVIORAL MUTANTS

One of the advantages of using *P. tetraurelia* as a model system is the ease with which its life cycle can be manipulated. The two sexual processes, autogamy and conjugation, are under laboratory control (see Sonneborn, 1974). Autogamy is a peculiar process of self-fertilization that leads to homozygosity in *all* loci. This greatly facilitates the recovery of recessive mutants after mutagen treatment. (Autogamy is unique to a few species of *Paramecium* and is not found in *P. caudatum* or *Tetrahymena*.) Conjugation involves meiosis and recombination and thus allows formal genetic analyses, as in other diploid forms.

Making use of autogamy and conjugation, Kung and co-workers have isolated over 400 lines of behavioral mutants in *P. tetraurelia*. Most of these lines have been analyzed genetically. The mid-1975 inventory of this collection is given in a review by Kung *et al.* (1975). While this collection continues to grow, Schein (1976a) has also isolated behavioral mutants in this species. Since the behavioral genetics of *Paramecium* has recently been reviewed (Byrne and Byrne, 1978a) and will soon be reviewed (Cronkite, in preparation; Kung, in preparation) elsewhere, only a brief summary of recent advances is given below. Although most of the work reviewed here is on *P. tetraurelia,* Takahashi (in preparation) has overcome many difficulties and succeeded in isolating behavioral mutants in *P. caudatum.* Some of her mutants have been studied electrophysiologically (Takahashi and Naitoh, 1978).

The behavioral mutants in *P. tetraurelia* fall into two classes; mutants with membrane defects and mutants with normal membrane and presumably ciliary defects.

3.7.1 Mutants with membrane defects

(a) *Ca-channel mutants*
These are the 'pawns' which cannot move backward. They are isolated using a behavioral method (Kung, 1971a,b; Chang and Kung, 1973a) or by their ability to survive Ba^{2+} (Schein, 1976a). All pawn mutations map on one of three unlinked loci: *pwA, pwB* or *pwC* (Kung, 1971b; Chang and Kung, 1973b; Chang *et al.,* 1974; Schein, 1976a). Allelic variants include temperature-sensitives. Pawns are identified as Ca-channel mutants because they have little or no excitation (Kung and Eckert, 1972; Satow *et al.,* 1974; Satow and Kung, 1976c; Schein *et al.,* 1976; Oertel *et al.,* 1977) or stimulated ^{45}Ca or ^{133}Ba influx (Browning, Nelson and Hansma, 1976; Ling and Kung, in preparation). Pawns have no defect in their cilia since they can swim forward normally and the demembranated models of pawns can swim backward when Ca^{2+} is applied (Kung and Naitoh, 1973).

(b) *K-channel mutants*

The TEA-insensitive mutant isolated by Chang and Kung (1976) has been identified electrophysiologically as a K-channel mutant (Satow and Kung, 1976a). The Fast-2 mutant also shows a relative increase in K^+ conductance (Satow and Kung, 1976b), although we do not know whether the lesion is on the K channel or the mechanism that controls it.

(c) *Membrane mutants whose defective components have not been identified*

The 'paranoiacs' are such mutants. 'Paranoiacs' swim backward for long periods in media containing Na^+. Although these mutants have been studied genetically (Van Houten *et al.,* 1977), electrophysiologically (Satow *et al.,* 1976), biochemically (Hansma and Kung, 1976), and electron-microscopically (Byrne and Byrne, 1978b), all with interesting results, we do not yet know in which channel(s) the primary lesion is. There are also mutants which show prolonged backing or spinning in Ba^{2+} solutions (Chang and Kung, in preparation). A mutant defective in chemotaxis has been described by Van Houten (1977). A class of K^+-resistant mutants has also been discovered recently. They have been isolated by adding 35 mM K^+ to the mutagenized, autogamized cultures (Shusterman, Thiede and Kung, in preparation). This kills the wild type, but the mutants can grow at 35 mM K^+ addition and can survive up to an 80 mM addition. Over 30 lines of such mutants are being studied. These mutants have little or no behavioral abnormalities in culture medium nor in various test solutions. However, they fail to 'adapt' (see above).

3.7.2 Mutants with normal membrane and presumably ciliary defects

Atalanta is such a mutant. This mutant can stop but cannot perform sustained backward swimming. It has been studied electrophysiologically (Satow and Kung, unpublished). It has normal membrane properties, but the action potential corresponds to stoppage rather than backing. Demembranated models of Atalanta fail to swim backward when Ca^{2+} is provided.

Although handicapped by the lack of autogamy and the low fecundity after conjugation in *P. caudatum.* Takahashi (in preparation) has isolated and analyzed 23 behavioral mutants of this species. Most of these mutants have their counterparts in *P. tetraurelia.* For example, the CNR (*caudatum non-reversal*) group is comparable to the pawns. However, there is also a K-sensitive mutant, a zigzag mutant and a temperature jump-sensitive mutant. These are types not yet reported in *P. tetraurelia.* Some of these mutants were analyzed physiologically and their defects were traced to ion channels (Takahashi and Naitoh, 1978).

3.7.3 The use of mutants

The behavioral mutants of *Paramecium* have been employed to solve a variety of behavioral or physiological problems. Pawns, acting as the null control for any processes which require membrane excitation, have been most useful. Some examples of how they have been used are given below.

Pawns have been used to show that the avoiding reaction is a necessary condition for most of the chemotactic responses (see above). The avoiding reaction is needed for thermotaxis as well, since pawns fail to avoid a heated wire (see above). However, not all taxes require the avoiding reaction. Pawns have normal geotaxis (Kung, 1971a and b). This finding shows that proper orientation in the gravitational field does not require a readjustment of body-axis through ciliary reversal.

Membrane currents can be measured when the membrane potential is abruptly changed and then held at a different level by a voltage clamp. This current is the total of the inward and outward currents, i.e., the sum of ion fluxes through all channels. By subtracting the leakage and rectification currents measured in a pawn mutant from the total current in wild type, Oertel *et al.* (1977) have isolated the Ca^{2+} current of wild type bathed in K-Ca buffer. In this experimental condition, the Ca^{2+} current subsides within 5 ms. This is interpreted to mean that the Ca channels close within a few ms after they are opened by the abrupt depolarization, even though the membrane remains depolarized under the conditions of this experiment ('time-dependent inactivation').

Pawn mutants have also been used to estimate the life time of the Ca channel by Schein (1976b). He has followed the progressive loss of Ca channel activity in successive fissions after the paramecia have been changed from heterozygotes (+/pw) to homozygotes (pw/pw) by autogamy. The active Ca conductance halves in each post-autogamous fission. Thus, the loss of Ca channels is almost completely due to dilution and not breakdown. Schein estimates that the channel half-life is 5 to 8 days.

Brehm and Eckert (in preparation) have used a pawn mutant to study the control of ciliary beat frequency. Upon depolarization, the normal cilia reverse their beat direction and increase their beat frequency. The pawn cilia cannot reverse and at the same time fail to beat faster. These and other experiments lead them to conclude that internal Ca^{2+} concentration controls the beat frequency during depolarization. The hyperpolarization-related increase in beat frequency is unimpaired in pawn. Brehm and Eckert conclude that this increase in frequency is apparently unrelated to the internal concentration of Ca^{2+}.

In a pawn, Satow (unpublished), Brehm (personal communication), or in a CNR mutant (the counterpart of pawn in *P. caudatum*), Takahashi and Naitoh (in press) independently show that the depolarization receptor potential can be observed unobscured by the action potential upon mechanical impact at the cell's anterior end. This observation makes possible the study of the ionic basis and physiological characters of this receptor potential.

3.8 PROSPECTS FOR THE FUTURE

As a model of excitable cells, *Paramecium* offers many advantages. It can be cloned, is easily grown, has a short doubling time, gives relatively large yields of cells, and requires little laboratory space. Intracellular recordings have unearthed a wealth of information on the bioelectric properties of the paramecium membrane. One can monitor the occurrence and duration of membrane excitation by direct observation of swimming behavior, bypassing the laborious electrophysiology. The genetics of *Paramecium* is well studied, and a collection of behavioral mutants has been established. The research we have reviewed here has exploited these advantages of the system and has provided a foundation for further investigations of excitability.

We and others have begun to attack several problems related to sensory biology in *Paramecium*. The comparison of ciliary membrane lipids and proteins of wild type and behavioral mutants may pinpoint components involved in excitation and allow their eventual isolation. Careful electron microscopic studies of ciliary structure may reveal the structural basis of ciliary reversal and provide information about the mechanism of reversal. It may be possible to correlate membrane particles seen in the microscope with ion channels or pumps. The voltage clamp technique now being used with *Paramecium* will allow a fuller characterization of ion channel activities in wild-type and mutant strains.

We hope that studies of *Paramecium* will yield basic information about the molecular bases of mechano-, thermo-, and chemoreception. Slow changes in excitability ('adaptation') may be a result of covalent modifications of membrane proteins, and our studies of protein phosphorylation and methylation in the ciliary membrane are aimed at discovering such changes.

This research on *Paramecium* is of interest beyond the realm of protozoology. Any information gained with *Paramecium* regarding the molecular nature of ion channels, the basis of sensory reception, the mechanism of 'adaptation', or the motile-sensory function of eucaryotic cilia, is likely to be relevant to the understanding of the behavior of higher forms. Indeed, the biochemical and biophysical universality underlying diversity in morphology, physiology, morphogenesis, and now behavior, is one of the main themes in modern biology.

REFERENCES

Andrews, D.W. (1977), M.S. Thesis, University of Wisconsin.
Andrews, D. and Nelson, D.L. (1977), *Fifth Int. Cong. Protozool. Abs.,* **315**.
Andrivon, C. (1970), *Protistologica,* **4**, 445.
Baugh, L.C., Satir, P. and Satir, B. (1976), *J. Cell Biol.,* **70**, 66a.
Browning, J.L. (1976), Ph. D. Thesis, University of Wisconsin.
Browning, J.L. and Nelson, D.L. (1976), *Biochim. biophys. Acta,* **448**, 338.
Browning, J.L., Nelson, D.L. and Hansma, H.G. (1976), *Nature,* **259**, 491.

Byrne, B.J. and Byrne, B.C. (1978a), *CRC Critical Reviews in Microbiology* (in press).

Byrne, B.J. and Byrne, B.C. (1978b), *Science,* **199**, 1091—1093.

Chang, S.Y. and Kung, C. (1973a), *Science,* **180**, 1197.

Chang, S.Y. and Kung, C. (1973b), *Genetics,* **75**, 49.

Chang, S.Y. and Kung, C. (1976), *Gen. Res.,* **27**, 97.

Chang, S.Y., Van Houten, J., Robles, L., Lui, S. and Kung, C. (1974), *Gen. Res.,* **23**, 165.

Dickinson, J.R., Graves, M.M. and Swoboda, B. (1976), *FEBS Letters,* **65**, 152.

Dryl, S. (1959), *Acta Biol. Exp.,* **19**, 53.

Dryl, S. (1973), In: *Behaviour of Micro-organisms* (Pérez-Miravete, A., ed), Plenum Press, New York, pp. 16—30.

Dryl, S. (1974), In: *Paramecium, A Current Survey* (Van Wagtendouk, W.J. ed), Elsevier Scientific Pub. Co., New York, pp. 165—218.

Dunlop, K. (1977), *J. Physiol.,* **271**, 119.

Dusenbery, D.B. (1973), *Proc. natn. Acad. Sci., U.S.A.,* **70**, 1349.

Dute, R. and Kung, C. (1977), *J. Cell Biol.,* **75**, 211a.

Eckert, R. (1972), *Science,* **176**, 473.

Eckert, R., Naitoh, Y. and Machemer, H. (1976), *Symp. Soc. exp. Biol.,* **30**, 233.

Fisher, G., Kaneshiro, E. and Peters, P.D. (1976), *J. Cell Biol.,* **69**, 429.

Fraenkel, S. and Gunn, D.L. (1961), *Orientation of Animals,* Dover, New York, pp. 10—23.

Gibbons, I.R. (1965), *Arch. Biol.,* (Liege), **76**, 317.

Gilula, N.B. and Satir, P. (1972), *J. Cell Biol.,* **53**, 494.

Glaser, O. (1924), *J. gen. Physiol.,* **7**, 177.

Grebecki, A. and Nowakowska, G. (1978), *Acta Protozoologica* (in press).

Hansma, H.G. (1974), Ph. D. Thesis, University of California-Santa Barbara.

Hansma, H.G. (1975), *J. Protozool.,* **22**, 257.

Hansma, H.G. and Kung, C. (1976), *Biochim. biophys. Acta,* **436**, 128.

Hildebrand, E. and Dryl, S. (1976), *Bioelectrochem. Bioenergetics,* **3**, 543.

Holtz, G.G. and Conner, R.L. (1973), In: *Biology of Tetrahymena.* (Elliott, A.M., ed), Dowden, Hutchinsin and Ross, Stroudsburg, Pa., p.99.

Jahn, T.L. and Bovee, E.C. (1967), In: *Research in Protozoology,* Vol. I (Chen, T.T., ed), Pergamon Press, New York.

Jennings, H.S. (1906), *Behavior of Lower Organisms.* Indiana University Press, Bloomington, Ind.

Kaneshiro, E.S., Beischel, L., Meyer, K. and Rhoads, D. (1977), *Fifth Int. Cong. Protozool. Abs.,* **316**.

Kung, C. (1971a), *Z. vergl. Physiologie,* **71**, 142.

Kung, C. (1971b), *Genetics,* **69**, 29.

Kung, C., Chang, S.Y., Satow, Y., Van Houten, J. and Hansma, H. (1975), *Science,* **188**, 898.

Kung, C. and Eckert, R., (1972), *Proc. natn. Acad. Sci. U.S.A.,* **69**, 93.

Kung, C. and Naitoh, Y. (1973), **179**, 195.

Levandowsky, M. and Hauser, D.C.R. (1978), *Int. Rev. Cytol.,* **55**, 145—210.

Machemer, H. and de Peyer, J. (1977), *Verh. Dtsch. Zool. Ges.* 86—110.

Machemer, H. and Eckert, R. (1973), *J. Gen. Physiol.,* **61**, 572.

Mendelssohn, M. (1902a), *J. Physiol. Path. Gen.*, **4**, 393.

Mendelssohn, M. (1902b), *J. Physiol. Path. Gen.*, **4**, 475.

Mendelssohn, M. (1902c), *J. Physiol. Path. Gen.*, **4**, 489.

Morofushi, H. (1973), *Biochim. biophys. Acta*, **327**, 354.

Morofushi, H. (1974), *Biochem. biophys. Acta*, **370**, 130.

Naitoh, Y. (1974), *Am. Zool.*, **14**, 883.

Naitoh, Y. and Eckert, R. (1968), *Z. vergl. Physiologie*, **61**, 427.

Naitoh, Y. and Eckert, R. (1969), *Science*, **164**, 963.

Naitoh, Y. and Eckert, R. (1974), In: *Cilia and Flagella.* (Sleigh, M.A., ed), Academic Press, New York, pp. 305–352.

Naitoh, Y. and Kaneko, H. (1972), *Science*, **176**, 523.

Nakaoka, Y. and Oosawa, F. (1977), *J. Protozool.*, **24**, 575.

Nowakowska, G. and Grebecki, A. (1978), *Acta Protozoologica* (in press).

Nozawa, Y. (1975), In: *Methods in Cell Biology,* Vol. 10 (Prescott, D.M. ed), Academic Press, New York, p. 105.

Oertel, D., Schein, S.J. and Kung, C., (1977), *Nature*, **268**, 120.

Ogura, A. and Takahashi, K. (1976), *Nature*, **264**, 170.

Preer, J.R. Jr. (1959), *J. Immunol.*, **83**, 387.

Preer, J.R. Jr. (1969), In: *Research in Protozoology.* Vol. 3 (Chen, T.T., ed), Pergamon Press, Oxford, pp. 129–278.

Plattner, H. (1975), *J. Cell Sci.*, **18**, 257.

Plattner, H. and Fuchs, S. (1975), *Histochemistry*, **45**, 23.

Rhoads, D., Meyer, K. and Kaneshiro, E.S. (1977), *Fifth Int. Cong. Protozool. Abs.* **436**.

Satir, B., Sale, W.S. and Satir, P. (1976), *Exp. Cell Res.*, **97**, 83.

Satow, Y. In: *Comparative Membrane Physiology of Invertebrate Organisms.* (Podesta, R.B., ed), Marcel Dekker, Inc., New York) (in preparation).

Satow, Y., Chang, S.Y. and Kung, C. (1974), *Proc. natn. Acad. Sci. U.S.A.*, **71**, 2703.

Satow, Y., Hansma, H.G. and Kung, C. (1976), *Comp. Biochem. Physiol.* **54A**, 323.

Satow, Y. and Kung, C. (1976a), *J. Exp. Biol.*, **65**, 51.

Satow, Y. and Kung, C. (1976b), *J. Neurobiol.*, **7**, 325.

Satow, Y. and Kung, C. (1976c), *J. Memb. Biol.*, **28**, 277.

Schein, S.J. (1976a), *Genetics*, **84**, 453.

Schein, S.J. (1976b), *J. exp. Biol.*, **65**, 725.

Schein, S.J., Bennett, M.V.L. and Katz, G.M. (1976), *J. exp. Biol.*, **65**, 699.

Sleigh, M.A. (1974), In: *Cilia and Flagella,* (Sleigh, M.A., ed), Academic Press New York, pp. 79–92.

Sonneborn, T.M. (1974), In: *Handbook of Genetics,* (King, R.C., ed), Plenum Press, New York, pp. 469–594.

Takahashi, M. and Naitoh, Y. (1978), *Nature*, **271**, 656.

Tawada, K. and Miyamoto, H. (1973), *J. Protozool.*, **20**, 289.

Tawada, K. and Oosawa, F. (1972), *J. Protozool.*, **19**, 53.

Thompson, G.A., Baugh, L.C. and Walter, L.F. (1974), *J. Cell Biol.*, **61**, 253.

Thompson, G.A. Jr. and Nozawa, Y. (1977), *Biochim. biophys. Acta*, **472**, 55.

Tsuchiya, T. (1976), *Experientia* (Basel), **32**, 1176.

Tsuchiya, T. and Takashi, K. *J. Protozool*, **23**, 523.

Van Houten, J. (1977), *Science,* **198**, 746.

Van Houten, J. *J. comp. Physiol.,* (in press).

Van Houten, J., Chang, S.Y. and Kung, C. (1977), *Genetics,* **86**, 113.

Van Houten, J., Hansma, H.G. and Kung, C. (1975), *J. Biochem. comp. Physiol. Ser. B,* **104**, 211.

Warner, M.A. (1976), In: *Cell Motility.* (Book 3) (Goldman, R., Pollard, T. and Rosenbaum, J., (eds.), Cold Spring Harbor Laboratory, pp. 891–914.

Winet, H. and Jahn, T.L. (1974), *J. Theoret. Biol.,* **46**, 449.

Yapp, W.B. (1941), *Nature,* **148**, 754.

4 Chemotaxis and Differentiation during the Aggregation of *Dictyostelium discoidium* Amoebae

MICHEL DARMON and PHILIPPE BRACHET

Acknowledgements

Authors are indebted to Drs L.H. Pereira da Silva, W.F. Loomis, A. Goldbeter and L. Segel for stimulating discussion and helpful criticism of the manuscript. They also thank Drs J. Gross, C. Klein, A. Ryter and B. Wurster for providing material for illustrations. They acknowledge the expert assistance of M. Lemoine and F. Petrou.

Taxis and Behavior
(*Receptors and Recognition,* Series B, Volume 5)
Edited by G.L. Hazelbauer
Published in 1978 by Chapman and Hall, 11 New Fetter Lane, London EC4P 4EE
© Chapman and Hall

4.1 INTRODUCTION

D. discoideum amoebae are eukaryotic cells which feed on bacteria living in the soil of temperate forests (Raper, 1935). They locate their preys by means of chemotaxis (Bonner *et al.*, 1966; Konijn, 1969) and engulf them by phagocytosis. They live and divide as unicellular amoebae as long as a food supply is available. In these organisms, lack of nutrients triggers a developmental program mainly characterized by its social aspect. After a certain time of starvation, called interphase (Bonner, 1963) the amoebae differentiate into cells able to aggregate (aggregation-competent amoebae) (Gerisch, 1968). At that time, a synchronous and highly organized aggregation of the individuals occurs, leading to the formation of a multicellular, rounded cell mass, surrounded by a polysaccharide sheath. This pseudoplasmodium gains a tip, and next affects the form of a slug, which is able to migrate as a function of environmental factors, and which finally differentiates into a fruiting body consisting of two different cell types: the stalk cells and the spores. The first type constitutes the somatic line while the spores represent the germinative line. They are relatively resistant to desiccation and germinate when good conditions are encountered. This developmental cycle presents several features conferring obvious selective advantages (Bonner, 1967).

Alternation of unicellular and multicellular phases as well as the relative simplicity of the morphogenetic process explains why social amoebae have been chosen as models for the study of morphogenesis and cell differentiation. Despite this relative simplicity as compared to embryogenesis of vertebrates, the co-ordinated aggregation of several thousand cells spread over a large surface implies sophisticated means of intercellular communication. Progression to aggregation-competence involves expression of a specific genetic program (Sussman *et al.*, 1967; Loomis, 1969a; Darmon *et al.*, 1975). The number of genes involved in aggregation has been estimated by Coukell (1975) and Williams and Newell (1976) from the frequency of complementation in diploids formed with pairs of aggregateless mutants; 30—50 genes are absolutely required for aggregation, and 100—200 more genes may be involved in fine tuning of the process.

It was shown very early that aggregation is under the control of chemo-attractants emitted by the cells (Runyon, 1942; Bonner, 1947). These attractants have been called acrasins (Bonner, 1947). In *Dictyostelium discoideum* aggregation is very efficient because of emission of acrasin in pulses (Shaffer, 1957) and because of relay from cell to cell of acrasin emissions over very long distances (Shaffer, 1957). Chemotactic tests (Shaffer, 1953; Konijn, 1965; Bonner, 1967) have permitted isolation of the acrasin of *D. discoideum* (Shaffer, 1953). This was later identified as being the cyclic nucleotide cAMP (Konijn *et al.*, 1967; Bonner *et al.*, 1969; Barkley, 1969). It is noteworthy that cAMP (Konijn *et al.*, 1969), along with folic acid

103

(Pan *et al.,* 1972) and related compounds, is one of the major chemo-attractants
emitted by bacteria and may attract amoebae during their vegetative life.

Since cAMP is a general intracellular effector of regulatory processes in prokaryotes
and eukaryotes, much work has focused on its role in *D. discoideum* aggregation,
where it behaves as an extracellular mediator (first messenger) (Konijn, 1972).
Several recent publications have reviewed the various aspects of development in
D. discoideum (Bonner, 1967, 1971; Konijn, 1972; Loomis, 1975; Gerisch *et al.,*
1975b,c; Newell, 1977). In the present report our aim is not to be exhaustive. We
will consider only some points which seem to us of major interest for understanding
the relationship between chemotaxis and cell differentiation during the aggregation
process of *D. discoideum.*

4.2 DESCRIPTION OF AGGREGATION

If vegetative amoebae are starved and spread on a solid surface, no evident changes
occur for five to six hours. The cells remain isolated and retain the same rounded
morphology and random motion as during growth. After this initial period of
starvation, called interphase (Bonner, 1963), cells undergo a series of morphological
and behavioural transformations. The cells lengthen, form cell-to-cell polar contacts
(Gerisch, 1968) and the resulting small chains of cells join to form streams which
converge at central points. After a certain time, all the cells of an aggregation
territory gather into an aggregate of $10^3 - 10^5$ cells. This sequence of events is
represented in Fig. 4.1.

Using two different methods, Runyon (1942) and Bonner (1947) were able to
show that attraction of amoebae to a central point was due to chemotaxis. Runyon
demonstrated that cells were attracted by aggregation centers and streams across
semi-permeable membranes. Bonner showed that if one establishes a stream of water
over an aggregation territory, only cells which are downstream are attracted by the
center. The attractant was called 'acrasin' from the name of a witch.

Aggregation is pulsatile (Bonner, 1944). Cells move by a series of inward steps
toward the center. They seem to respond to periodic waves which propagate from
the center to the periphery of the territory. Periodicity is about 5 min (Shaffer,
1962; Gerisch, 1968). A concentric wave pattern may be easily observed under a
low-power microscope (Fig. 4.2) and has been studied using time-lapse films
(Bonner, 1944; Shaffer, 1957; Gerisch, 1968; Alcantara and Monk, 1974). Shaffer
(1957) proposed that this pattern was due to a relay of acrasin gradients which were
emitted by the centre. He observed (1962) that cells may alternatively respond to two
different aggregation centers, suggesting that the observed periodicity of movement
was actually due to a periodic emission of pulses of attractant and not to a periodic
response to a continuous emission of attractant. In order to explain the unidirectionality of wave propagation, he also suggested the existence of a refractory period
during which cells are not able to relay the signal. Gerisch (1965; 1968) drew the

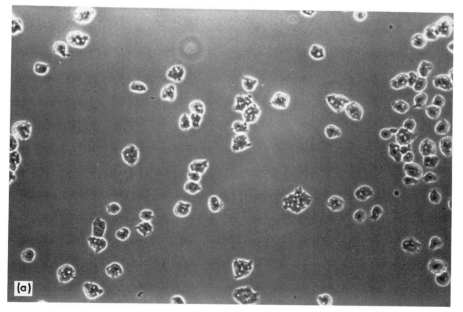

(a) Growth phase cells (× 200 phase contrast).

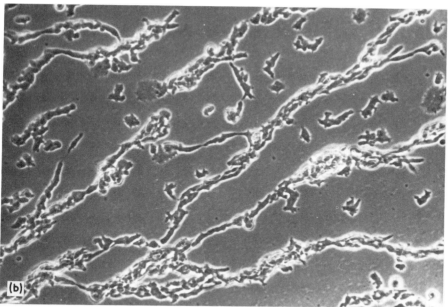

(b) Starved cells elongate and orient themselves into streams after 5–6 h
(× 200 phase contrast).
Fig. 4.1 Stages of aggregation of *D. discoideum*.

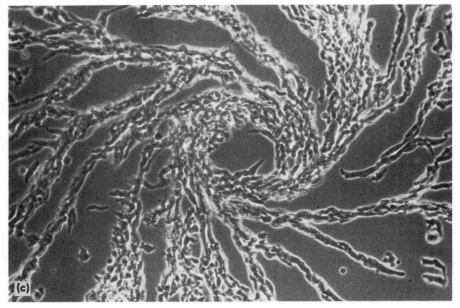

(c) Streams merging toward a center (x 200 phase contrast).

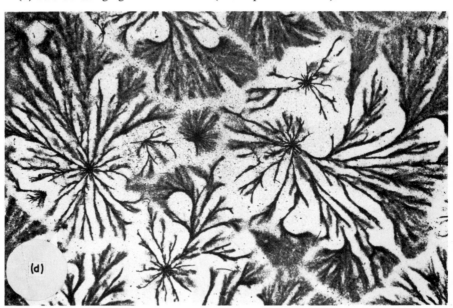

(d) Low magnification of aggregating amoebae. Discrete territories are seen (x 10).

Fig. 4.1 Stages of aggregation of *discoideum*.

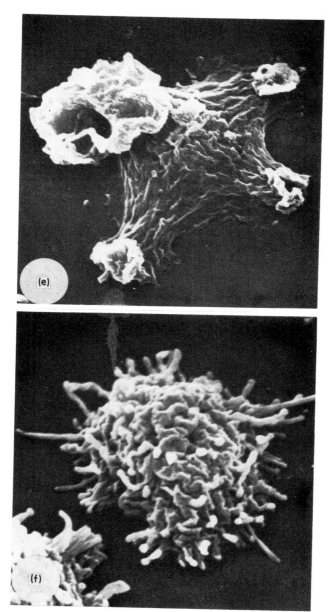

(e, f) Important changes in cell morphology are seen in scanning e.m. The wrinkled membrane and the phagocytic cups observed early during starvation (e) disappear once cells become aggregation-competent (f). At that stage, they develop many filopods (Ryter and Brachet, 1978). (Reproduced with permission, A. Ryter and *Biol. Cellulaire*).

Fig. 4.1 Stages of aggregation of *D. discoideum*.

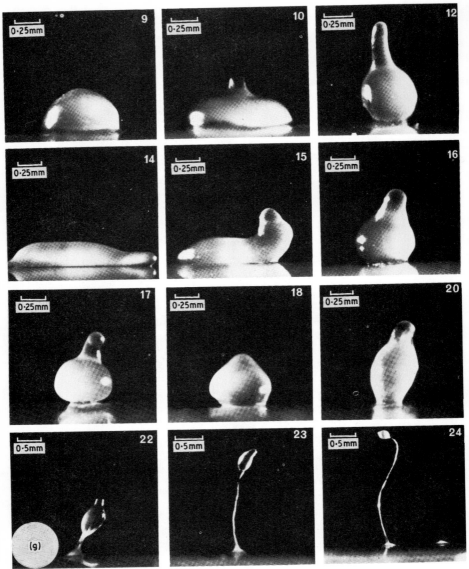

(g) The sequence of morphological changes of an aggregate observed on an agar support. The numbers indicate the approximate time in hours after initiation of development. (Reproduced with permission, W.F. Loomis and Academic Press).

Fig. 4.1 Stages of aggregation of *D. discoideum*.

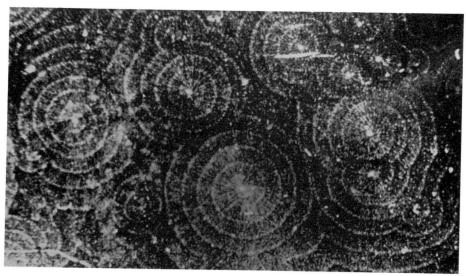

Fig. 4.2 Relaying fields of amoebae showing concentric or spiral wave patterns. (Dark field optics, reproduced with permission, courtesy of M.J. Peacey).

same conclusions about relay and the refractory period for relay. He also observed that conduction of stimuli does not require immediate cell-to-cell contact and measured the speed of the propagating waves. From this measure of velocity of acrasin waves, Cohen and Robertson (1971a) suggested that the rate-limiting factor in velocity of propagation was not intercellular diffusion but an intracellular delay for relay.

Recent analysis of time-lapse films has allowed a refined description of aggregation. The concentric wave pattern is due to an alternation of light and dark bands of cells (Fig. 4.2). Alcantara and Monk (1974) observed that the light bands are formed by elongated moving cells and the dark bands by rounded non-moving cells. They showed that the width of the band of moving cells corresponds to the zone of influence of a signal propagating outwards from the center of the aggregation territory. Width of the movement band is independent of the frequency of the signals and only depends upon movement duration and velocity of signal propagation (v):

$$v = \frac{\text{width of movement band}}{\text{movement duration}}$$

By measuring the width of the movement band ($\simeq 470\ \mu$m) and the duration of movement (100 s) they calculate the velocity of signal propagation ($\simeq 4.7\ \mu$m s^{-1}). The width of the band of non-moving cells corresponds to the distance of propagation of the wave between two successive signals. Consequently, that width decreases when the frequency of signalling increases. The authors also measured the range of

Table 4.1 Parameters of aggregation. From Alcantara and Monk (1974).

For densities ranging from 10^5 to 5×10^5 amoebae/cm^2

Period	Decreases from 10 to 3 min
Movement band width (independent of period)	500 to 700 μm
Interband width (decreases when period decreases)	400 to 2000 μm
Movement duration	100 s
Velocity of signal propagation	4.7 μm s^{-1}
Range of the relayed signal	57 μm
Delay of relay	12 s

the relayed signal ($\simeq 57$ μm) by estimating the width of a block of cells responding at the same time. Delay for relay (12 s) is measured as the time elapsing between the response of two successive blocks of amoebae. Table 4.1 lists values for the parameters of aggregation measured by Alcantara and Monk. These authors also attempted to detect a refractory period for movement response by measuring the minimum uni-directional path-time of cells which were being signalled successively from different directions. They conclude from that study that the refractory period for movement, if it exists, should be less than 12 s.

Observations made by Durston (1974) are an important complement to the work of Alcantara and Monk, since they provide information about the nature of pace-makers (the loci from which waves propagate). Durston studied the two wave shapes which had previously been noticed in *D. discoideum* aggregation (Gerisch, 1965): concentric rings and spirals (Fig. 4.2). He concludes that spiral waves are maintained by continuous wave propagation around a central core by signal relaying alone (without autonomous signalling). The period of the spiral waves is thought to be equal to the refractory period for signal relaying. These observations fit well with the Keller and Segel model for equilibrium instability (1970), which predicts that aggregation does not require that any particular cells be distinguished, but rather assumes a homogeneous population. However, autonomous periodic signals (period $\simeq 5$ min) exist. They initiate circular waves of relaying and are generally believed to be generated by cells capable of sustained autonomous synthesis of acrasin.

Bimodal concentric pacemakers have been observed. Sharp transitions from a period of 10 min to a period of 5 min (Durston, 1974) or from 4 to 2 min have been reported (Gross *et al.,* 1977). The longer period takes place while cells are still scattered. Transitions occur when the cells form tight streams and aggregates. These phenomena could be explained by the existence of a refractory period for signal relaying initially exceeding the period of the autonomous signal and then decreasing with the developmental age (Durston, 1974). The conclusions of

Durston are consistant with the fact that concentric waves with periods shorter than the period of spiral waves located in the vicinity are never observed (Gross *et al.,* 1976). Data presented by Durston also suggest that the tip which forms in a mature aggregate is a continuous signal source which nevertheless induces waves in the outer population with a period equal to the refractory period for signal relaying.

4.3 CONTROL OF AGGREGATION BY EXOGENOUS cAMP PULSES

Robertson *et al.* (1972) were able to mimic the attracting power of an aggregation center by electrophoretically releasing cAMP pulses with a periodicity of 4.5 min. This important experiment shows that cAMP pulses control both chemotaxis and signal relaying in the same fashion as in the spontaneous aggregation toward an aggregation center. Monitoring responses of the cell population by time-lapse films allowed the authors to study the sequence of development of the components of the aggregation system. First, cells increase their chemotactic responsiveness to cAMP, then become capable of relaying signals, then autonomous signalling appears and finally cell contacts form.

Using the same microelectrode system, Robertson and Drage (1975) were able to measure directly the refractory period for relaying and confirmed the work of Durston (1974). If pulses are delivered every 3 min, cells respond first to every third, then to every second, and finally to each pulse. So the refractory period declines with developmental age from a value between 6 and 9 min to a value less than 3 min. This experiment was the first direct evidence of the existence of a refractory period for relaying. The authors also showed that a continuous cAMP signal can cause periodic signal relaying, presumably by stimulating amoebae as soon as they emerge from the refractory state. Near the source, chemotactic motion is continuous. This result confirms the prediction of Durston (1974) of continuous secretion at the tip. In their experiments, Robertson and Drage also confirmed that the threshold for chemotaxis is about two orders of magnitude less than the threshold for signal relaying.

4.4 AGGREGATION-COMPETENCE

If aggregating cells are dissociated and spread over a solid surface they resume the aggregation process immediately. The cells have developed an ability to aggregate which does not depend on their position in the field. This differentiated state, which has been called aggregation-competence, can also be attained if cells are starved in agitated suspensions (Gerisch, 1968). This important observation shows that oriented motion is not necessary for development of aggregation-competence. Under such conditions, Beug and his colleagues were able to demonstrate

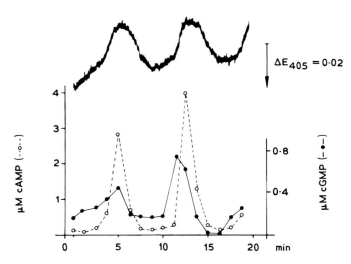

Fig. 4.3 Sustained oscillations of aggregation-competent amoebae. The population was monitored by light-scattering measurement (upper curve). Intracellular levels of cAMP and cGMP were assayed concomitantly. (Reproduced with permission, B. Wurster and *FEBS Letters*).

development of new contact sites (contact sites A) different from contact sites which exist during growth (contact sites B) (Beug *et al.*, 1970, 1973). Unlike contact sites B, A-sites are involved in cohesion resistant to high concentrations of EDTA. They are implicated in polar contacts characteristic of aggregation-competent cells, since specific univalent antibodies directed against them prevent the cells from forming end-to-end contacts. Aggregates formed in stirred suspensions are able to give rise to normal fruiting bodies provided that they are transferred onto a solid-air interface.

Development of aggregation-competence in stirred suspensions was first interpreted as an expression of the developmental abilities of single cells. It was thought that starvation would trigger development of the chemotactic signalling system and of the membrane changes involved in cohesiveness independently. Formation of aggregates in cell suspensions was interpreted as the result of passive agglutination of cells which had differentiated individually. The chemotactic system was thus thought to be unnecessary for the differentiation process. It would be functional (and necessary) only when cells had to orient their motion on a solid surface.

However three observations showed that these conclusions were probably incorrect:

(1) If cells are starved below a critical density, aggregation does not occur (Konijn and Raper, 1961). This was interpreted to mean that at such low densities intercellular distances are greater that the range of signal diffusion allowing

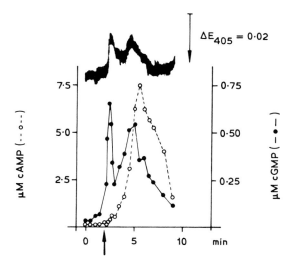

Fig. 4.4 Biphasic response evoked by a pulse of cAMP. The biphasic response is detected by light-scattering measurement (upper curve). Intracellular levels of cAMP and cGMP were measured concomittantly. The experiment was performed at $10°$C. (Reproduced with permission, B. Wurster and *FEBS Letters*).

suprathreshold concentrations for relay (Alcantara and Monk, 1974). However, if cells starved at less than the critical density were concentrated, they did not exhibit aggregation-competence at a time when control cultures were fully differentiated (Brachet, Klein and Darmon, unpublished observations). This observation suggests that, for the differentiation process itself, cells need to be close to their neighbours, as if some kind of cell communication were necessary.

(2) If starvation triggers the development of chemotactic behavior and of membrane cohesiveness independently, one might expect to find mutants unable to aggregate on a solid surface but able to do so in stirred suspensions. However, all aggregation-defective mutants isolated as defective in aggregation on a solid surface are also unable to aggregate when starved in homogeneous conditions (Darmon, Brachet, Pereira da Silva, unpublished results).

(3) The third observation was made by Gerisch and Hess (1974) concerning periodic changes of light scattering that can be recorded in suspensions of differentiating cells (Fig. 4.3). Those changes appear to be equivalent to propagated waves observed in cell layers. Oscillations develop after a certain time of starvation with a period of 7 min; cAMP pulses (10^{-8}–10^{-9} M) interfere with the spontaneous oscillations (precocious oscillations, delays, phase-shifts). A single pulse of cAMP added to starved cells, which have not begun to oscillate, provokes one change in light scattering which resembles those observed in spontaneous oscillations.

However the response is biphasic (Fig. 4.4). Sensitivity of cells to such an added pulse increases with time of starvation. Continuous applications of cAMP have no effect up to a certain rate, at which oscillations are suppressed. These exciting results showed that in stirred suspensions cells actually behave as a synchronous population, in which intercellular communication occurs, possibly in the form of cAMP signals.

To test the possibility that cell differentiation to aggregation-competence was itself mediated by diffusible molecules, Darmon *et al.* (1975) adapted the technique of Runyon (1942) to the study of developmental mutants. Wild type cells and mutant cells were starved on Petri dishes in such a way that the two cell layers were separated by a cellophane membrane. In addition to the two expected classes (no response and chemotactic response, already described by Ennis and Sussman (1958)), they found a third class of mutants, which exhibited not only a chemotactic response but which were also induced to differentiate up to the stage of mature aggregates (i.e. cell masses capable of developing into fruiting bodies with viable spores of the mutant genotype). These results indicated that a diffusible molecule of small molecular weight produced by the wild type was able to bypass the differentiation-defective phenotype of some mutants. To test whether this induction of cell differentiation was due to emission of cAMP by wild type cells, the authors submitted these mutants to pulses of cAMP ($10^{-8}-10^{-7}$ M) delivered at a 5 min intervals. Not only could aggregation-competence be induced but the complete development cycle could be achieved; the aggregates formed in stirred suspensions became fruiting bodies when transferred onto a solid-air interface. If cAMP pulses were delivered to the wild-type, aggregation-competence could be achieved precociously (after four hours of starvation instead of six hours for the control). Pulses of cGMP, which is a much poorer chemo-attractant than cAMP, were active at high concentration only. Continuous flow of cAMP appeared to be less efficient than pulses, since with continuous flow, EDTA-resistant contacts were induced in the mutants, but mature aggregates could not be obtained. These experiments suggested that cAMP in the form of pulses was able to induce all the properties of aggregation-competent cells. Gerisch and his colleagues (1975a) used a different approach to demonstrate that cAMP was the agent initiating differentiation as well as the chemotactic signal bringing differentiated cells together; they took advantage of the fact that cells of axenic strains are unable to differentiate upon transfer to starvation buffer if they have reached the stationary phase of growth in axenic semi-defined medium. However, in such cells, pulses of cAMP are able to induce the production of contact sites A (used as an index of differentiation) as well as the ability to aggregate. The authors also showed that cAMP pulses provoke a slight acceleration of differentiation in cells harvested in the exponential phase of growth. However, they found that continuous flow at the same average rate delayed aggregation.

These experiments have important implications. Not only do cAMP pulses control the short-term responses of cells (i.e. formation of a pseudopod, relay of the signal) but they also control long-term functions such as synthesis and activation of new molecules (i.e. contact sites A). cAMP pulses also induce synthesis of phosphodiesterase (Klein and Darmon, 1975) and cAMP receptors (Gerisch *et al.*, 1975b) and repress production of phosphodiesterase inhibitor (Klein and Darmon, 1977).

It is unclear why efficient signals should be in the form of pulses. This might suggest that cells sense only transient increases in cAMP concentration followed by decrease. In that case, the sharpness of the gradient with respect to time should be of importance. However, the relative inefficiency of continuous flows in inducing aggregation-competence might result from the fact that only a narrow range of concentrations are effective in causing cell differentiation. Such a window however would be systematically crossed by each cAMP pulse.

Although the chemotactic apparatus appears to be necessary for development of cell cohesiveness the reverse is not true:

(1) Mutants can be found which migrate rhythmically toward centers without forming cell contacts (Gross *et al.*, 1977; Barrand, Brachet and Darmon, unpublished observation).

(2) Univalent Fab antibodies directed against contact sites A block formation of contacts but do not impair chemotactic migration (Beug *et al.*, 1970).

4.5 BIOCHEMICAL APPROACHES TO THE STUDY OF INTERCELLULAR COMMUNICATION

4.5.1 Emission of cAMP

It was known from early studies that aggregating cells emit large amounts of acrasin (Bonner *et al.*, 1969). Assays of cAMP in developing populations showed that mean intra- and extracellular levels were maximal at the time of aggregation (Malkinson and Ashworth, 1973). These experiments, however, did not provide detailed information on the kinetics of cAMP synthesis, since they were performed on cells starved on solid surfaces, which consequently belonged to several out-of-phase populations. The first direct evidence that cAMP is periodically released from differentiated cells came from the refined work of Gerisch and Wick (1975). The authors assayed cellular and extracellular cAMP during the spontaneous oscillations of light scattering observed in cells starved in agitated suspensions. They found that the light-scattering oscillations are associated with sharp rises of both intra- and extracellular cAMP (Fig. 4.3). The intracellular concentration reaches its maximal value (20 μM, about 10-fold above the basal level) 1–2 min after the beginning of the increase. The rise of extracellular cAMP begins to be detectable about 30 s after the intracellular one. The value of the peak is 1 μM. Decrease to basal levels (0.1 μM) takes 1–2 min. The cAMP peaks coincide with the minima of optical density oscillations.

These results suggest that the oscillatory activity is due to periodic variations in adenylate cyclase activity. They also argue against storage of cAMP for an extended period of time. Maeda and Gerisch (1977) observed with electron microscopy formation of short-lived vesicles and vacuoles fusing to the membrane at the presumed time of the release of cAMP. This process was also induced during the relay response (see below); it is thought to correspond to secretion of cAMP through the plasma membrane, and could be analogous to acetylcholine secretion by nerve cells.

4.5.2 Relay

Biochemical evidence for the relay of a signal of cAMP by emission of cAMP has been presented by Shaffer (1975) and Roos *et al.* (1975). Shaffer added pulses of 10^{-6} M cold cAMP to aggregation-competent amoebae starved in Petri dishes containing ^{3}H-adenine. Peaks of secreted ^{3}H-cAMP occurred less than one min after the delivered cAMP pulse. Peak duration was 2–3 min. Roos *et al.* used approximately the same technique to measure relay in cells starved in suspensions. Cells stimulated with pulses of 6×10^{-8} M cAMP responded by secreting cAMP 30 s later, with a maximum at 90 s and a duration of about 3 min. Signal amplification was estimated to be of a factor of 40. The peak was coincident with the slow response of the biphasic recording of light scattering (Fig. 4.4).

4.5.3 cAMP receptors

The large amount of phosphodiesterase (PDE) present during differentiation makes it difficult to assay binding of radioactive cAMP to the plasma membrane. Using the fact that cGMP is a good substrate for PDE but a poor chemotactic attractant (three orders magnitude less active than cAMP), Malchow and Gerisch (1974) were able to demonstrate specific binding of tritiated cAMP molecules at the surface of the cell in the presence of an excess of cGMP. The nucleotide bound was rapidly and almost entirely recovered in the extracellular medium as 5'AMP. cAMP binding sites were not detected in vegetative cells but increased throughout starvation up to 5×10^5 binding sites per cell (dissociation constant: 100–200 nM). This developmental regulation of binding sites parallels the increase in chemotactic sensitivity of the cells and is not observed in an aggregation-defective mutant. Furthermore, affinity of binding sites for cAMP analogs increases with their chemotactic activity. These observations suggested that cAMP binding sites play a role in the chemotactic response.

Green and Newell (1975) overcame the problem of PDE by performing the binding assay in 2 mM dithiotreitol. Scatchard plots of binding were strongly curvilinear. Such kinetic data, common to many hormonal receptors, could be interpreted in terms of negative cooperativity or by the existence of two classes of binding sites. Green and Newell calculated that their data were consistent with the existence of two classes of sites: low affinity sites (2×10^5/cell, K_d 150–200 nM) and high affinity sites (2×10^4/cell, K_d 10 nM). They suggested that these two sites could correspond to two different receptor systems, one for chemotaxis and one for signal relay. Their view was supported by the observation that a mutant aggregating with small territories (presumably unable to relay) lacks the high affinity sites. Henderson (1975) independently developed an assay based on the use of DTT. She found 10^5 binding sites of K_d 36 nM at the time when aggregation-competent cells exhibit maximum binding. She also found that, when cells were maintained in shaken suspensions, this high level of binding was retained but that, if formation of mature aggregates was allowed to occur, binding of cAMP decreased during tip formation. In parallel studies, Mato and Konijn (1975) showed that binding of cAMP is limited to slime mold species which utilize this nucleotide as a chemotactic agent.

Gerisch *et al.* (1975b) found that cAMP receptors are induced by cAMP pulses. This effect probably accounts for the increase in chemotactic sensitivity during differentiation, which has been shown to be under the control of cAMP pulses (Darmon *et al.*, 1975). Induction of cAMP receptors by cAMP pulses is one aspect of the effect of cAMP pulses on cell differentiation and is a good example of the highly co-operative character of the aggregation process. However cAMP has also been shown to down-regulate the number of cAMP binding sites (Klein and Juliani, 1976). This process is commonly observed for several receptors in the presence of excess hormone. The step down in the presence of cAMP as well as the reappearance of high binding levels after elimination of excess nucleotide appears to be independent of protein synthesis and takes place even in the presence of metabolic inhibitors.

In liquid suspension, synchronized cells share periodic variations of cAMP binding, which correlate with changes in light scattering. Maximal binding is obtained just before the wave of cAMP synthesis (Klein *et al.*, 1977). King and Frazier's data (1977) support the idea that this is due to rhythmic changes of receptor affinity. They also show that the decrease of cAMP binding is accompanied by an enhanced level of phosphorylation of membrane components. Thus it appears possible that down regulation of cAMP receptors is mediated through their phosphorylation. A phosphatase activity would then be responsible for restoration of maximal binding as proposed in other systems.

4.5.4 Phosphodiesterase and its inhibitor

Shaffer (1956a, 1962) pointed out that an acrasinase could be important for preventing the gradient from being masked by noise, and he reported such an activity in *D. discoideum* (Shaffer, 1956b). Phosphodiesterases activities are associated with both cytoplasmic (Panbacker and Bravard, 1972) and membrane fractions (Malchow *et al.*, 1972) and are found also in the extracellular media (Chang, 1968; Chassy *et al.*, 1969). Regulation of phosphodiesterase (PDE) activity during aggregation is very complex. Synthesis of the enzyme is induced by cAMP pulses (Klein and Darmon, 1975) so that levels of activity increase in aggregating cells (Malchow *et al.*, 1972; Klein and Darmon, 1975); high levels of activity are found in cytoplasmic and membrane fractions of aggregation-competent cells. During differentiation the enzyme is steadily secreted (Klein and Darmon, 1975) but is extensively neutralized

by an inhibitor excreted earlier during starvation (Riedel and Gerisch, 1971).
Some of the extracellular activity is resistant to the inhibitor (Brachet *et al.,* 1977).
Synthesis of inhibitor is probably induced by starvation and stopped by cAMP pulses
at the time of differentiation to aggregation-competence (Klein and Darmon, 1977).
Because of its membrane localization (Malchow *et al.,* 1972) and its negative
cooperativity kinetics (Malchow *et al.,* 1975), the membrane-bound enzyme has
been ascribed a major role in signal reception (i.e. as an element coupled with the
cAMP receptor). However, the very limited amount of enzyme exposed on the cell
membrane of living cells (Malchow *et al.,* 1972) as well as kinetic experiments
(Darmon and Klein, 1976; Klein and Darmon, 1975) suggest that membrane-bound
PDE is mostly an intermediate of enzyme excretion.

The role of extracellular PDE in aggregation seems to be more clear. Alcantara and
Bazill (1976) have been able to accelerate the onset of aggregation-competence of
wild type cells starved at low densities in agitated suspensions by adding phosphodiesterase. They showed that rat brain PDE was as efficient as *D. discoideum* PDE.
At the same time, Darmon *et al.* (1976) identified a differentiation-stimulating
factor (DSF) which was able to induce aggregation of cells starved on dishes at a
density below the critical one for aggregation. This factor, which was shown to act
synergistically with cAMP pulses (Klein and Darmon, 1976), turned out to be
identical with inhibitor-resistant PDE (Brachet *et al.,* 1978).

Many aggregateless mutants are PDE-defective (Darmon *et al.,* 1977), but this
defect is only one aspect of the general negative pleiotropy of their mutations. For
the mutants whose morphogenetic block can be suppressed by cAMP pulses, induction
of PDE parallels induction of the other parameters of aggregation-competence
(Darmon *et al.,* 1977). Recently a mutant specifically blocked in synthesis of phosphodiesterase, HP X235, has been isolated (Barra, 1977; Brachet *et al.,*1977; Darmon
et al., 1978). The mutant is aggregation-defective, but cells recover the wild-type
ability to aggregate if the medium is supplemented with PDE from slime moulds or
rat brain. The size of the aggregation territories increases with the amount of enzyme
activity added to mutant HP X235 until, at 2 units ml^{-1}, wild-type aggregation is
achieved (Darmon *et al.,* 1978). No inhibition of aggregation is found up to added
enzyme activities of 32 units ml^{-1}. The enzyme is necessary not only for differentiation to aggregation-competence but also for aggregation itself. If added PDE
is washed away, cells do not aggregate and, moreover if cells are washed during
aggregation, the process stops completely in a few minutes. Even during aggregation
mediated by exogenous PDE the mutant does not produce a significant amount of
cytoplasmic or membrane-bound enzyme. This argues against an absolute requirement
for cytoplasmic PDE in the generation of chemotactic signals, and shows that
membrane-bound activity is not required for the functioning of the receptor. The
latter conclusion is strengthened by the fact that direct contact of the enzyme
with the membrane of mutant cells is not necessary for inducing aggregation. Moreover, aggregation of mutant HP X235 can occur without any extra enzyme, under
conditions facilitating the diffusion of cAMP. Release of cAMP from its receptors

appears, therefore, independent of hydrolysis. This situation is analogous to the case of the cholinergic receptor (Changeux *et al.*, 1976).

Theoretical models of aggregation argue that increasing the PDE level would decrease the size of aggregation territories (Parnas and Segel, 1978) and increase the critical density for aggregation (Gingle, 1976). Actually, experimental findings are the opposite (Alcantara and Bazill, 1976; Klein and Darmon, 1976; Darmon *et al.*, 1978). This discrepancy probably depends on the range of concentrations considered. At low PDE activities, increasing activity might have the net effect of increasing the cAMP signal-to-noise ratio. The consequences would be an increase of territory size and a decrease of the critical density, due to an increase of the range of the relayed signal. On the contrary very high PDE activity should lower the amplitude of the signal below the threshold for relay.

The recent work on PDE suggests that it is not involved in generation or recognition of cAMP signals, but is essential in control of cAMP signal steepness, as was pointed out in the early studies (Shaffer, 1962). The role of PDE inhibitor in aggregation is still unclear. Existence of an inhibitor-resistant PDE (Brachet *et al.*, 1977) makes aggregation possible even in the presence of an excess of inhibitor. In any case, it seems that extracellular, inhibitor-resistant PDE is not absolutely required for aggregation, since Gerisch (1976) described a strain for which no extracellular PDE can be detected during aggregation. However, it is impossible to determine whether hydrolysis of the cAMP signals in that strain is due to the membrane-bound enzyme or to the inhibitor-sensitive extracellular enzyme. Since PDE is steadily secreted in the medium (Klein and Darmon, 1975) and since the kinetics of neutralization of PDE by its inhibitor is relatively slow (half-neutralization time is approximately 5 min) (Riedel and Gerisch, 1971; Darmon and Blondelet, unpublished data), it is highly probable that actual enzyme activity is much higher than activity assayed in equilibrium conditions.

4.5.5 Adenylate cyclase

Rossomando and Sussmann (1972) reported the existence of an adenylate cyclase activity in cell lysates of *D. discoideum*. The activity assayed at 37°C was absolutely dependent on the presence of 5'AMP and was partially purified (50–100 fold) by chromatography. The authors found that adenylate cyclase activity was constant throughout development. The increase in cAMP production occuring during aggregation (Bonner *et al.*, 1969; Malkinson and Ashworth, 1973) remained unexplained by their findings since, at that time, PDE activity is also increasing (Malkinson and Ashworth, 1973; Malchow *et al.*, 1972; Klein and Darmon, 1975).

Using a different assay, Klein (1976) found an adenylate cyclase activity presenting strikingly different features. It is maximal at 27°C and is abolished at 37°C; 5'AMP is a potent inhibitor. Klein found a 40-fold increase in enzyme activity, beginning two hours after starvation and maximal after four, which could account for increased production of cAMP by starved cells. Therefore, the increase in adenylate cyclase activity precedes all the changes associated with aggregation-competence (Klein, 1977; Klein and Darmon, 1977) and seems to be due to new protein synthesis, since it is completely prevented by cycloheximide (Klein, 1977).

Darmon and Klein (1978) showed that a complete mixture of amino acids (used at concentrations described by Marin (1976) as inhibitory to cell differentiation) prevented the increase in adenylate cyclase synthesis. This result suggests that starvation initiates the developmental cycle by inducing synthesis of adenylate cyclase. Other experiments showed that the enzyme may be active in cell-free extracts but nevertheless be inactive *in vivo* (Klein and Darmon, 1977). For instance, cells collected from stationary growth phase do not aggregate even after 12 hours of starvation (Gerisch *et al.,* 1975a) and do not synthesize cAMP (Klein and Darmon, 1977), yet the specific activity of adenylate cyclase measured in extracts is as high as that of aggregating cells (Klein and Darmon, 1977, and unpublished observations). A similar situation is encountered when cells are incubated in buffer with high concentration of glucose. The cells do not synthesize cAMP but have normal levels of adenylate cyclase (Darmon and Klein, 1978; Rahmsdorf *et al.,* 1976). Pulses of cAMP can induce aggregation-competence in glucose-treated cells (Darmon and Klein, 1978), presumably by activating adenylate cyclase, since aggregation can proceed autonomously after 4 hours of treatment with cAMP pulses.

Roos and Gerisch (1976) demonstrated short-term, transient activation of adenylate cyclase after a pulse of cAMP. Such an activation probably reflects the relay mechanism, since it appears to be receptor-mediated; it is evoked 30 s after the stimulating pulse and persists for only 1 min. Roos *et al.* (1977b) found that cAMP pulses are also able to increase basal activity. Such an effect was not found by Klein and Darmon (1977), whose interpretation was that cAMP pulses do not affect adenylate cyclase synthesis but rather its activation. It is not yet known if the short-term response and the long-term activation of adenylate cyclase by cAMP pulses involve the same biochemical mechanism.

Oscillations of adenylate cyclase have been recently detected by Roos *et al.* (1977a) and Klein *et al.* (1977) (see Fig. 4.5). Both groups found that, in synchronized populations of aggregation-competent cells, an increase in adenylate cyclase activity correlates with synthesis of cAMP. Roos *et al.* (1977a) also reported that no concomitant changes of cellular ATP level were found.

A biochemical study of the phenotypic defects of aggregateless mutants provides additional information about regulation of adenylate cyclase and the functions controlled by cAMP pulses. Most completely aggregateless mutants appear identical; they display a complete negative pleiotropy for all elements and functions of the aggregation program. However, detailed physiological and biochemical studies (Darmon *et al,,* 1975; Darmon *et al.,* 1977; Juliani and Klein, 1978) indicate that they differ and may be classified into three distinct classes according to their responses to cAMP pulses. Mutants of group I are totally insensitive to cAMP pulses. Only one mutant of this category, Agip 43, has been studied in detail. This mutant is able to synthezise PDE inhibitor, but does not synthezise adenylate cyclase or any of the

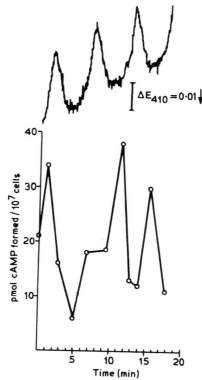

Fig. 4.5 Oscillations of adenylate cyclase activity. The upper curve is a light-scattering measurement. (Reproduced with permission, C. Klein and *FEBS Letters*).

biochemical markers which are under the control of cAMP pulses. cAMP pulses have no effect on the behavior of the mutant or on the time course of expression of the biochemical markers.

Mutants of group II are partially responsive to cAMP pulses. These mutants are unable to develop any of the characteristics of aggregation-competence by themselves, but they are able to synthesize adenylate cyclase and PDE inhibitor. Assays of cAMP indicate that, in these mutants, adenylate cyclase is not functional. Exogenous cAMP pulses are able to induce a full chemotactic response to cAMP as well as EDTA-resistant contacts. Cell elongation, formation of polar contacts and formation of mature aggregates able to develop further into fruiting bodies do not occur. If pulse treatment is interrupted no autonomous aggregation occurs. cAMP pulses induce formation of cAMP receptors and synthesis of PDE, and also repress production of PDE inhibitor. Such mutant cells co-aggregate with wild-type cells when both populations are mixed together. However, spores with a mutant genotype are not

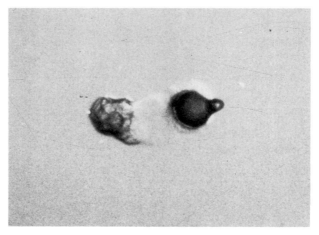

Fig. 4.6 Sorting-out of wild-type and mutant cells. Both cell types were allowed to aggregate together. Mutant cells are excluded from the aggregate once this one starts differentiating into a fruiting body.

formed; rather, mutant amoebae are excluded from the mixed aggregate once it forms a slug (Fig. 4.6).

In group III mutants, the morphogenetic block is fully suppressed by cAMP pulses. These mutants do not develop any of the characteristics of aggregation-competent cells nor synthezise adenylate cyclase. However cAMP pulses induce an increase in adenylate cyclase activity and development of all the physiological and biochemical parameters of aggregation-competence. The increase of adenylate cyclase could be either an induction of synthesis or an activation by cAMP pulses. cAMP pulses permit formation of mature aggregates which further develop into normal fruiting bodies. If cAMP pulses are interrupted late in the development, group III mutants are able to aggregate to some extent by themselves. Their aggregation is rudimentary, but cells are able to form polar contacts and stream to form aggregates which will mature. This behavior could be due to the permanent increase in adenylate cyclase induced by cAMP; the mutants may acquire the ability to generate their own cAMP pulses after a sufficient time of treatment by exogenous pulses. However this autonomous ability is probably weak, since the mutants are unable to form large aggregation territories (Darmon *et al.,* 1975, 1977) and spontaneous periodic oscillations do not develop in agitated suspensions even after prolonged treatment by cAMP pulses (Darmon, unpublished observations; Wurster, personnal communication).

4.6 MECHANISMS FOR INTRACELLULAR REGULATION

Even if the development of *D. discoideum* requires complex interrelationships in a cell population, in the last analysis, regulation of cell behavior and metabolism must have its expression at the level of the single cell. cAMP plays the role of an extracellular mediator (i.e. a hormone) during aggregation of *D. discoideum.* This is an unusual function for cAMP since, in both prokaryotes and eukaryotes, it is an intracellular effector. Moens and Konijn (1974) showed that cAMP does not have to penetrate the cell membrane to exert its chemotactic effect. Thus, an important question is: what are the second messengers which mediate the cell responses intracellularly after interaction of cAMP with its receptor? Two kinds of cell responses should be considered, short-term or behavioral responses (i.e. detection of chemoattractants, cell movements) and long-term or differentiation responses (i.e. activation or synthesis of new enzymes and membrane components).

4.6.1 Differentiation responses to cAMP

Several lines of evidence indicate that differentiation of amoebae to aggregation-competence requires cAMP synthesis and, hence, activation of adenylate cyclase. Treatment with 1 mM EDTA and 5 mM $MgCl_2$, or with micromolar amounts of ionophore A 23187 causes cells to develop aggregation-competence precociously. Direct and indirect measurements indicate that both treatments increase cAMP production (Klein and Brachet, 1975; Brachet and Klein, 1977). Adenylate cyclase activity appears stimulated by a factor of 2—3 (Brachet and Klein, unpublished results). Conversely, cells treated with progesterone, an inhibitor of cell differentiation, fail to accumulate cAMP, adenylate cyclase activity remains low, and cells appear totally unresponsive to treatment with exogenous cAMP pulses (Brachet and Klein, 1977) at least during the first 12 hours of starvation. Experiments of Darmon and Klein (1978) lead to similar conclusions. Amino acids, which prevent the increase in adenylate cyclase activity, also make the cell totally unresponsive to externally applied cAMP pulses. There is no induction of aggregation-competence, nor any significant activation of adenylate cyclase. In both cases, the lack of cellular responses should be attributed to a lack of endogenous synthesis of cAMP rather than to a defect in signal reception, since the basal level of cAMP binding remains detectable in such treated cells. Furthermore, data of Darmon and Klein (1978), Juliani and Klein (1978) and Brachet (unpublished) show that cAMP pulses are able to induce an increase of cAMP binding if (and only if) the increase in adenylate cyclase has taken place. It appears likely, therefore, that functioning of adenylate cyclase is an essential step in differentiation to aggregation-competence. Some aspects of this assumption may be tested with mutant cells. Aggregateless mutants in which the mutant phenotype is specifically supressed by exogenous cAMP pulses may be expected to be stimulated to synthesize cAMP in response to the treatment. This seems to be the case in the two strains tested (Wurster, personal communication).

Low concentrations of cAMP, if delivered in pulses induce cell differentiation (Darmon *et al.,* 1975; Gerisch *et al.,* 1975a). This involves an increase in chemotactic susceptibility (Darmon *et al.,* 1975), development of contact sites A (Gerisch *et al.,* 1975a), induction of phosphodiesterase (Klein and Darmon, 1975) and induction of cAMP receptors (Gerisch *et al.*, 1975b). Induction of PDE may also be obtained with a steady concentration of cAMP. However, under these conditions, very high cAMP concentrations are required (10^{-3}–10^{-4} M) (Klein, 1975). Klein and Darmon (1975) interpreted that difference in concentrations to mean that, at high concentrations of cAMP, the effect is not mediated via the receptor (which would be jammed by such a high concentration) but via cAMP penetrating into the cell. High cAMP, when applied at the beginning of starvation, has no inducive effects on cell cohesiveness and rather appears to delay aggregation competence. The same treatment applied after two hours, however, causes precocious appearance of contact sites A (Brachet, unpublished; Sampson *et al.*, 1978). Therefore if an increase in intracellular cAMP level is an essential event, this must occur after a certain time of starvation. At present there are no clear data indicating that cAMP is an intracellular control element of gene activation or protein synthesis in *D. discoideum*. Sampson (1977), however, described two developmentally regulated cAMP-dependent protein kinases. The early appearance of these activities, which parallels the increase of adenylate cyclase (Klein, 1977), would be consistent with the idea that they mediate the effects of cAMP on gene expression. cAMP stimulation of some kinase activities, but inhibition of others, might explain cAMP induction of PDE but repression of inhibitor synthesis. Adenylate cyclase and protein kinases appear after a lag (Klein, 1976, 1977; Sampson, 1977) equaling the latent period necessary for development of sensitivity to the differentiation inducing activity of cAMP pulses (Darmon *et al.*, 1975) or to high extracellular cAMP levels (Town and Gross, 1978; Brachet, unpublished). Mato and Konijn (1976) reported that ATP enhances aggregation in *D. discoideum* and that this is associated with phosphorylation of two proteins.

4.6.2 Behavioral responses to cAMP

That cAMP is not the intracellular mediator for the chemotactic response could be deduced from Gerisch and Wick's work (1975). The intracellular peak of cAMP evoked after an added pulse of cAMP appears only after a delay of 30 s–1 min, i.e. long after the beginning of the chemotactic response of the cell (Alcantara and Monk, 1974; Gerisch *et al.*, 1975). Wurster *et al.* (1977) and Mato *et al.* (1977a,b) independently presented evidence that a peak of intracellular cGMP was associated with the chemotactic response. Only 2 s after an added pulse of cAMP or of folic acid (a chemo-attractant specific for growth phase cells), an increase of cGMP was observed, with a maximum after 10–20 s. Thus, the cGMP peak just precedes the chemotactic response. A second cGMP peak was observed by Wurster *et al.* (1977) after 3 min, just prior to the intracellular cAMP peak (Fig. 4.4). The second cGMP peak may be due to the chemotactic response to the relayed cAMP signal, but could also be interpreted as evidence of a function of cGMP in adenylate cyclase activation (Wurster *et al.*, 1977). The two cGMP peaks correspond to the biphasic deflection of light scattering, supporting the assumption that they are related to the chemotactic responses evoked by the added cAMP (fast response) and by the relayed cAMP signal (slow response). The broadness of the second cGMP peak and the second (slow) light scattering response may be caused by signal relaying that is slightly out of phase. Spontaneous cGMP oscillations are also correlated with spontaneous oscillations of light scattering and seem to occur just prior to cAMP emissions (Fig. 4.3). In that case, the width of the cGMP pulse also corresponds to the width of the light scattering deflection. Cells which have been starved for only 1/2 hour are a hundred times less sensitive to the chemotactic power of cAMP than aggregation-competent cells; in such cells cAMP does not elicit cGMP accumulation (Mato *et al.*, 1977a). Conversely, an added pulse of folic acid induces a pulse of intracellular cGMP in those cells but without an increase of cAMP; this strongly supports the idea that cGMP is an intra-cellular mediator involved in the chemotactic response. Similarly Mato *et al.* (1977a) showed that an addition of *D. lacteum* acrasin to these amoebae provokes an increase of intracellular cGMP concentration without modifying cAMP levels.

Folic acid pulses have been shown to accelerate differentiation of *D. discoideum* amoebae to aggregation-competence (Wurster and Schubiger, 1977). This could be due to the fact that, after a certain time of starvation, folic acid pulses induce not only a fast cGMP synthesis, but also a rise in intracellular cAMP (Mato *et al.*, 1977b; Wurster *et al.*, 1977). However, since folic acid pulses are already active in inducing cell differentiation at a time when they are not yet able to induce cAMP synthesis it might be that cGMP functions independently of cAMP as an intracellular mediator of cell differentiation (Wurster *et al.*, 1977). The equal effectiveness of high concentra-tions of cGMP or cAMP in inducing cAMP–PDE (Blondelet, Darmon, Brachet, unpublished results; Town and Gross, 1978) supports this interpretation. No extra-cellular cGMP has been assayed during the cellular response to a cAMP pulse (Mato *et al.*, 1977b); eGMP in *D. discoideum* plays only the role of an intracellular (second) messenger. A guanylate cyclase activity has recently been assayed *in vitro* by Ward and Brenner (1977).

It would be very interesting to determine whether the membrane and cytoskeletal modifications involved in pseudopod formation are triggered by phosphorylation of proteins by cGMP-dependent protein kinases. Mato *et al.* (1977c) studying the aggregateless mutant Agip 55 (Darmon *et al.*, 1975; Darmon *et al.*, 1977) showed that this mutant, which is deficient in chemotaxis, is also deficient in cGMP accu-mulation in response to cAMP. cAMP pulses can reverse the chemotactic response of Agip 55 (see also Darmon *et al.*, 1975, 1977). Mato and his colleagues show that under these conditions a normal cGMP accumulation in response to cAMP is also reversed. It is possible that cAMP pulses induce development of a normal chemotactic response and cGMP accumulation because of their effect in increasing the number of cAMP receptors of mutant Agip 55 (Mato *et al.*, 1977c; Juliani and Klein, 1978).

Mato *et al.* (1977a) found that cGMP formation was dependent on the concentra-tion of cAMP added. Half maximum cGMP formation occured at about 10^{-8} M cAMP. They also showed a desensitized period of 1–5 min during which a second cAMP pulse does not elicit a second peak of cGMP accumulation. This desensitized period is dependent on the magnitude of the cAMP signal or more exactly on the ratio of the first to the second signal.

4.6.3 Calcium and divalent ions

In a number of systems, hormone-mediated cAMP or cGMP accumulation depends on stimulation of Ca^{2+} transport across the cellular membrane (Rasmussen *et al.*, 1975). Although several reports indicate that Ca^{2+} also plays a role in the differentiation of *D. discoideum*, the situation remains unclear, due to a great number of apparently contradictory results. Mason *et al.* (1971) reported that EGTA increases cAMP synthesis but blocks aggregation. Data of Gerisch and co-workers (1975b) support this observation, since these authors observed that EGTA blocks spontaneous oscillations of light scattered by aggregation-competent cells starved in liquid suspensions. However, Ca^{2+} chelators do not impair the chemotactic response to a single pulse of cAMP (Gerisch *et al.*, 1975b; Mato *et al.*, 1977a). Other data stress the relationship of divalent ions to cyclase activity. Incubation of cells with EDTA overtitrated with Mg^{2+} or with micromolar amounts of ionophore A23187 increases the rate of calcium leakage by starved cells (Brachet, 1976). These treatments, which accelerate the aggregation process by increasing adenylate cyclase activity, were also shown to cause aggregation of morphogenetic mutants, in which aggregation-competence may be induced with cAMP pulses. Conversely, high doses of progesterone, which inhibit cell differentiation, lower calcium release by starved cells. These data are consistent with the Chi and Francis (1971) experiments in which treatment of amoebae with a high concentration pulse of cAMP was shown to cause a wave of expulsion of calcium about 15 min later. Recent experiments by Wick and colleagues (1978) have shown that low concentration pulses of cAMP induce a transient influx of calcium into the cells within a few seconds, causing a short pause in calcium leakage. In other studies, Malchow and colleagues (1978) showed that in pre-aggregation amoebae low concentration pulses of cAMP induced a biphasic pH change of the extracellular medium, due to the expulsion of protons. The biphasic pattern mimics the changes observed by light scattering measurements as well as changes of the intracellular levels of cAMP and cGMP. Presence of calcium, but not magnesium, in the extracellular buffer was shown to decrease proton leakage by the cells.

The preceeding results indicate that calcium is involved not only in signal generation but also in the ability to respond to successive chemotactic signals. However, Mato and his co-workers (1977a) did not observe any significant effect of extracellular calcium either on chemotaxis and cGMP synthesis or on cell aggregation. These discrepancies could be explained if signal transduction is effected by displacement of Ca^{2+} between intracellular pools; the influx of calcium observed by Wick and colleagues would not be an essential step of the cell response but a way of reequilibrating intracellular Ca^{2+} pools. Moreover, additions of calcium, chelators of calcium, or calcium ionophores might have opposite effects, depending on experimental conditions, if they affect fluxes of calcium between extracellular and intracellular spaces or between two intracellular compartments.

It is probable that cells are able to respond to a positive temporal gradient of cAMP (Gerisch and Hess, 1974). However cells are also able to move in a spatial gradient of cAMP. This could be due to either a determination of spatial differences of concentration (Mato and Konijn, 1975) or to the temporal gradient created by the extension of pseudopods (Gerisch *et al.*, 1975c). At present there is no explanation for the mechanism of orientation of movement toward a source of attractant, continuous or pulsatile. Observations about calcium fluxes may be related to the data of Condeelis and Taylor (1977) who showed the importance of calcium ions in geling of *D. discoideum* cytosol. Such a geling could be involved in pseudopod formation. Also, Juliani and Klein (1977) have shown that Ca^{2+} causes a rapid increase of the level of cAMP binding. Whether or not this effect is important for the chemotactic response remains unclear.

4.6.4 Early control of cell differentiation, effect of starvation

Some proteins are induced from the beginning of starvation; this is the case with α-mannosidase and with *N*-acetyl-glucosaminidase (Loomis, 1969b, 1970). However, their involvement in aggregation is doubtful. Critical elements which participate in the differentiation program to aggregation-competence are induced before the cells are able to synthezise cAMP, but after a lag of 1.5–2 hours of starvation. This is the case with adenylate cyclase (Klein, 1976, 1977), cAMP-dependent protein kinases (Sampson, 1977) and the phosphodiesterase inhibitor (Klein and Darmon, 1975). This two hour period probably corresponds to the time necessary for the metabolic compounds produced by starvation to activate specific genes. It should be noted that cAMP pulses have no effect in advancing the onset of aggregation during that period of time (Darmon *et al.*, 1975), which has been called the latent period. Darmon and Klein (1978) have shown that the inhibitory effect of amino acids can be correlated with an inhibition of adenylate cyclase synthesis. Since the absence of amino acids from an otherwise complete growth media allows initiation of differentiation (Marin, 1976), it is probable that amino acid starvation is the trigger for adenylate cyclase synthesis. The mechanism for such an activation is unknown but could present some analogies with stringent control in bacteria since ppGpp or a closely related compound accumulates in the cells very early during starvation (1–2 hours) (Klein, 1974). Unfortunately this observation is still not confirmed. Lodish *et al.* (1976) showed that a few minutes after the beginning of starvation 70% of the polysomes dissociate. They proposed that the control of differentiation might depend on the higher probability of protein synthesis initiation of 'differentiation' mRNA versus 'vegetative' mRNA. However, polysome dissociation seems to depend only on cessation of growth since it is observed for cells in growth media at stationary phase and also for cells treated with amino acids in buffer (Darmon and Monier, unpublished observation), neither condition allowing cell differentiation. It is still possible that polysome dissociation, even if not sufficient for promoting cell differentiation, might be a necessary initial event in development.

Glucose inhibits cell differentiation of *D. discoideum* by preventing adenylate cyclase activation (Darmon and Klein, 1978). It is very tempting to compare this effect of glucose on cAMP synthesis to catabolic repression in bacteria. However the situation is not clear, since Darmon and Klein found similar effects with non-metabolizable sugars, while Rhamsdorf *et al.* (1976) found that only metabolizable sugars are effective in preventing cAMP synthesis and cell differentiation.

4.6.5 The end of aggregation: regulation by cell contacts

Cell contacts do not play any role in development of aggregation-competence since they only develop after the elements of the chemotactic system (Robertson *et al.*, 1972). However, cell contacts seem to be involved in termination of the differentiation program for aggregation (Darmon, 1976; Okamoto and Takeuchi, 1976; Gross *et al.*, 1977). At the time compact aggregates form, there is a sharp decrease in PDE synthesis (Henderson, 1975; Darmon, 1976; Okamoto and Takeuchi, 1976; Gross *et al.*, 1977), receptor synthesis (Henderson, 1975; Klein, 1977) and adenylate cyclase synthesis (Klein, 1977) and an increase in the frequency of oscillations (Gross *et al.*, 1977) which precede their disappearance. For mutants unable to form tight intercellular contacts these changes are not observed (Darmon, 1976; Okamoto and Takeuchi, 1976; Gross *et al.*, 1977). If cells are agitated vigourously the decrease in PDE (Darmon, 1976; Okamoto and Takeuchi, 1976; Gross *et al.*, 1977) and cAMP receptor (Henderson, 1975) are not seen. If the cells are dissociated after the decrease in PDE a new round of enzyme synthesis may be observed (Darmon, 1976; Okamoto and Takeuchi, 1976). These data favor a role of cell contacts in termination of the program of differentiation to aggregation-competence. At the time aggregates form, new enzymes which will later participate in the spore or stalk differentiation are induced, and it has been shown for some of them that cell contacts direct their synthesis (Newell *et al.* 1971; Okamoto and Takeuchi, 1976; Gross *et al.*, 1977). This new enzyme synthesis is probably under transcriptional control (Lodish *et al.* 1977; Alton and Lodish, 1977). It would be of great interest to determine the mechanism of control of gene activity by intercellular contacts. It is possible that membrane reassortments triggered by cell contact mechanically alter the efficiency of adenylate cyclase, guanylate cyclase or the cAMP receptor, thus modifying intracellular levels of cAMP or cGMP which could alter translation or transcription. Town and Gross (1978) and Klein and Brachet (unpublished observations) were able to stop PDE accumulation and increase synthesis of post-aggregation enzymes by adding a high concentration of cAMP to vigourously shaken cultures of cells which were starved for 6 hours. cAMP can thus replace the requirement for stable cell-to-cell contacts in the transition from aggregation to post-aggregation programs. Town and Gross interpret these results to mean that large agglomerates are probably necessary to establish a new mode of signalling (see Gross *et al.*, 1977) which would be involved in the control of enzyme synthesis after aggregation.

4.7 THEORETICAL MODELS FOR cAMP GENERATION

Aggregation of *D. discoideum* is a very attractive subject for theoretical work because of its relationship to dissipative structures and excitable systems. A number of studies have been concerned with these problems (Keller and Segel, 1970; Cohen and Robertson, 1971a,b). Here, we will discuss only the models dealing with mechanisms of periodic generation of cAMP pulses. Goldbeter (1975) presented a model for intracellular oscillations and periodic release of cAMP based on the regulatory properties of adenylate cyclase and pyrophosphohydrolase which had been reported by Rossomando and Sussman (1973). Several features of the model have not been verified by experimental work. For instance 5'AMP is not an activator of adenylate cyclase (Klein, 1976; Roos and Gerisch, 1976) but an inhibitor (Klein, 1976). Cellular or membrane-bound PDE are not required for pulsatile aggregation (Darmon *et al.,* 1978). Goldbeter noted that periodic generation of cAMP pulses occurs in this model even if one postulates regulatory properties for adenylate cyclase only. From such an observation, Goldbeter and Segel (1977) devised a model accounting both for relay and periodic oscillations. The model is based on adenylate cyclase activation by extracellular cAMP, mediated via the cAMP receptor (Roos and Gerisch, 1976), and subsequent excretion of the cAMP formed. Depending on critical injection rates of ATP, relay or autonomous generation of cAMP pulses are obtained. According to that model a periodic decrease of ATP levels should occur in phase with the cAMP pulses. Such a variation has not been observed (Roos *et al.,* 1977) but could occur in a membrane compartment and not be apparent in the total ATP cell pool. However since adenylate cyclase may be either activated or unactivated (Klein *et al.,* 1977; Roos *et al.,* 1977; Roos and Gerisch, 1976) in *in vitro* conditions where ATP is in excess it is unlikely that enzyme activity is controlled by ATP levels. Other parameter changes than the rate of ATP entry might in principle bring about the transitions predicted in Goldbeter and Segel's calculations. M. Cohen (1977) has presented a model which has approximately the same mathematical structure as that of Goldbeter and Segel, but is based on catabolite regulation of cAMP synthesis. It remains to be seen which, if either, of these models correctly incorporates the major features of the relay-oscillator system, but it is noteworthy that the models show how the observed slow change of development parameters can successively bring about three transitions in cellular behaviour, from indifference to cAMP stimulation to relay, to autonomous oscillation and finally to fast steady cAMP secretion.

In the Goldbeter—Segel model, the refractory period after a pulse of cAMP or during oscillations is also based on the shortage of ATP resulting from cyclase activation. The refractory period and the period of signalling are equal in spiral pacemakers (Durston, 1974) or in cells stimulated by continuous sources of cAMP (Robertson and Drage, 1975) but this is not the case in the concentric wave patterns (Durston, 1974). One explanation for this discrepancy would be that in the latter case the autonomous center cell signals with a period equal to its refractory period but that the responding cells of the field have a higher refractory period (because

Table 4.2 Parameters of pulse generation and aggregation. From Parnas and Segel (1977)

Periods of autonomous signal	5 min
Amount of chemical per signal pulse per amoebae (concentration equivalent)	10^7 molecules (40 μM)
Secretion duration per pulse	0.01 min
Concentration threshold for relay	3 μM
Relay delay	12 s
Refractory period for relay	7 min
Duration of absolute movement refractory period	12 s
Duration of relative movement refractory period	100 s
Primary $\frac{\delta C}{\delta t}$ threshold for movement signal	0.002 μM/0.01 min
Speed of cell movement	15 μM/min^{-1}
Michaelis constant for phosphodiesterase	0.5 μM

oscillatory parameters of relaying cells are different from those of cells oscillating autonomously) so that they respond only to 1 out of 2 or 3 pulses of the autonomous center. Alternatively, it could be argued that the refractory period is not directly linked to cyclase oscillation but is due to a transition at the receptor level which could correspond to a decreased affinity (Klein *et al.,* 1977; King and Frazier, 1977).

If the existence of a refractory period for relay can explain the unidirectionality of propagation of the cAMP signal, it cannot account for the unidirectionality of movement. A cell which has been stimulated by a neighbour proximal to the center moves towards it and relays the signal in all directions, but, because of the refractory period for relay, only the cells which are distal to it will emit cAMP, so that the cell in question should move back toward the distal cells. A refractory period for movement should then exist and it should be of a duration approximately equal to that of the peak of extracellular cAMP. Parnas and Segel (1977) described a model for pulse generation and aggregation which was simulated on a computer. They consider one spatial dimension. With parameter values taken from the literature (see Table 4.2), the simulation provides outward moving waves of attractant and organized inward pulsatile steps of cell movement. However, the authors assume a cAMP signal of very short duration (0.01 min) and an absolute refractory period for movement of 12 s followed by a relative refractory period for movement of 100 s. Alcantara and Monk (1974) in their study of time-lapse films tried to demonstrate the existence of a refractory period for movement. They concluded that this refractory period must be less than 12 s. Gerisch *et al.* (1975b) found an even shorter refractory period ($\simeq$ 5 s) for emission of a second pseudopod after a second addition of cAMP. If cAMP signals last 60 to 90 s, as appears from the work of Roos *et al.,* (1975), very short refractory periods cannot account for unidirectionality of movement. However, it is possible that actual secretion by single cells is of much shorter duration since Roos *et al.* (1975) studied populations of cells which could have been somewhat out of phase. Moreover, it is possible that at low cAMP concentrations a relative refractoriness for movement would exist (Parnas and Segel, 1977). In their second paper, Parnas and Segel (1978) also consider the long secretion case, if the parameters are tuned carefully a relative refractory period can also explain unidirectionality of movement. Mato *et al.* (1977a) showed a period of desensitization for cGMP accumulation following a pulse of cAMP. This period which lasts for 1 to 5 min could account for the relative refractoriness of movement since cGMP is implicated in the chemotactic response (Wurster *et al.,* 1977, Mato *et al.,* 1977a,b,c).

4.8 CONCLUSIONS

Observations concerning differentiation to aggregation-competence can be ordered in a sequential model of regulation. The cells seem to differentiate not only according to a temporal clock but also following a chronology of crucial events. Three successive steps can be defined.

STEP I: *No intercellular communication via cAMP is required*
The synthesis of new proteins is under the direct control of starvation (probably starvation for amino acids).The inhibitor of PDE, protein kinases and adenylate cyclase are synthezised. Adenylate cyclase is in an inactive form.

STEP II: *Intercellular communications via cAMP are required*
This step corresponds to initiation and functioning of oscillatory mechanisms. The cell population is in an unstable equilibrium, so that any spontaneous perturbation can trigger aggregation. Some cells will spontaneously activate adenylate cyclase (aleatory process) so that emissions of cAMP will be generated and will activate adenylate cyclase of neighboring cells; cAMP pulses will be amplified and propagated (relay system). Even in the absence of autonomous centers, pacemakers will be generated. cAMP pulses induce cAMP receptors and PDE in a parallel way; the result is an increase of cell sensitivity to cAMP. At all levels this process is highly co-operative. cAMP pulses also induce formation of elements not involved in signal transmission, namely polar contact sites, which favor formation of streams and increase efficiency of aggregation.

STEP III: *Intercellular contacts are required*
In step III intercellular contacts which have been formed in the aggregate turn off elements which have been participating in aggregation: adenylate cyclase, cAMP receptors, PDE. In other words, completion of aggregation directs termination of the functioning of these elements. Simultaneously, functions involved in further steps of the developmental cycle are induced.

One of the most striking feature of *D. discoideum* aggregation is that both cell differentiation and cell movements are controlled by the same signal. It is possible that such dual controls account for 'the morphogenetic cell movements' which occur during embryogenesis of vertebrates.

REFERENCES

Alcantara, F. and Bazill, G.W. (1976), Extracellular cyclic AMP-phosphodiesterase accelerates differentiation in *Dictyostelium discoideum. J. gen. Microbiol.,* **92**, 351–368.

Alcantara, F. and Monk, M. (1974), Signal propagation during aggregation in the slime mould *Dictyostelium discoideum. J. gen. Microbiol.,* **85**, 321–334.

Alton, T.H. and Lodish, H.F. (1977), Synthesis of developmentally regulated proteins i *Dictyostelium discoideum* which are dependent on continued cell-cell interaction *Dev. Biol.,* **60**, 207–216.

Barkley, D.S. (1969), Adenosine-3′-5′-phosphate:identification as acrasin in a species of cellular slime mold. *Science,* **165**, 1133–1134.

Barra, J. (1977), Synergie entre mutants d'agrégation de *Dictyostelium discoideum. C.R. Acad. Sci. Paris,* **284**, 689–692.

Beug, H., Gerisch, G., Kempf, S., Riedel, V. and Cremer, G. (1970), Specific inhibition of cell contact formation in *Dictyostelium* by univalent antibodies. *Exp. Cell Res.,* **63**, 147–158.

Beug, H., Katz, F.E. and Gerisch, G. (1973), Dynamics of antigenic membrane sites relating to cell aggregation in *Dictyostelium discoideum. J. Cell Biol.,* **56**, 647–6

Bonner, J.T. (1944), A descriptive study of the development of the slime mold *Dictyostelium discoideum. Am. J. Bot.,* **31**, 175–182.

Bonner, J.T. (1947), Evidence for the formation of cell aggregates by chemotaxis in the development of the slime mold *Dictyostelium discoideum. J. exp. Zool.,* **110**, 259–271.

Bonner, J.T. (1963), Epigenetic development in the cellular slime molds. *Symp. Soc. Exp. Biol.,* **17**, 341–358.

Bonner, J.T. (1967), *'The Cellular Slime Moulds'* 2nd edn., Princeton University Press.

Bonner, J.T. (1971b), Aggregation and differentiation in the cellular slime molds. *A. Rev. Microbiol.,* **25**, 75–92.

Bonner, J.T., Barkley, D.S., Hall, E.M., Konijn, T.M., Mason, J.W., O'Keefe, G. and Wolfe, P.B. (1969), Acrasin, acrasinase and the sensitivity to acrasin in *Dictyostelium discoideum. Dev. Biol.,* **20**, 72–87.

Bonner, J.T., Kelso, A.P. and Gillmor, R.G. (1966), A new approach to the problem of aggregation in the cellular slime molds. *Biol. Bull.,* **130**, 28–42.

Brachet, P. (1976), Effet d'un ionophore sur l'agrégation de *Dictyostelium discoideum C.R. Acad. Sci. Paris,* **282**, 377–380.

Brachet, P., Barra, J., Darmon, M. and Barrand, P. (1977), A phosphodiesterase-defective mutant of *Dictyostelium discoideum.* In: *Development and Differentiation in Cellular Slime Moulds.* (Cappuccinelli and Ashworth, J., eds), Elsevier-North Holland. pp. 125–134.

Brachet, P., Darmon, M. and Blondelet, M.H. (1978), Sensitivity of extracellular phosphodiesterase to its inhibitor during aggregation of *D. discoideum*. *Exp. Cell Res.*, in press.

Brachet, P. and Klein, C. (1977), Cell responsiveness to cAMP during the aggregation phase of *Dictyostelium discoideum*. *Differentiation*, **8**, 1–8.

Chang, Y.Y. (1968), Cyclic 3'-5'-adenosine monophosphate phosphodiesterase produced by the slime mold *Dictyostelium discoideum*. *Science*, **161**, 57–59.

Changeux, J.R., Benedetti, L., Bourgeois, J.P., Brisson, A., Cartaud, J., Devaux, P., Grunhagen, H., Moreau, M., Popot, J.L., Sobel, A. and Weber, M. (1976), Some structural properties of the cholinergic receptor protein in its membrane environment relevant to its function as a pharmacological agent. *Cold Spring Harbor Symp. Quant. Biol.*, **40**, 211–230.

Chassy, B.M., Love, L.L. and Krichevsky, M.I. (1969), Purification properties and biological role of an extracellular nucleoside 3'-5' cyclic phosphate phosphodiesterase from *Dictyostelium discoideum*. *Fedn Proc., Fedn Am. Socs exp. Biol.*, **28**, 842.

Chi, Y.Y. and Francis, D. (1971), Cyclic AMP and calcium exchange in a cellular slime mold. *J. Cell Physiol.*, **77**, 169–174.

Cohen, M.H. (1977), The cyclic AMP control system in the development of *Dictyostelium discoideum*. *J. theor. Biol.*, **69**, 57–85.

Cohen, M.H. and Robertson, A. (1971a), Wave propagation in the early stages of aggregation of cellular slime molds. *J. theor. Biol.*, **31**, 101–118.

Cohen, M.H. and Robertson, A. (1971b), Chemotaxis and the early stages of aggregation of cellular slime molds. *J. theor. Biol.*, **31**, 119–135.

Condeelis, J.S. and Taylor, D.L. (1977), The contractile basis of amoeboid movement. V. The control of gelation, solation and contraction in *D. discoideum*. *J. Cell Biol.*, **74**, 901–927.

Coukell, B. (1975), Parasexual genetic analysis of aggregation-deficient mutants of *Dictyostelium discoideum*. *Mol. gen. Genet.*, **142**, 119–135.

Darmon, M. (1976), Rôle possible des contacts cellulaires dans l'arrêt d'un programme de différenciation chez *Dictyostelium discoideum*. *C.R. Acad. Sci. Paris*, **282**, 1993–1896.

Darmón, M., Barra, J. and Brachet, P. (1978), The role of phosphodiesterase in aggregation of *Dictyostelium discoideum*. *J. Cell Sci.*, **31**, 233–243.

Darmon, M., Barrand, P., Brachet, P., Klein, C. and Pereira da Silva, L. (1977), Phenotypic suppression of morphogenetic mutants of *Dictyostelium discoideum*. *Dev. Biol.*, **58**, 174–184.

Darmon, M., Brachet, P. and Pereira da Silva, L.H. (1975), Chemotactic signals induce cell differentiation in *Dictyostelium discoideum*. *Proc. natn. Acad. Sci. U.S.A.*, **72**, 3163–3166.

Darmon, M. and Klein, C. (1976), Binding of concanavalin A and its effect on the differentiation of *Dictyostelium discoideum*. *Biochem. J.*, **154**, 743–750.

Darmon, M. and Klein, C. (1978), Effects of amino acids and glucose on adenylate cyclase and cell differentiation of *Dictyostelium discoideum*. *Dev. Biol.*, **63**, 377–389.

Darmon, M., Klein, C. and Brachet, P. (1976), Evidence for a macromolecular effector of cell differentiation in *Dictyostelium discoideum* amoebae. In: *Surface Membrane Receptors*, (Bradshaw, R.A., ed), Plenum, New York, pp. 317–327.

Durston, A. (1974), Pacemaker activity during aggregation in *Dictyostelium discoideum*. *Dev. Biol.*, **37**, 225–235.

Ennis, H.L. and Sussman, M. (1958), Synergistic morphogenesis by mixtures of *Dictyostelium discoideum* wild-type and aggregateless mutants. *J. gen. Microbiol.*, **18**, 433–449.

Gerisch, G. (1965), Stadienspezifische aggregationsmuster von *Dictyostelium discoideum*. *Roux' Arch. Entwicklungsmech. Org.*, **156**, 127–144.

Gerisch, G. (1968), Cell aggregation and differentiation in *Dictyostelium discoideum*. *Curr. Top. Dev. Biol.*, **3**, 157–197.

Gerisch, G. (1976), Extracellular cyclic-AMP phosphodiesterase regulation in agar plate cultures of *Dictyostelium discoideum*. *Cell differentiation*, **5**, 21–25.

Gerisch, G., Fromm, H., Huesgen, A. and Wick, U. (1975a), Control of cell contact-sites by cyclic AMP pulses in differentiating *Dictyostelium discoideum*. *Nature*, **255**, 547–549.

Gerisch, G. and Hess, B. (1974), Cyclic-AMP controlled oscillations in suspended *Dictyostelium discoideum*. Their relation to morphogenetic cell interactions. *Proc. natn. Acad. Sci. U.S.A.*, **71**, 2118–2122.

Gerisch, G., Hülser, D., Malchow, D. and Wick, U. (1975c), Cell communication by periodic cyclic AMP pulses. *Phil. Trans. R. Soc. Lond. Ser. B.*, **272**, 181–192.

Gerisch, G., Malchow, D., Huesgen, A., Nanjundiah, V., Roos, W., Wick, U. and Hüsler, D. (1975b), Cyclic-AMP reception and cell recognition in *Dictyostelium discoideum* In: *Developmental Biology* (MacMahon, D. and Fox, C.F., eds.), ICN-UCLA Sym. Mol. Cell Biol., **2**, 76–88.

Gerisch, G. and Wick, U. (1975), Intracellular oscillations and release of cyclic AMP from *Dictyostelium* cells. *Biochem. biophys. Res. Comm.*, **65**, 364–370.

Gingle, A.R. (1976), Critical density for relaying in *Dictyostelium discoideum* and its relation to phosphodiesterase secretion into the extracellular medium. *J. Cell. Sci.*, **20**, 1–20.

Goldbeter, A. (1975), Mechanism for oscillatory synthesis of cyclic AMP in *Dictyostelium discoideum*. *Nature*, **253**, 540–542.

Goldbeter, A. and Segel, L.A. (1977), Unified mechanism for relay and oscillation of cyclic AMP in *Dictyostelium discoideum*. *Proc. natn. Acad. Sci. U.S.A.*, **74**, 1543–1547.

Green, A.A. and Newell, P.C. (1975), Evidence for the existence of two types of cAMP binding sites in aggregating cells of *Dictyostelium discoideum*. *Cell*, **6**, 129–136.

Gross, J., Kay, R., Lax, A., Peacey, M., Town, C. and Trevan, D. (1977), Cell contact, signalling and gene expression in *Dictyostelium discoideum*. Embo workshop on Development and Differentiation in cellular slime moulds n° 13. (Cappuccinelli, ed), pp. 135–148, Elsevier North-Holland Publishing Company, Amsterdam.

Gross, J.D., Peacey, M.J. and Trevan, D.J. (1976), Signal emission and signal propagation during early aggregation in *Dictyostelium discoideum*. *J. Cell Sci.*, **22**, 645–656.

Henderson, E.J. (1975), The cyclic adenosine $3'$-$5'$-monophosphate receptor of *Dictyostelium discoideum*. *J. biol. Chem.*, **250**, 4730–4736.

Juliani, M.H. and Klein, C. (1977), Calcium ion effects on cyclic adenosine 3′-5′-mono-phosphate binding to the plasma membrane of *Dictyostelium discoideum*. *Biochim. biophys. Acta*, **497**, 369–376.

Juliani, M.H. and Klein, C. (1978), A biochemical study of the effects of cAMP pulses on aggregateless mutants of *Dictyostelium discoideum*. *Dev. Biol.*, **62**, 162–172.

Keller, E.F. and Segel, L.A. (1970), Initiation of slime mold aggregation viewed as an instability. *J. theor. Biol.*, **26**, 399–415.

King, A.C. and Frazier, W.A. (1977), Reciprocal periodicity in cAMP binding and phosphorylation of differentiating *Dictyostelium discoideum* cells. *Biochem. biophys. Res. Comm.*, **78**, 1033–1099.

Klein, C. (1974), Presence of magic spot in *Dictyostelium discoideum*. *FEBS Letters*, **38**, 149–152.

Klein, C. (1975), Induction of phosphodiesterase by cyclic adenosine 3′-5′-mono-phosphate in differentiating *Dictyostelium discoideum* amoebae. *J. biol. Chem.*, **250**, 7134–7138.

Klein, C. (1976), Adenylate cyclase activity in *Dictyostelium discoideum* amoebae and its changes during differentiation. *FEBS Letters*, **68**, 125–128.

Klein, C. (1977), Changes in adenylate cyclase during differentiation of *Dictyostelium discoideum*. *FEBS Letters*, **1**, 17–20.

Klein, C. and Brachet, P. (1975), Effects of progesterone and EDTA on cyclic AMP and phosphodiesterase in *Dictyostelium discoideum*. *Nature*, **254**, 432–433.

Klein, C., Brachet, P. and Darmon, M. (1977), Periodic changes in adenylate cyclase and cAMP receptors in *Dictyostelium discoideum*. *FEBS Letters*, **76**, 145–147.

Klein, C. and Darmon, M. (1975), The relationship of phosphodiesterase to the developmental cycle of *Dictyostelium discoideum*. *Biochem. Biophys. Res. Commun.*, **67**, 440–447.

Klein, C. and Darmon, M. (1976), A differentiation stimulating factor induces cell sensitivity to 3′-5′-cyclic AMP pulses in *Dictyostelium discoideum*. *Proc. natn. Acad. Sci. U.S.A.*, **73**, 1250–1254.

Klein, C. and Darmon, M. (1977), Effects of cAMP pulses on adenylate cyclase and the phosphodiesterase inhibitor of *D. discoideum*. *Nature*, **268**, 76–77.

Klein, C. and Juliani, M.H. (1976), cAMP-induced changes in cAMP binding sites on *Dictyostelium discoidcum* amoebae. *Cell*, **10**, 329–335.

Konijn, T.M. (1965), Chemotaxis in the cellular slime mold. I. The effect of temperature. *Dev. Biol.*, **12**, 487–497.

Konijn, T.M. (1969), Effect of bacteria on chemotaxis in the cellular slime molds. *J. Bact.*, **99**, 503–509.

Konijn, T.M. (1972), Cyclic AMP as a first messenger. *Adv. Cyclic Nucleotide Res.*, **1**, 17–31.

Konijn, T.M. and Raper, K.B. (1961), Cell aggregation in *Dictyostelium discoideum*. *Dev. Biol.*, **3**, 725–756.

Konijn, T.M., Van de Meene, J.G.C., Bonner, J.T. and Barkley, D.S. (1967), The acrasin activity of adenosine 3′-5′-cyclic phosphate. *Proc. natn. Acad. Sci. U.S.A.*, **58**, 1152–1154.

Konijn, T.M., Van de Meene, J.G.C., Chang, Y.Y., Barkley, D.S. and Bonner, J.T. (1969), Identification of adenosine-3′-5′-monophosphate as the bacterial attractant for myxamoebae of *Dictyostelium discoideum*. *J. Bact.*, **99**, 510–512.

Lodish, H.F., Alton, T., Dottin, R.P., Weiner, A.M. and Margolskee, J.P. (1976), Synthesis and translation of messenger RNA during differentiation of the cellular slime mold *Dictyostelium discoideum* In: *The Molecular Biology of Hormone Action*, pp. 75–103, Symposium of the Society for Developmental Biology. Academic Press, New York.

Loomis, W.F. (1969a), Temperature-sensitive mutants of *Dictyostelium discoideum*. *J. Bact.*, **99**, 65–69.

Loomis, W.F. (1969b), Acetylglucosaminidase, an early enzyme in the development of *Dictyostelium discoideum*. *J. Bact.*, **97**, 1149–1154.

Loomis, W.F. (1970), Developmental regulation of α-mannosidase in *Dictyostelium discoideum*. *J. Bact.*, **103**, 375–381.

Loomis, W.F. (1975), *Dictyostelium discoideum*. A developmental system. Academic Press, New York.

Maeda, Y. and Gerisch, G. (1977), Vesicle formation in *Dictyostelium discoideum* cells during oscillations of cAMP synthesis and release. *Exp. Cell Res.*, **110**, 119–126.

Malchow, D., Fuchila, J. and Nanjundiah, V. (1975), A plausible role for a membrane-bound cyclic AMP phosphodiesterase in cellular slime mold chemotaxis. *Biochim. biophys. Acta*, **385**, 421–428.

Malchow, D. and Gerisch, G. (1974), Short-term binding and hydrolysis of cyclic 3'-5'-adenosine monophosphate by aggregating *Dictyostelium* cells. *Proc. natn. Acad. Sci. U.S.A.*, **71**, 2423–2427.

Malchow, D., Nägele, B., Schwartz, H. and Gerisch, G. (1972), Membrane-bound cyclic AMP phosphodiesterase in chemotactically responding cells of *Dictyostelium discoideum*. *Eur. J. Biochem.*, **28**, 136–142.

Malchow, D., Nanjundiah, V., Wurster, B., Eckstein, F. and Gerisch, G. (1978), Cyclic AMP induced pH changes in *Dictyostelium discoideum* and their control by calcium. *Biochim. biophys. Acta,* in press.

Malkinson, A.M. and Ashworth, J.M. (1973), Adenosine 3'-5'-cyclic monophosphate concentrations and phosphodiesterase activities during axenic growth and differentiation of cells of the cellular slime mould *Dictyostelium discoideum*. *Biochem. J.*, **134**, 311–319.

Marin, F.T. (1976), Regulation of development in *Dictyostelium discoideum*. Initiation of the growth to development transition by amino acid starvation. *Dev. Biol.*, **48**, 110–117.

Mason, J.W., Rasmussen, H. and Dibella, F. (1971), 3'-5'-cyclic AMP and Ca²⁺ in slime mold aggregation. *Exp. Cell Res.*, **67**, 156–160.

Mato, J.M., Frans, A.K., Van Haastert, P.J. and Konijn, T.M. (1977a), 3'-5'-cyclic AMP dependent 3'-5'-cyclic GMP accumulation in *Dictyostelium discoideum*. *Proc. natn. Acad. Sci. U.S.A.*, **76**, 2348–2351.

Mato, J.M. and Konijn, T.M. (1975), Chemotaxis and binding of cyclic AMP in cellular slime molds. *Biochim. biophys. Acta*, **385**, 173–179.

Mato, J.M. and Konijn, T.M. (1976), The activation of cell aggregation by phosphorylation in *Dictyostelium discoideum*. *Exp. Cell Res.*, **99**, 328–332.

Mato, J.M., Krens, F.A., Van Haastert, P.J. and Konijn, T.M. (1977c), Unified control of chemotaxis and cAMP mediated cGMP accumulation by cAMP in *Dictyostelium discoideum*. *Biochem. biophys. Res. Comm.*, **77**, 399–402.

Mato, J.M., Van Haastert, P.J., Krens, F.A., Rhijnsburger, E.H., Dobbe, F.O. (1977b), Cyclic AMP and folic acid mediated cyclic GMP accumulation in *Dictyostelium discoideum. FEBS Letters,* **79,** 331–336.

Moens, P.B. and Konijn, T.M. (1974), Cyclic AMP as a cell surface activating agent in *Dictyostelium discoideum. FEBS Letters,* **45,** 44–46.

Newell, P.C. (1977), Aggregation and cell surface receptors in cellular slime molds. In: *Microbial Interactions,* pp. 3–49. Receptors and Recognition, Series B, Volume 3. (Reissig, J.L., ed), Chapman and Hall, London.

Newell, P.C., Longlands, M. and Sussman, M. (1971), Control of enzyme synthesis by cellular interaction during development of the cellular slime mold *Dictyostelium discoideum. J. mol. Biol.,* **58,** 541–554.

Okamoto, K. and Takeuchi, I. (1976), Changes in activities of two developmentally regulated enzymes induced by disaggregation of the pseudoplasmodia of *Dictyostelium discoideum. Biochem. biophys. Res. Comm.,* **72,** 739–746.

Pan, P., Hall, E.M. and Bonner, J.T. (1972), Folic acid as secondary chemotaxic substance in the cellular slime molds. *Nature New Biol.,* **237,** 181–182.

Pannbacker, R.G. and Bravard, L.J. (1972), Phosphodiesterase in *Dictyostelium discoideum* and the chemotactic response to cyclic adenosine monophosphate. *Science,* **175,** 1014–1015.

Parnas, H. and Segel, L.A. (1977), Computer evidence concerning the chemotactic signal in *Dictyostelium discoideum. J. Cell Sci.,* **25,** 191–204.

Parnas, H. and Segel, L.A. (1978), A computer simulation of pulsatile aggregation in *Dictyostelium discoideum. J. theor. Biol.,* in press.

Rahmsdorf, H.J., Cailla, H.L., Spitz, E., Moran, M.J. and Rickenberg, H.V. (1976), Effect of sugars on early biochemical events in development of *Dictyostelium discoideum. Proc. natn. Acad. Sci. U.S.A.,* **73,** 3183–3187.

Raper, K.B. (1935), *Dictyostelium discoideum* a new species of slime mold from decaying forest leaves. *J. Agric. Res.,* **50,** 135–147.

Rasmussen, H., Jensen, P., Lake, W., Fiedmann, N. and Goodman, D.B.P. (1975), Cyclic nucleotides and cellular calcium metabolism *Adv. Cyclic Nucleotide Res.,* **5,** 375–394.

Riedel, V. and Gerisch, G. (1971), Regulation of extracellular cyclic-AMP-phospho-diesterase activity during development of *Dictyostelium discoideum. Biochem. biophys. Res. Comm.,* **42,** 119–124.

Robertson, A. and Drage, D.J. (1975), Stimulation of late interphase *Dictyostelium discoideum* amoebae with an external cAMP signal. *Biophys. J.,* **15,** 765–775.

Robertson, A., Drage, D.J. and Cohen, M.H. (1972), Control of aggregation in *Dictyostelium discoideum* by an external periodic pulse of cyclic adenosine monophosphate. *Science,* **175,** 333–334.

Roos, W. and Gerisch, G. (1976), Receptor-mediated adenylate cyclase activation in *Dictyostelium discoideum. FEBS Letters,* **68,** 170–172.

Roos, W., Malchow, D. and Gerisch, G. (1977b), Adenylyl cyclase and the control of cell differentiation in *Dictyostelium discoideum. Cell differentiation,* **6,** 229–239.'

Roos, W., Nanjundiah, V., Malchow, D. and Gerisch, G. (1975), Amplification of cyclic-AMP signals in aggregating cells of *Dictyostelium discoideum. FEBS Letters,* **53,** 139–142.

Roos, W., Scheidegger, C. and Gerisch, G. (1977a), Adenylate cyclase activity oscillations as signals for cell aggregation in *Dictyostelium discoideum*. *Nature*, **266**, 259–261.

Rossomando, E.F. and Sussman, M. (1972), Adenylate cyclase in *Dictyostelium discoideum*. A possible control element of the chemotactis system. *Biochem. biophys. Res. Comm.*, **47**, 604–610.

Rossomando, E.F. and Sussman, M. (1973), A 5'-adenosine monophosphate-dependent adenylate cyclase and an adenosine 3'-5'-cyclic monophosphate-dependent adenosine triphosphate pyrophosphohydrolase in *Dictyostelium discoideum*. *Proc. natn. Acad. Sci. U.S.A.*, **70**, 1254–1257.

Runyon, E.H. (1942), Aggregation of separate cells of *Dictyostelium* to form a multicellular body. *Collecting Net*, **17**, 88.

Ryter, A. and Brachet, P. (1978), Cell surface changes during early development stages of *Dictyostelium discoideum*. A scanning electron microscopic study. *J. biol. Cell.* In press.

Sampson, J. (1977), Developmentally regulated cyclic AMP dependent protein kinases in *Dictyostelium discoideum*. Cell, **11**, 173–180.

Sampson, J., Town, C. and Gross, J. (1978), High extracellular levels of cyclic AMP and cyclic GMP induce aggregation competence in *Dictyostelium discoideum*. *FEBS Letters*, in press.

Shaffer, B.M. (1953), Aggregation in cellular slime moulds: *In vitro* isolation of acrasin. *Nature*, **171**, 975.

Shaffer, B.M. (1956a), Acrasin, the chemotactic agent in cellular slime moulds. *J. exp. Biol.*, **33**, 645–657.

Shaffer, B.M. (1956b), Properties of acrasin. *Science*, **123**, 1172–1173.

Shaffer, B.M. (1957), Aspects of aggregation in cellular slime molds. I Orientation and chemotaxis. *Am. Nat.*, **91**, 19–35.

Shaffer, B.M. (1962), The acrasina. *Adv. Morph.*, **2**, 109–182.

Shaffer, B.M. (1975), Secretion of cyclic AMP induced by cyclic AMP in the cellular slime mold *Dictyostelium discoideum*. *Nature*, **255**, 549–552.

Sussman, M., Loomis, W.F., Ashworth, J.M. and Sussman, R.R. (1967), The effect of actinomycin D on cellular slime mold morphogenesis. *Biochem. biophys. Res. Comm.*, **26**, 353–359.

Town, C. and Gross, J. (1978), The role of cyclic nucleotides and cell agglomeration in post aggregation enzyme synthesis in *Dictyostelium discoideum*. *Dev. Biol.*, in press.

Ward, A.M. and Brenner, M. (1977), Guanylate cyclase from *Dictyostelium discoideum*. *Life Sci.*, **21**, 997–1008.

Wick, U., Malchow, D. and Gerisch, G. (1978), Cyclic-AMP stimulated calcium influx into aggregating cells of *Dictyostelium discoideum*. *Cell Biology international reports*. In press.

Williams, K.L. and Newell, P.C. (1976), A genetic study of aggregation in the cellular slime mould *Dictyostelium discoideum* using complementation analysis. *Genetics*, **82**, 287–306.

Wurster, B. and Schubiger, K. (1977), Oscillations and cell development in *Dictyostelium discoideum* stimulated by folic acid pulses. *J. Cell Sci.*, **27**, 105–114.

Wurster, B., Shubiger, K., Wick, U. and Gerisch, G. (1977), Cyclic GMP in *Dictyostelium discoideum*. Oscillations and pulses in response to folic acid and cyclic AMP signals. *FEBS Letters,* **76**, 141–144.

5 Nematode Chemotaxis and Chemoreceptors

SAMUEL WARD

Taxis and Behavior
(*Receptors and Recognition,* Series B, Volume 5)
Edited by G.L. Hazelbauer
Published in 1978 by Chapman and Hall, 11 New Fetter Lane, London EC4P 4EE
© Chapman and Hall

5.1 INTRODUCTION

A small sightless worm crawling among particles of soil and decaying vegetation must have a variety of chemical senses to locate bacteria for food and to avoid poisons and predators. What chemicals are sensed? How many different kinds of receptor molecules are there? On which neurons are the receptors located? How sensitive are these neurons? How is the detection of a chemical communicated to the worm's central nervous system and converted into a behavioral response?

All of these questions have been addressed in studies of the soil nematode *Caenorhabditis elegans*. This organism has recently become the subject of intensive genetic, behavioral and anatomical studies (Brenner, 1973, 1974; reviewed in Ward, 1977b). The behavior that has been examined in most detail is chemotaxis. This chapter will review what is known about *C. elegans* chemotaxis and will present a number of new observations. The results will be interpreted in terms of a specific model of chemoreceptor function. The problem of analysis of central nervous system processing of chemosensory neuron information will be discussed briefly.

5.2 CHEMOSENSORY RESPONSES

Three assays have been used to study nematode chemotaxis. The first uses radial gradients of attractants established in thin slurries of Sephadex gel beads spread on Petri plates. When worms are added to the periphery they accumulate at the peak of the gradient in such a way that the fraction of the population in the center is a function of the attractant concentration (Ward, 1973). The second assay uses radial gradients of attractants established in thin layers of agarose. Worms applied to the periphery cut a groove in the agar leaving a track behind (Fig. 5.1). Analysis of these tracks shows that the worm's behavioral response includes orientation up the gradient, movement toward the peak of the gradient, accumulation at the peak and then apparent 'habituation' (Ward, 1973, 1976). In the third assay, worms are injected into a counter-current apparatus with two solutions flowing over one another in opposite directions (Dusenbery, 1973). When attractant is added to either solution the worms accumulate there preferentially. This causes them to be swept out of the apparatus so that they can be counted. The fraction in the attractant solution is dependent on attractant concentration.

The first assay is rapid and easy to use with many samples. The second assay is the most sensitive and it gives information about the worm's behavioral response to gradients. The third assay is the most quantitative and it is equally suited for

143

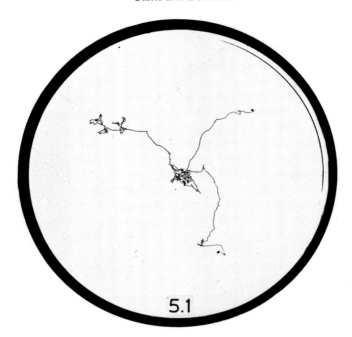

Fig. 5.1 Tracks of three wild-type adults responding to gradients of $NH_4 Cl$. Three worms were applied near the edge of the plate and allowed to track for 20 min. Note the orientation up the gradient and the accumulation at the center.

Table 5.1 Attractants
Chemicals that attract *C. elegans* are listed. They are grouped into classes by competition experiments and by mutant phenotypes as discussed in Section 5.4. Within each class, attractants are listed in order of decreasing attractiveness. The third column list the threshold of detection of the first attractant in each class for each of the three chemo-tactic assays (orientation, accumulation and counter-current). (Data combined from Ward, 1973; Dusenbery, 1974, 1975, 1976 and unpublished observation of P.St. John and S. Ward). NT means not tested).

Class	Attractants	Threshold (mM)		
		Orient.	Accum.	C-C.
1. Anions	Cl^-, SO_4^{2-}, NO_3^-, Br^-, I^-	0.01	2	0.1
2. Cations	Na^+, Li^+, K^+, Mg^{2+}, Ca^{2+}	0.01	2	0.1
3. Cyclic nucleotides	cAMP, cGMP	0.005	0.2	est. 0.01
4. Base	OH^-	NT	0.001	0.01
5. Bacterial filtrate	?	?	?	?
6. Pyridine	Pyridine	NT	NT	0.1
7. CO_2 (borate)	HCO_3^- or CO_3^{2-} ?	NT	NT	0.005
8. Acetate	$CH_3 COO^-$	$\simeq 1$	50	10

Table 5.2 Repellents
The repellents of *C. elegans* that have been studied quantitatively by counter-current distribution are listed. Other repellents are discussed in text. (Data from Dusenbery, 1974, 1975)

Class	Repellent	Threshold (mM) C-C.
1. Acid	H^+	0.01
2. CO_2 (phosphate)	CO_2, H_2CO_3, HCO_3^- ?	0.03
3. D-Tryptophan	D-tryptophan	0.1

studying either attractants or repellents. It is also the easiest to scale up for mutant isolation.

Using these assays a large number of chemicals have been identified as attractants and repellents. These are listed in Tables 5.1 and 5.2. The classification of these chemicals into groups that represent the classes of receptors necessary to detect them is discussed in Section 5.4.

The biological significance of the responses to most of the chemicals in Table 5.1 is puzzling. cAMP is a logical candidate for a bacterial attractant although it is not the major attractant released by *E. coli* (Ward, 1973). The sensitive responses to inorganic ions, pH changes and pyridine do not seem to make sense for an organism that lives in the soil and eats bacteria. Studies of the worms' responses in more natural habitats and analysis of the micro-distribution of ions in soil would be helpful to understanding the adaptive significance of these responses (Dusenbery, 1974).

Other attractants and repellents have been found in natural sources, but these have not been identified or studied extensively. There are species of fungi which are nematode predators and other species that are endozootic nematode parasites (reviewed in Pramer, 1964, and Duddington, 1962). Reasoning that these fungi might release attractants or repellents, fungal mycellia from 16 different species were incubated in water for several hours. The treated water was tested for attraction and repulsion. The endozootic parasite *Harposporium anguillae* released an attractant, whereas three species of predacious fungi released repellents (N. Kennedy and S. Ward, unpublished). No chemistry has been done to characterize these responses further except to show they are not due to inorganic salts or cAMP. These fungal secretions are an intriguing example of the evolution of predator—prey chemical warfare.

Other substances found to be repellent include zinc ions (10^{-5} M), extracts of garlic, camphor, menthol and α-terthieyl. The last is a trithiophene released by marigold roots (Uhlenbroek and Bijloo, 1958). α-Terthienyl is toxic to some plant-parasitic nematodes and is one of the chemicals in marigold root secretions that kills plant parasitic nematodes. It does not kill *C. elegans* but repels it strongly. The repellent effect is not specific, however; thiophene itself and other aromatic compounds will also repel.

The attractants present in filtrates of *E. coli* have not been identified. They are released in the greatest quantity as growing cells enter the stationary phase. Some of the activity is heat-labile. Interestingly, filtrates of the bacterium *Bacillus subtilis,* which is a sufficient food for *C. elegans,* are not attractive (Y. Argon and S. Ward, unpublished).

We have attempted to demonstrate a sexual attractant in *C. elegans* since sex pheromones are common in other nematode species (e.g., Green, 1971). Hermaphrodites confined in dialysis tubing do attract males preferentially, but no attractant activity could be identified after removing the hermaphrodites (R. Cawthon and S. Ward, unpublished). Perhaps there is a labile or volatile attractant. No evidence for an attractant is found when observing male mating behavior on petri plates. Males appear to encounter hermaphrodites randomly and do not alter their motion when crossing fresh hermaphrodite tracks. Males will also attempt to copulate with each other.

5.3 CHEMOTAXIS-DEFECTIVE MUTANTS

Mutants altered in their chemotactic responses have been sought in order to provide variants that could be compared to wild type behaviorally, anatomically and eventually biochemically. By analyzing the range of chemotactic defects in each mutant it should be possible to deduce the number of classes of chemoreceptors. By correlating anatomical and behavioral defects it should be possible to assign specific functions to identified neurons and to trace the neural pathways that lead from the sensory neurons to the behavioral response.

Seventeen chemotaxis-defective mutants were obtained by Dusenbery *et al.* (1975) in a screening for altered response to NaCl using the counter-current apparatus. These mutants fall into at least six complementation groups named *tax-1* to *tax-6*. Mutants in all complementation groups are defective in their responses to Na$^+$ and Cl$^-$, but differ in their response to other attractants and repellents as shown in Table 5.3.

Twenty-one other chemotaxis-defective mutant strains were isolated by Lewis and Hodgkin (1977) and two more by Ward (1976). Several of these were isolated initially because their males were sterile and were subsequently found to be non-chemotactic. Others were selected as strains that would swim away from the peak of an attractant gradient, and some were identified by morphological defects in the head. These mutants have been assigned to at least nine different complementation groups named *che-1* and *che-9* distributed among all the chromosomes (Lewis and Hodgkin, 1977). Like the *tax* mutants, various *che* mutants differ in the range of their chemo-tactic-defective responses (Table 5.3). Except for *che-1* and *tax-1* which are the same gene, complementation tests have not been reported between the *tax* and *che* mutants. Some may well be in the same complementation groups. There is no reason to suppose they are fundamentally different; the different names simply reflect isolation by different workers. The mutants have not all been tested in the three assays for chemotactic responses; but those that have fail to respond in all three.

The use of mutant phenotypes to estimate the number of different classes of receptors is discussed in the following section. The identification and interpretation of anatomical defects in the *che* mutants is discussed in Section 5.5.

Table 5.3 Mutant phenotypes

The chemotaxis mutants are listed. + = normal response, (+) = partial response, 0 = no response, R = reversed response. Blank entries mean not tested. The strains S1 and DD76 have not been assigned to genes. *Tax-1* and *che-1* are the same gene. Other *tax* and *che* genes have not been complemented. In addition to the responses tabulated, *che-1* mutants retain a normal response to acetate. (Data from Dusenbery, 1976; Lewis and Hodgkin, 1977; Ward, 1976)

Gene or strain	Chemotactic responses									
	Attractants							Repellents		
	Na^+	Cl^-	OH^-	cAMP	bact.	CO_2 (bor.)	Pyr.	CO_2 (phos.)	H^+	D-try
tax-1	0	0	0	0		0	+	+	+	0
che-1	0	0	0	0	+					
tax-3	+	(+)	0	0		0	+	+	+	0
che-4	(+)	+		+						
tax-2	0	0	0	0		0	0	+	+	0
tax-4	0	R	R	0		0	0	(+)	(+)	0
tax-5	0	(+)	0	R		0	+	+	+	+
tax-6	0	0	0	0		0	0	(+)	(+)	0
che-2	0	0	0	0	0					
che-3	0	0	0	0	0					
(S1)	0	0	0	0	(+)					
(DD76)	+	(+)	0	0		0	0	+	+	0

5.4 HOW MANY RECEPTORS ARE THERE?

Two kinds of experiments have been used to estimate how many different chemo-receptors the nematode must have. The first of these tests for competion between chemicals and is similar to experiments used in the study of bacterial chemotaxis (Adler, 1975). The behavioral response to a gradient of one attractant is assessed in the presence of a uniform high concentration of a second attractant. If the worm can still respond to the gradient of the first chemical, it is likely that the two attractants are being detected by different receptors. Otherwise, the high concentration of the second attractant should saturate or adapt the receptor and prevent detection of the gradient of the first attractant. If the worms can also detect a gradient of the second attractant in the presence of a uniform high concentration of the first, then the inter-pretation of two distinct receptors is strengthened. This interpretation does not require that the two chemicals actually compete for identical binding sites on the receptor molecule, but only that the binding of one chemical to the receptor prevents the receptor from responding to changes in concentration of the second.

If the result of the competition experiment is that one chemical abolishes the response to the second, and vice versa, then the interpretation is more difficult. It might be that both chemicals bind to the same receptor and thus compete, but there are several alternatives. One chemical might inhibit the response indirectly by acting at a site elsewhere than the receptor; distinct receptors on the same neuron might compete if saturation of one prevented the neuron from responding to the other; receptors on different neurons might compete if response of one neuron overrode the central nervous processing of the other; and there might be indirect effects of one chemical on the worms' general physiology. These alternatives cause difficulties in interpreting competition experiments. In practice, the difficulties in interpretation appear to be minimal because most attractants do not compete with one another unless they are chemically related (Ward, 1973 and Table 5.1).

The second method of estimating the number of different receptors is to classify the sensory mutants by the number of chemicals to which they fail to respond. For example, if a mutant cannot detect cations but still responds normally to a bacterial filtrate it can be concluded that the receptor for cations and those for the attractants in the bacterial filtrate must be different. Note that this argument is nearly independent of the nature of the mutant defect. The receptor is by definition the first step in chemical detection so the most specific type of mutant obtainable would be a mutant altering the receptor*. Mutants elsewhere in the machinery that converts the receptor's response into the worms' behavior and mutants affecting the morphology of the sensory neurons should be less specific. So if a mutant strain retains a response while losing another, the two responses must have, at the least, different receptors. Nothing

---

* An exception could arise if specificity of detection depended on the integration of input from several neurons each with similar receptors. Then a mutant affecting the integration could be most specific.

can be concluded about the receptors for a mutant that has simultaneously lost two responses. The receptors could be the same or different because the mutant defect could be anywhere along the chain of events that act after receptor binding.

Dusenbery (1976a,b) has combined analysis of both mutant phenotypes and competition experiments to conclude that one must postulate at least six classes of receptors to explain the mutant phenotypes and the competition experiments. Additional data included in Tables 5.1, 5.2, and 5.3 suggests that at least nine classes are necessary. Not all mutants have been tested for response to every attractant and repellent, nor have all pairwise competitions been done. Nonetheless, examination of the data in Tables 5.1, 5.2, and 5.3 leads one to postulate the following minimum classes of receptors: Cations, anions, cAMP, hydroxyl ions, pyridine, CO_2 (borate), D-tryptophan, bacterial filtrate. Hydrogen ions and CO_2 (phosphate) need not have separate receptors. There are some ambiguities in some of the assignments. Moreover, it is difficult to know what to do with the mutants with reversed responses. They probably retain the receptor but have altered their response to receptor binding either in the sensory neuron or in the central nervous response to the neuron.

The analysis of receptor classes does not reveal how these classes are distributed among the individual sensory neurons. From the sensory anatomy described in the following section there are 28 anterior sensory neurons that have dendritic terminals exposed to the external medium. These include eleven pairs of ampidial neurons and one inner labial neuron present in each of the six inner labial papillae. The anatomical analysis of chemotaxis-defective mutants described below does not help assign receptors to specific neurons. The defects found in some mutants are in the amphidial and inner labial neurons but they are not specific enough or reproducible enough to allow specific assignments of neuron function (Lewis and Hodgkin, 1977; Ward, 1977a). Unfortunately, the anatomical defects in the *tax* mutants have not been described.

It is possible that one class of receptor is confined to one class of sensory neuron, but this is certainly not necessary. There could be multiple receptors on a single neuron. Such a neuron would be able to respond in a competition experiment between attractants if it adapted to the high concentration of one chemical in such a way that it could still respond to the second.

The behavioral studies so far have not revealed any differences in behavioral response to attractants that could not be explained by differences in sensitivity. Therefore it is not known whether or not it is important to the worm to discriminate among the attractants. Perhaps the worm only divides its chemical milieu into attractants and repellents and it swims toward the attractants and away from the repellents. If so, there would be no need to discriminate among attractants and no reason to limit receptors to specific neurons. It would be helpful to see how the worm responds to choices between various attractants or between repellents and attractants. Dusenbery has tested some of the salts and deduced an order of preference that comes out the same as ordering by threshold sensitivity (Dusenbery, 1974). The choice between repellents and attractants has not been examined.

5.5 SENSORY ANATOMY

5.5.1 Wild type

The arrangement of sensory neurons in the tip of *C. elegans* head resembles that of other nematodes (Ward *et al.*, 1975; Ware *et al.*, 1975). There are 58 neurons in the tip of the head, 52 of these are arranged in sensilla. The neurons are summarized in Table 5.4 and their arrangement in the head is summarized by Fig. 5.2. The symmetrical arrangement of identical sensilla reduces the number of different types of neuron to only 21.

Table 5.4 Anterior neurons
Neurons all make synaptic contact to other cells in the central nervous system. Each neuron type reflects a symmetrical grouping of neurons with nearly identical fine structure at their endings. The symmetry of these groupings is indicated (1 = lateral; v = sub-ventral; d = sub-dorsal). There are two additional anterior neurons which innervate the pharynx about 12 μm from the tip of the head. The male has four additional cephalic neuron processes. (Data from Ward *et al.*, 1975)

Sensillum	Neuron labels	Number of neuron types	Symmetry	Total neurons
	1, 2	2	six	12
Inner Labial (I)	m, n	2	two (l)	4
	−	1	two (v)	2
Outer Labial (0)	0	1	six	6
Cephalic (C)	C	1	four (d, v)	4
Amphid (A)	a−1	12	two (l)	24
Not in sensilla	x	1	two (d)	2
	y	1	four (d, v)	4
	Total types	21	Total neurons	58

Each sensillum has the same general structure: one or more ciliated sensory neurons surrounded by a channel created by an encircling socket cell and an enclosing sheath cell. The socket cell corresponds to the support cell described in other nematodes and the amphidial sheath cell corresponds to the amphidial gland cell. The anatomy of four wild-type animals was found to vary only in the finest details. The number of neurons, their specialization, their position and organization into sensilla were invariant.

In both the amphids and the inner labial papillae, the neuron channel opens to the outside and thus these sensilla are likely to contain chemosensory neurons. The structure of an amphid is shown diagrammatically in Fig. 5.3. Eight neurons extend dendrites to the very tip of the channel while four others end in complex wings or sheets embedded in the sheath cell. One of these hardly contacts the channel at all.

In addition to reconstruction of the sensory terminals, every sensory neuron has been followed in its entirety to determine its axonal projection in the central nervous system. The positions of all the cell bodies are described by Ward *et al.*

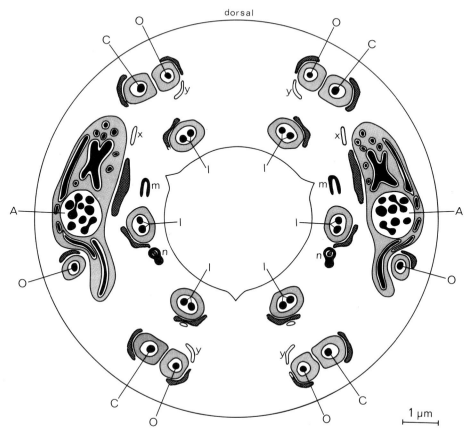

Fig. 5.2 Summary of the arrangement of neurons and sensilla in the head. All of the sensilla are shown as neurons surrounded by sheath cells (lightly shaded) with socket cells (darkly shaded) adjacent. Ciliated neurons are black, unciliated neurons are unshaded. Labelling is a Table 5.4. (From Ward *et al.*, 1975.)

(1975), who note that one of the neurons of the inner labial sensilum makes a direct synapse on a muscle, making this a sensory-motor neuron.

5.5.2 Mutants

Because the wild-type sensory anatomy is largely invariant and is known in such complete detail, it is relatively easy to detect anatomical alterations in the sensory endings of mutant animals. Lewis and Hodkin (1977) have reconstructed the sensory terminals of most of *che* mutants and Ward (1976) has reconstructed two others. Mutants in gene *che-1* are abnormal in the amphidial neuron 'd', which normally ends with finger-like extentions in the sheath cell and does not contact the channel. In all three alleles of this gene the mutant cell has many less fingers than normal. The

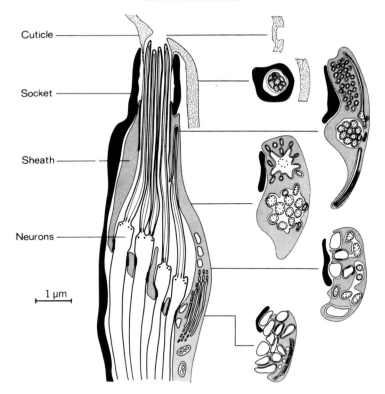

Cuticle

Socket

Sheath

Neurons

1 µm

Fig. 5.3 Amphid. A right amphid is shown diagrammatically in radial and transverse section. The shapes of the cells were simplified slightly for clarity. Dense vesicles are shown near the basal bodies of the neurons. A large golgi apparatus and mitochondria are shown in the base of the sheath cell. The scale of the transverse sections is one-half that shown for the longitudinal sections. (From Ward *et al.*, 1975.)

other neurons in the amphid are normal as are the other sensilla, except the lateral inner labial sensilla in which the terminal of one neuron is shorter in some of the mutant individuals but not in others.

In the *che-4* mutant, three of the amphidial neurons do not reach the end of the amphidial channel. Instead, they veer off and end in the amphidial sheath cell. In several mutant individuals examined, the final position of these neurons varied, but apparently the same three neurons were defective in each case.

Mutants in genes *che-2* and *che-3* were defective in all the ciliated sensory neurons except amphidial neuron 'd'. The neurons have their basal bodies but no cilia project from them. The neurons terminate in amorphous blobs rather than their normal extensions. The 'fingers cell' appears normal in these individuals. The neurons in the mutant S1, which has not yet been assigned to a gene, appear normal in the one individual which has been sectioned.

Unlike the mutants described above, other mutants have defective sensory endings, but the extent of the defects varies substantially among individuals of identical mutant genotype.

The identification of anatomical lesions in these chemotaxis-defective mutants indicates that behavioral mutants are commonly in genes specifying the development or maintenance of the nervous system rather than just its function. Similar results have been found by analysis of some of the uncoordinated mutants: most mutants were found to have anatomical alterations in their motor ganglion (Brenner, 1973).

5.5.3 Interpretation of mutant anatomical defects

The anatomical defects in the *che* mutants can not be correlated simply with their behavioral defects. Mutants in *che-1, che-3* and *che-4* are all unable to sense NaCl but they are defective in a non-overlapping set of sensory neurons. In addition, variation in the extent of neuro-anatomical defects in *che-1* alleles was not correlated with variability in behavior: all alleles were equally defective (Ward, 1976, 1977a). It may be that the anatomical defects visible at the tip of the head are not the only defects caused by the *che* mutations. There may be other, so far undetected, defects that cause the behavioral phenotypes.

As other sensory mutants are analyzed anatomically, better correlation of anatomical and behavioral defects may be found. It may have just been bad luck that the first mutants analyzed were difficult to interpret because they were in genes that affected the development of the neurons in complex ways.

Half of the mutants analyzed by Lewis and Hodgkin had visible defects in their dendritic terminals. The other half may contain mutations altering the chemoreceptors on the neuron terminals without altering their final structure. Note that none of the mutant strains obtained so far are defective in only a single class of response. Our attempts at selection of non-responders to cAMP yielded only slightly defective strains.

5.6   ANALYSIS OF THE ORIENTATION RESPONSE

Orientation in a chemical gradient requires that the nematode compares the concentration of attractant at different points to determine the direction of the gradient. This determination could be done in at least three ways:

(1) single or multiple chemosensors could compare concentrations successively in time, at points separated by the forward movement of the nematode;

(2) successive comparisons in time could be made at points separated by side-to-side (actually dorsoventral) displacement of chemosensors; or

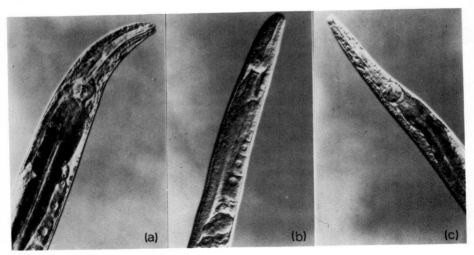

Fig. 5.4 Light micrographs of adult head-defective mutants. (a) E611, 'bent-head'; (b) E30, 'short-head'; (c) E25, 'head muscle-degenerate'. Differential interference contrast optics.

(3) concentrations could be compared in space by simultaneous use of two receptors separated on the body. These receptors could be separated anteriorly and posteriorly or dorsally and ventrally. The orientation behavior of several mutants shows that the second mechanism, side-to-side sampling, is used by *C. elegans* to detect the direction of a chemical gradient.

If the first mechanism were involved in the orientation response, then the accuracy of orientation should depend on the worm's forward velocity. The forward velocity can be varied by using a progressive muscle-degeneration mutant strain (E444) in which the body muscles degenerate before the head muscles. Animals can be chosen that move forward very slowly, although their head nods from side to side nearly normally. Tracks of two such animals are shown in Fig. 5.5 along with tracks of E444 juveniles that have normal musculature. The adult tracks resemble the tracks of a wild-type adult although they required two hours to reach the center rather than the 15 minutes required by the wild-type adult or the juveniles. In shallower gradients E444 adults still orient as well as wild-type. This result suggests that the orientation is not affected by the forward velocity of the worm so that the first mechanism of orientation is unlikely.

The wild-type sensory anatomy makes it unlikely that dorso-ventral paired receptors are used for orientation. The two amphids could not detect a chemical gradient by simulatneous comparisons because they are located laterally. Since the animal swims on its side there would be no difference in attractant concentration between amphids. In principle, the animal could detect a difference in attractant concentration between the sub-dorsal and sub-ventral inner labial papillae. However, these are separated by only 10 μm. In the gradients used in the orientation studies, such separation would give a difference in concentration of less than 0.1% between the two receptors. It is unlikely that an organism as small as a nematode could detect this small a concentration difference rapidly enough.

Orientation by simultaneous comparisons between the amphids in the head and the phasmids in the tail is unlikely because mutants with cuticle blisters covering the phasmids in the tail orient normally (Ward, 1973). Orientation by head-tail comparisons is ruled out even more decisively by the tracks of bent-headed worms of the morphological mutant, E611. The mutation of this strain causes a small fraction of the adult population to have a distinct bend in the head. Dorsal and ventral bends occur at equal frequency. A moderately bent individual is shown in Fig. 5.4a and the tracks of similar bent-headed animals are shown in Fig. 5.6. The spiral track is caused because the animal orients with its head pointing up the gradient. When it does so, its body is at an angle to the gradient. Its forward movement is determined by the body so it is at an angle to the direction of the gradient. This generates the logarithmic spiral track. The angle of orientation corresponds roughly to the angle of bend of the head and is much greater that would be expected if orientation were determined by comparison of head and tail receptors. This mutant shows that the direction of orientation is determined solely by the orientation of the head.

The arrangement of anterior sensilla together with the tracks of the bent-headed, blistered and slow-moving mutants appear to rule out orientation mechanisms (1) and (3). This leaves mechanism (2): orientation by successive comparisons in time using the side-to-side displacement of chemosensors. The tracks of other head-defective mutants support this mechanism. The short-headed mutant, E30, which is shown in Fig. 5.4b, does not orient as directly as the wild-type. Typical tracks are shown in Fig. 5.7. This defect is consistent with the orientation being dependent on the side-to-side span of the head motion because the span is reduced by the shortened head of this mutant. A similar effect is seen in juveniles, which are smaller than adults. As illustrated by the E444 juveniles (Fig. 5.5), the juveniles stop and turn more frequently than adults. This effect is quantified in Table 5.5 which compares tracks of adults, juveniles and two head-defective mutants. This stopping and turning may be a mechanism of improving the precision of orientation by sampling larger areas in spite of their shorter heads.

In the wild-type, the end of the head moves from side-to-side in co-ordination with waves of movement down the body. There is also a fine side-to-side twitching of the tip of the head, which is independent of body movements. That this fine head movement is not essential for orientation is shown by a mutant with defective head musculature, E25 (Fig. 5.4c). This mutant does not have the fine head motion yet it can still orient, although not as directly as the wild type (Fig. 5.8). When E25 is observed moving in a gradient, its head moves from side-to-side as the waves of motion are initiated at the neck — the body wags the head.

The analysis of orientation with the above mutants establishes that (1) the head

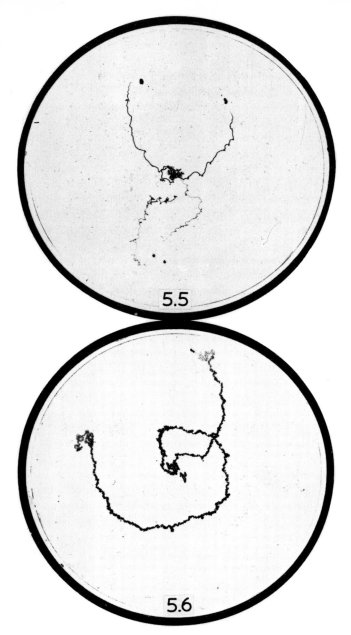

Fig. 5.5 Tracks of mutant E444. The two darker tracks were made by adults whose body muscles had degenerated. More than 2 hours were required for the adults to reach the center. The lighter tracks are two juveniles whose musculature is normal. They were removed after reaching the center in 20 min.

Fig. 5.6 Tracks of two 'bent-head' mutants responding to NH_3Cl.

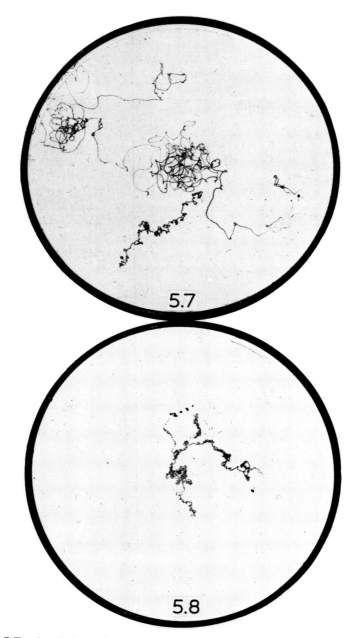

Fig. 5.7 Tracks of three 'short-head' mutants responding to NH₃ Cl.

Fig. 5.8 Tracks of four 'head muscle-degenerate' mutants responding to NH₃ Cl.

Table 5.5 Comparison of mutant and wild-type tracks
Tracks as in Fig. 5.1, 5.4 and 5.6 were analyzed to determine the fraction of worms
that reached the center in 45 min, the number of stops visible as tails on the tracks,
and the directness of the path to the center

Genotype	Stage	Number tracked	Number in center (%)	Number of stops	Actual path / Direct path
Wild type	Adult	26	25 (96)	4 ± 1.6	1.4 ± 0.3
Wild type	Juvenile	21	21 (100)	9 ± 4	1.5 ± 0.2
E30	Adult	32	18 (56)	13 ± 8	2.8 ± 1
E25	Adult	21	17 (81)	9 ± 4	2.1 ± 1

determines the direction of orientation, (2) rapid forward motion is unnecessary for
orientation, (3) fine control of head motion is unnecessary for orientation, (4) the
span of the head from side to side affects orientation.

5.7 THE SENSITIVITY OF GRADIENT DETECTION

In order to analyze the mechanism of orientation in more detail, I have filmed worms
moving on thin films of agarose containing a gradient of attractant. These films have
been analyzed frame-by-frame to record the position of the tip of the head. Fig. 5.9
shows examples of the head motion of worms moving in a gradient of potassium ions.
Each dot represents the position of the tip of the head every 0.25 s. The highest
concentration is at the top.

The gradient present during filming was generated by applying attractant in a thin
line at the top of the plate at two different times before adding worms. The shape of
the gradient was determined by measuring the diffusion of ^{32}P-orthophosphate in
identical films of agarose. (The time allowed for diffusion of the potassium ions was
adjusted to correct for the difference in diffusion coefficient between potassium and
phosphate ions.) In the region filmed the gradient is essentially a simple exponential
as expected from theory.

The average side-to-side span of the head movement of an adult was 0.15 mm.
The maximum span was 0.28 mm. From the known slope of the gradient, the concentration change experienced by a worm moving at right angles to gradient would
be 3% on the average and 6.2% maximum. In similar gradients, juvenile worms also
oriented but their smaller size would cause them to experience only a 1% change in
concentration from side-to-side. Gradients less steep have not been tested so it is
not known whether this represents the minimal concentration change that the worm
can detect.

Observation of wild type, the slow-moving mutant, and the bent-headed mutant
moving in gradients showed that they sometimes change their orientation to point
more directly up the gradient after a single swing of the head. This suggests that they

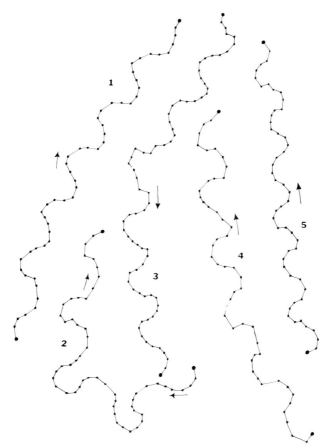

Fig. 5.9 Motion of the tip of the head in exponential gradients of concentration. The position of the tip of the head every 0.25 s is shown for 5 different intervals of movement (3 different worms). Gradient maximum toward the top.

can detect the gradient in a single side-to-side excursion. From the film analysis, such an excursion takes about a second. Therefore, it appears that the worm must be able to detect a 1–3% change in concentration in about one second.

By placing worms at various distances from the center of radial gradient of attractant with slope similar to that used for the filming, it was found that the worm would orient over a concentration range of salts from 100 mM to 0.05 mM (Ward, 1973). Subjective examination of the tracks suggests that the orientation may not be as direct at the lowest concentrations (see the initial tracks in Fig. 5.1), but this has not be quantified. In any case it is clear that orientation occurs over at least three and probably four orders of magnitude change in absolute concentration.

5.8 A MODEL FOR A MECHANISM OF GRADIENT DETECTION

The previous sections have shown that a model for gradient detection must explain the following:

(1) gradient detection depends on comparisons of concentration by receptors at the tip of the head;

(2) the comparisons are made successively in time at points separated by side-to-side excursions of the head;

(3) the receptors must be able to operate over 3–4 orders of magnitude change in absolute concentration;

(4) the estimated sensitivity of detection is a 1–3% change in concentration experienced in about 1 s.

The structure of the amphid and the fact that several of the chemotaxis-defective mutants have defective amphidial neurons indicates that the amphid contains chemosensory neurons. Eight of the twelve amphidial neurons reach to the tip of the amphidial channel which is exposed to the outside but three others contact the channel at its base (Fig. 5.3). These three could still participate in chemotaxis because the channel is only 5 μm deep. Calculation of the rate of diffusion into such a channel indicates that a change in concentration at the opening of the channel would be experienced at the base in 20 ms or less.* Since the nematode's head takes about 1 s to move from side to side, the neurons at the base of the channel should have ample time to experience the same concentration change as those that reach to the tip. Therefore it is possible that eleven amphidial neurons and not just the eight that reach the tip of the head could be primary chemosensory neurons. The one neuron that could not be a primary chemosensory neuron is the neuron 'd', the fingers cell, which hardly contacts the channel.

The requirement that the receptors respond to small concentration changes in time over a range of absolute concentration is strikingly similar to the requirements for bacterial chemotaxis (Mesibov *et al.,* 1973; MacNab and Koshland, 1972; Brown and Berg, 1974; Berg and Purcell, 1977). Therefore, a model similar to that used for *E. coli* chemotaxis can be used to explain nematode chemotaxis with the following assumptions. There are receptor molecules for each class of attractant and repellent. These are distributed in the membranes of the endings of eleven of the amphidial neurons. Each class of receptor might be confined to a single neuron but it is more

---

* The problem of chemical diffusion into a closed channel is equivalent to the problem of heat diffusion into a short insulated rod. The diffusion equation for this situation is solved in Carslaw and Jaeger (1947, equation 3.5). By substituting a diffusion coefficient of 2×10^{-5} cm^2 s^{-1} (approximately that of cAMP) for the diffusivity of heat and substituting concentration for temperature, this equation can be evaluated. It is found that it takes 20 ms for a point 4 μm down the channel (about where the neurons end) to experience 90% of a concentration change at the opening of the channel.

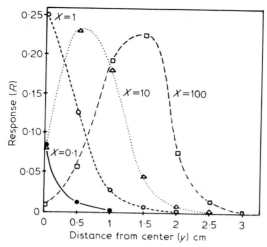

Fig. 5.10 Graphs of response, R, in arbitrary units versus distance, y, from peak of a gradient predicted by equation 5.5. Different values of X are shown.

likely that each is distributed among several neurons. The receptors have a specific binding affinity for each attractant inversely proportional to the dissociation constant of binding K_d. The response of the neuron to changes in concentration of attractant or repellent is proportional to the rate of change of the fraction of receptor sites occupied by an attractant or repellent.

As shown by Brown and Berg (1974) and Mesibov *et al.* (1973), with the above assumptions, the response, R, of a cell to changes in concentration of an attractant will be

$$R = c\frac{dA}{dT}\frac{K_d}{(K_d + A)^2} \tag{5.1}$$

Where A is the concentration of attractant and T is time and c is a proportionality constant.

In the orientation assays used for nematode chemotaxis the shape of the gradient of concentration was approximately

$$A = A_o e^{-3.5y} \tag{5.2}$$

where A_o is the concentration at the peak of the gradient and y is the distance from the peak in centimeters. In such a gradient

$$\frac{dA}{dT} = -3.5A_o e^{-3.5y}\frac{dy}{dT}. \tag{5.3}$$

Substituting equations 5.2 and 5.3 into 5.1 gives

$$R = -3.5cA_oe^{-3.5y} \frac{K_d}{(K_d + A_oe^{-3.5y})^2} \frac{dy}{dT}. \qquad (5.4)$$

If A_o is expressed as a fraction of the attractant that causes the receptors to be half-saturated, that is K_d, then $A_o = XK_d$ so equation 5.4 becomes

$$R = -3.5c \frac{Xe^{-3.5y}}{1 + Xe^{-3.5y}} \frac{dy}{dT}. \qquad (5.5)$$

Graphs of R as a function of y, assuming dy/dt is independent of y are shown in Fig. 5.10 for various values of X.

There are many difficulties in trying to determine whether or not the curves in Fig. 5.10 agree with experimental observations. First of all, the response measured in orientation assays is not the response of a sensory neuron but the result of the worm's nervous system processing the response of the sensory neuron to generate the behavioral response (see following section). Second, the ability to orient at various points in the gradient is difficult to quantify. Third, the worm has control of dy/dt which is the velocity of head movement in the direction of the gradient. The data presented in Section 5.6, showing variation in stopping frequency for different mutants suggests that this is one variable the worm might use to improve precision of orientation at low attractant concentrations. Nonetheless, the model could account for the worm's orientation response if the sensory neurons can detect a small enough fractional change in receptors occupied to cover the range of attractant concentrations detected. The fall off in response predicted at low y values is not seen because all the orientation assays are probably well below K_d as discussed below.

If one examines the predictions of the model when applied to the accumulation and counter-current assays, more critical tests may be made. In the accumulation assay it is the response at small values of y near the peak of the gradient that is important. The gradients formed in the counter-current apparatus have not been determined but they are likely to be roughly exponential and steeper than those used for accumulation assays because less time for diffusion is allowed, but the model could also apply to the counter-current assay. Fig. 5.11 shows R at the peak of a gradient as a function of X, which is a measure of attractant concentration. Such a graph is a concentration-response curve similar to those generated in the capillary assay of bacterial chemotaxis (Mesibov *et al.*, 1973). Fig. 5.12a,b and c shows examples of nematode concentration response curves from both accumulation and counter-current assays for the attractant cAMP, pyridine and the combination NaCl. The cAMP response corresponds to the model if the K_d for cAMP is 4 mM or greater. Pyridine shows a peaked response that would correspond to a K_d of 1 mM. Dusenbery showed carefully that the fall off in response at high pyridine concentration is not due to toxic effects so it might indeed reflect saturation of the receptors for pyridine. The NaCl response does not fall off at high concentration as predicted by theory. This might be because the response is to the combination of two classes of receptors.

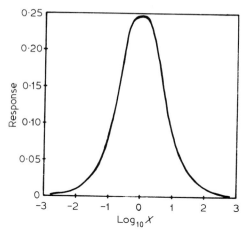

Fig. 5.11 Theoretical concentration response curve. Response at $y = 0$ is plotted as a function of X, the ratio of the attractant concentration to K_d.

The response does fall off a concentrations above 0.2 M but this is due, in part at least, to repulsion by high osmotic strength.

Although the concentration response curves can be explained by the model and can be used to estimate the K_d of each receptor class, they are not a very sensitive test of the model nor do they yield a very precise value for K_d. Almost any response model that is dependent on the fraction of binding sites occupied by ligand will be most sensitive in the concentration range around the K_d and will fall off at higher concentrations as the receptors become saturated. To estimate K_d more precisely, 'sensitivity curves' could be generated as has been done with bacteria (Mesibov *et al.*, 1973). This could be most easily done using the counter-current apparatus by studying the response while maintaining a fixed ratio of attractant concentrations in the two solutions and varying the absolute concentration.

All of the assays used so far to study nematode chemotaxis have the disadvantage for quantitative analysis that the worm's movement determines the concentration change that it experiences. An assay for responses in an isotropic solution would allow much more precise control of stimulation. Preliminary observations suggest that the worm makes a deep dorsal bend when it encounters an attractant in solution and this behavior might be used to measure responses. Methods analogous to those used by Brown and Berg (1974) to control stimulation of *E. coli* or stopped flow methods (MacNab and Koshland, 1972) could then be employed to control stimulation precisely. It should be possible to generate changes in cAMP concentration by enzymatically synthesizing it from dibutyrl-cAMP or degrading it to 5'-AMP, both of which are non-attractants. Salt concentrations might be varied uniformly by dissolving sparingly soluble salts. Only when such methods are developed will it be possible to establish precisely what parameters of concentration change the worm

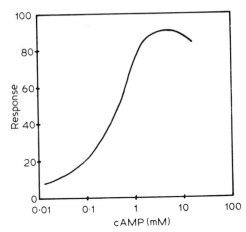

Fig. 5.12(a) Concentration response curves. Accumulation assay to cAMP (redrawn from Ward, 1973).

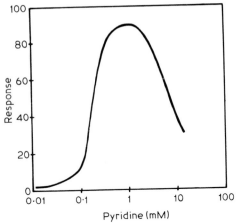

Fig. 5.12(b) Concentration response curves. Counter-current assay of pyridine (redrawn from Dusenbery, 1976).

detects. It is clear from the present results however, that it is sufficient for the response to be dependent on the rate of change to the fraction receptors occupied to explain the behavior.

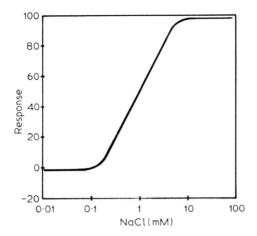

Fig. 5.12(c) Concentration response curves. Counter-current assay of NaCl (redrawn from Dusenbery, 1974).

5.9 GENERATION OF THE BEHAVIORAL RESPONSE

The previous section proposed a model for chemical gradient detection that requires the sensory neurons to respond to the rate of change of occupancy of their receptors as the worm moves across the gradient. Presumably, this response would be translated into a receptor potential and communicated to the central nervous system either in analog form as a graded potential or in digital form as a train of action potentials. The information from the sensory neuron must be translated into the behavioral response of turning up the gradient. How might this be done?

It can be seen from the tracks in Fig. 5.1 that the worm can change direction in several ways. It can make a smooth turn as the one filmed in Fig. 5.9 (2). Presumably, this is caused by contracting muscles more strongly on one side than the other during a wave of contraction. The worm can also turn abruptly by stopping, bending its head sharply to one side and starting again in a new direction following the head. The worm also stops and reverses its direction for one or two wavelengths and then begins again in a new direction. These reversals leave little tails on the tracks which are visible in Figs. 5.1, 5.5 and 5.8.

Clearly, the sensory input must modify the motor output to alter the pattern of muscle contraction. The motor system must receive information to tell it to turn and tell it which way to turn. One way this could be done is by the use of proprioreceptors that communicate the position of the head while the chemoreceptors are responding. Several of the sensilla have dendritic terminals that lie embedded in the cuticle and these could be proprioreceptors (Ward *et al.*, 1975; Ware *et al.*, 1975). The orientation of the bent-headed mutant makes such a mechanism unlikely, however, because the bend in the head should cause a proprioreceptor to respond continually and cause the worm to move in circles. If the proprioreceptor adapted, however, and only responded to changes in head position it might still function in the bent head, so this argument against proprioreceptors is not decisive.

It is not necessary to postulate proprioreceptors if the sensory neurons only respond as the head moves up a gradient. If the motor system were programmed to continue bending the head when sensory neurons responded this would cause a turn in the direction of head movement up a gradient. Thus the time dependence of the sensory neuron response would reveal the direction of the gradient.

The central nervous connections of all the sensory neurons have been determined by J. White, E. Southgate, N. Thomson and S. Brenner using serial-section electron microscopy (personal communication). The twelve amphidial neurons synapse primarily onto four central nerve ring interneurons. Additional synapses are made onto three other interneurons. The interneurons receiving input from the amphidial neurons synapse in turn onto each other, onto motoneurons that drive the head muscles and onto the four major interneurons that drive the body muscles (White *et al.*, 1976).

There is no obvious correlation between the pattern of synaptic connections and the terminal morphology of the neurons. Neither the 'fingers cell' which does not contact the outside nor the other three neurons that end embedded in the sheath cell have a pattern of connections distinctly different from the eight neurons that penetrate to the tip of the amphid. If the individual neurons are functionally distinct, this distinction is not revealed by their anatomical connectivity.

It is not easy to interpret the wiring pattern of the sensory neurons. The information from the amphidial neurons is communicated to the motor neurons by way of two sets of interneurons. It is not known how these interneurons integrate and process the information they receive. This makes it difficult to specify further how the system might work. It is probably better to work backwards first and try to understand how the motoneuron controls wave generation and propagation before attempting to interpret the modification of this control imposed by sensory input. Whether this analysis can be successful without physiological recording from individual interneurons remains to be determined.

5.10 SUMMARY AND CONCLUSIONS

The results presented here have shown that the nematode has a complex repertoire of chemical senses. Analysis of competition experiments and mutant phenotypes implies that there are at least nine classes of receptors that mediate the worm's attraction to or avoidance of chemicals. In gradients of attractants the initial response of the worm is to orient up the gradient. This orientation is dependent on the side-to-side motion of the tip of the head and requires a concentration change of about 1% experienced in 1 s.

The sensitivity of gradient detection by the nematode resembles that of bacteria. A model for receptor function similar to that used to explain bacterial chemotaxis is one that generates a response proportional to the rate of change of the fraction of receptor sites occupied by ligand. This model is sufficient to account for the nematode's response, but quantitative analysis of nematode chemotaxis is not yet precise enough to test the model critically.

Chemotactic mutants with a wide range of phenotypes have been obtained. These mutants have helped to establish the number of receptor classes and to show that chemoreceptive neurons are in the amphid. The interpretation of anatomical defects in these mutants has not been straighforward, however. There is not a simple correlation between anatomical changes in the dendritic terminals of the sensory neurons and the range of behavioral defects.

A limitation of the studies on the nematode so far is the total absence of biochemical information about the chemoreceptors themselves. Their specificity indicates that they must be proteins and the sensory anatomy suggests they must be distributed on the amphidial neuron endings. Since these endings represent only a miniscule fraction of the worm's tissue, the difficulty of isolation of receptors has deterred biochemical characterization.

A promising direction for further work is to analyze the behavioral response to attractants in more detail to specify precisely the sensitivity of detection and to describe the motor response exactly. Then analysis of the wiring diagram to determine the potential pathways by which the information from the amphidial neurons is translated by the interneurons into the motor response may be possible. The nematode is one of the few organisms in which all of the connections of the neurons in the nervous system is known. Analysis of the response to changes in chemical stimulation is one pattern of behavior that can be used to see if unique models of central nervous system function can be predicted without detailed electrophysiology.

REFERENCES

Adler, J. (1975), Chemotaxis in bacteria. *A. Rev. Biochem.*, **44**, 341–356.

Berg, H.C. and Purcell, E.M. (1977), Physics of chemoreception. *Biophys. J.*, **20**, 193–219.

Brenner, S. (1973), The genetics of behavior. *Br. med. Bull.*, **29**, 269–271.

Brenner, S. (1974), The genetics of *Caenorhabditis elegans. Genetics*, **77**, 71–94.

Brown, D.A. and Berg, H.C. (1974), Temporal stimulation of chemotaxis in *E. coli. Proc. natn. Acad. Sci. U.S.A.*, **71**, 1388–1392.

Dusenbery, D.B. (1973), Countercurrent separation: A new method for studying behavior of small aquatic organisms. *Proc. natn. Acad. Sci. U.S.A.*, **70**, 1349–1352.

Dusenbery, D.B. (1974), Analysis of chemotaxis in the nematode *Caenorhabditis elegans* by countercurrent separation. *J. exp. Zool.*, **188**, 41–48.

Dusenbery, D.B. (1975), The avoidance of D-tryptophan by the nematode *Caenorhabditis elegans*. *J. exp. Zool.*, **193**, 413–418.

Dusenbery, D.B. (1976a), Attraction of the nematode *Caenorhabditis elegans* to pyridine. *Comp. Biochem. Physiol.*, **53C**, 1–2.

Dusenbery, D.B. (1976b), Chemotactic behavior of mutants of the nematode *Caenorhadbitis elegans* that are defective in their attraction to NaCl. *J. exp. Zool.*, **198**, 343–352.

Dusenbery, D.B., Sheridan, R.E. and Russell, R.L. (1975), Chemotaxis-defective mutants of the nematode *Caenorhabditis elegans*. *Genetics*, **80**, 297–309.

Duddington, C.L. (1962), Predacious fungi and the control of elworms. *Viewpoints in Biol.*, **1**, 151–200.

Green, C.D. (1971), Mating and host finding behavior of plant nematodes. *Plant Parasitic Nematodes*, **2**, 247–266.

Lewis, J.A. and Hodgkin, J.A. (1977), Specific neuroanatomical changes in chemosensory mutants of the nematode *Caenorhabditis elegans*. *J. comp. Neurol.*, **172**, 489–510.

Macnab, R.M. and Koshland, D.E. (1972), The gradient-sensing mechanism in bacteria chemotaxis. *Proc. natn. Acad. Sci. U.S.A.*, **69**, 2509–2512.

Mesibov, R., Ordal, G.W. and Adler, J. (1973), The range of attractant concentration for bacterial chemotaxis and the threshold and size of response over this range. *J. gen. Physiol.*, **62**, 203–223.

Pramer, D. (1964), Nematode trapping fungi. *Science*, **144**, 382–387.

Uhlenbroek, J.H. and Bijloo, J.D. (1958), Investigations on nematacides. I. Isolation and structure of a nematacidal principle occurring in *Tagetes roots*. *Rec. Trav. Chim. Pays-Bas*, **77**, 1004–1009.

Ward, S. (1973), Chemotaxis by the nematode *Caenorhapditis elegans:* Identification of attractants and analysis of the response by use of mutants. *Proc. natn. Acad. Sci. U.S.A.*, **70**, 817–821.

Ward, S. (1976), The use of mutants to analyze the sensory nervous system of *Caenorhabditis elegans*. In: *The Organization of Nematodes*, (Croll, N., ed), Academic Press, New York.

Ward, S. (1977a), The use of nematode behavioral mutants for analysis of neural function and development. *Neurosci. Res. Symp.* **II**, 1–26.

Ward, S. (1977b), Invertebrate Neurogenetics. *A. Rev. Genetics*, **II**, 415–450.

Ward, S., Thomson, J.N., White, J.G. and Brenner, S. (1975), Electron microscopical reconstruction of the anterior sensory anatomy of the nematode *Caenorhabditis elegans*. *J. comp. Neurol.*, **160**, 313–338.

Ware, R.W., Clark, D., Crossland, K. and Russell, R.L. (1975), The nerve ring of the nematode *Caenorhabditis elegans:* Sensory input and motor output. *J. comp. Neurol.*, **162**, 71–110.

White, J.G., Southgate, E., Thomson, J.N. and Brenner, S. (1976), The structure of the ventral nerve cord of *Caenorhabditis elegans*. *Phil. Trans. Roy. Soc. Ser. B.*, **275**, 327–348.

6 Sexual Chemotaxis and Chemotropism in Plants

JOSEPH P. MASCARENHAS

Taxis and Behavior
(*Receptors and Recognition,* Series B, Volume 5)
Edited by G.L. Hazelbauer
Published 1978 by Chapman and Hall, 11 New Fetter Lane, London EC4P 4EE

The general role of chemotaxis (movement towards a chemical substance) and chemotropism (growth towards a chemical substance) in bringing together sexual cells of plants was recognized in the latter part of the nineteenth century (see review of early literature by Machlis and Rawitscher-Kunkel, 1967). During the last few years, the chemical nature of several of these compounds has been elucidated. The subject matter of this review concerns the absolutely fascinating mechanisms by which different groups of plants actively promote the meeting of the male and female sex cells so that this contact is not just a matter of chance. A few representative experimental systems from both higher and lower plants that have been best studied will be considered in this review, and the reader is referred to other recent articles which treat individual groups of plants in more detail (Bu'Lock, 1976; Gooday, 1975; Horenstein and Cantino, 1969; Machlis and Rawitscher-Kunkel, 1967; van den Ende, 1976; Wiese, 1969). Certain other lower plants, e.g. the yeasts and slime molds have been treated in this volume and other volumes of the series.

6.2 FUNGI

There is much variation among fungi in the kinds of structures that contain gametic nuclei and the manner in which the gametic nuclei are brought into close proximity for fertilization to occur. In this section three groups of fungi, in which the chemical nature of the attractive substances has been determined, have been selected for discussion.

6.2.1 *Allomyces*

Allomyces is a coenocytic, filamentous, aquatic fungus in the class Chytridiomycetes, which reproduces both asexually and sexually (Butler, 1911; Emerson, 1941). The gamete-bearing generation (Fig. 6.1) consists of a branching mycelium that bears many small, orange, male gametangia and larger, colorless, female gametangia. The gametes which are released from the gametangia in the presence of water are motile, uni-flagellate cells, lacking cell walls and containing a double membrane-bound organelle, the nuclear cap (unique to the order Blastocladiales), which contains all of the 80S ribosomes of the cell at this stage of the life cycle (Blondel and Turian, 1960; Lovett, 1963; Turian, 1955). The male gametes are highly motile, orange cells which are smaller in size than the less actively motile colorless, female gametes. Fusion of the gametes occurs shortly after their release from the gametangia. The biflagellate,

171

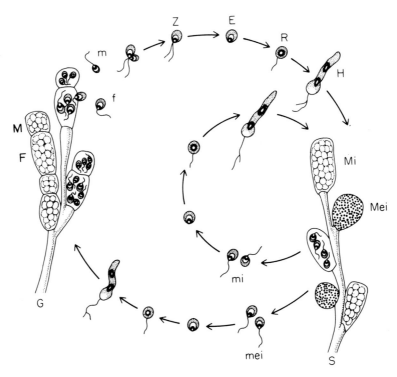

Fig. 6.1 The life cycle of *Allomyces macrogynus*. *S*: Sporophyte hyphae;
Mi: mitosporangium; *mi*: mitospore (zoospore); *Mei*: meiosporangium
(resistant sporangium); *mei*: meiospore; *G*: gametophyte hyphae; *M*: male
gametangium; *m*: male gamete; *F*: female gametangium; *f*: female gamete;
Z: zygote; *E*: encysted zygote; *R*: germling with rhizoidal germ tube;
H: germling with hyphal germ tube (not drawn to scale).

actively motile zygote thus formed is the product of the complete fusion of the two
gametes (Hatch, 1938; Pommerville and Fuller, 1976). The environment of the
zygote of *Allomyces* can be manipulated experimentally to maintain the zygotes as
actively motile cells which undergo no visible morphological change or, alternatively,
to induce them to germinate synchronously into sporophyte germlings (Bruce and
Mascarenhas, 1977). Under the microscope the male gametes can be observed to
cluster in the vicinity of unopened female gametangia. Male gametes are also strongly
attracted to female gametes which results in the clustering of male gametes around
the female gametes. The first proof that the clustering of male gametes was a response
to a chemical agent was obtained by Machlis (1958a), who showed that male gametes
were attracted to female gametangia that had been embedded in agar. Male gametes
would also approach and cluster against a dialyzing membrane that separated them

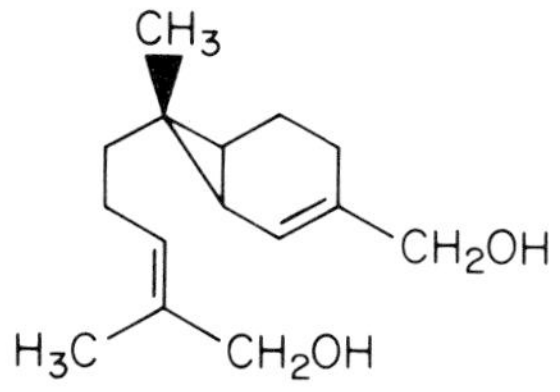

Fig. 6.2 Structure of *l*-sirenin.

from a supernatant in which female gametangia had discharged female gametes. This hormone produced by the female gametes which attracts the male gametes was aptly given the name, sirenin, after the sirens of Greek mythology (Machlis, 1958b). In order to produce and purify enough sirenin for its chemical analysis and identification, hybrid strains derived from crosses between *Allomyces arbuscula* and *A. javanicus* (Emerson and Wilson, 1954) were made. The hybrids produced a minimum of 95% male or female gametangia, and were essentially entirely male or female plants. The female plants were used to produce sirenin and the male plants for the production of large numbers of sperm for use in assaying for sirenin. A quantitative bioassay for sirenin was developed in which test solutions were placed on one side of a membrane, whose other side was in contact with a suspension of male gametes. The male gametes attach to the membrane in direct proportion to the concentration of sirenin above the membrane (Machlis, 1958a, 1958c). The availability of male and female strains and a quantitative bioassay enabled Machlis and his collaborators to produce and isolate sufficient sirenin to determine its chemical structure (Machlis *et al.*, 1966; Machlis *et al.*, 1968). Sirenin was the first plant sex hormone to be chemically characterized. It is a colorless, optically active, viscous liquid with the structure shown in Fig. 6.2. In addition to *l*-sirenin, *d*-sirenin, *dl*-sirenin and several analogues have been synthesized (Plattner *et al.*, 1969; Plattner and Rapoport, 1971). All these compounds (Fig. 6.3) have been tested for their sperm-attracting activity in the bioassay (Machlis, 1973a). The most active compound was synthetic *l*-sirenin. The number of sperm attracted to a unit area of the membrane in the bioassay was directly proportional to the concentration of *l*-sirenin in the range 0 to 7.5 nM. Above 7.5 nM there was significant deviation from linearity. None of the analogues (compounds **1–6**) showed any chemotactic activity, indicating that the side-chain allylic alcohol function is essential and that the stereochemistry of the side chain on the cyclopropyl ring is also important for activity. Compound **1** (*d*-sirenin) showed no activity at a concentration of 5 nM and some activity at higher concentrations which could possibly have been due to a slight contamination with *l*-sirenin.

When sirenin is added to a suspension of male gametes it is rapidly taken up by the gametes with first-order kinetics. No sirenin was detectable by extraction in the male gametes, however, implying that the sirenin on being taken up by the sperm was transformed into a chemotactically inactive compound (Machlis, 1973a). When sperm have taken up all the sirenin from a 5 nM solution, their ability to absorb more

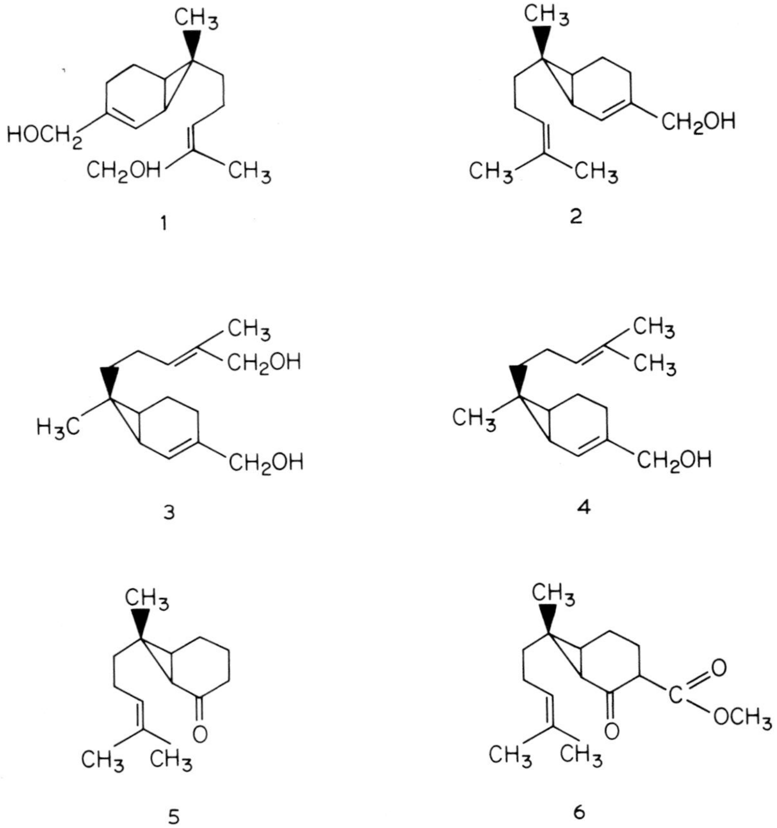

Fig. 6.3 Structures of several sirenin analogues tested for activity. **1**, *d*-sirenin; **2**, *l*-monodeoxysirenin; **3**, *dl*-isosirenin; **4**, *dl*-monodeoxyisosirenin; no trivial name given for compounds **5** and **6**.

added sirenin remains unaltered. However, the ability of gametes which had taken up sirenin from a 5 nM solution for 30 min, to respond in the bioassay to a 5 nM test solution was significantly diminished and full recovery to respond to a gradient of sirenin required almost 50 min. This appears to indicate that some process must take place after the uptake of sirenin before the sperm are again fully responsive. Optimum response of *Allomyces* sperm to sirenin requires the calcium ion (3 mM CaCl$_2$) and chelated trace elements (Machlis, 1973b). Machlis (1973a) has suggested that since sirenin appears to control the direction of swimming of the sperm it must ultimately, possibly in a metabolized form of sirenin, affect flagellar action. All the very interesting work concerning receptors for sirenin on the male gametes and the mechanisms by which the sirenin signal is converted into directional movement still remains to be done.

In a recent report, Pommerville (1977), using a newly devised bioassay, has shown that sirenin is produced not only during the final stages of female gametogenesis, but also by motile female gametes for at least 5 h after their release from the gametangia. Using the same bioassay, evidence is also presented for a female attractant produced by the male gametes. This is a very interesting and unexpected finding.

In addition to the chemotaxis exhibited by male gametes to sirenin and the recent report of chemotaxis of female cells to sperm, the motile mitospores, meiospores and zygotes of *Allomyces* (see Fig. 6.1) respond chemotactically to certain amino acids (Carlile and Machlis, 1965; Machlis, 1969a,b). Zoospores and zygotes of *Allomyces macrogynus* and *A. arbuscula* respond chemotactically to a mixture of L-leucine and L-lysine (each at 5×10^{-4} M) with the response enhanced by the addition of L-proline. Neither the male nor the female gametes respond to the amino acids. It is indeed amazing that the chemotactic capability to respond to amino acids seems to occur almost coincidentally with the act of fertilization (Machlis, 1969b). Again, the mechanisms by which the activation of the chemotactic system is achieved on fertilization, or how amino acids control the direction of movement of the cells, remain unanswered.

6.2.2 Chemotropic phenomena in the watermold *Achlya*

Achlya is a water mold in the family Saprolegniaccae. Like other members of this family, it grows as a profusely branched coenocytic mycelium. Septa or walls are formed in the mycelium to separate the reproductive organs from the vegetative hyphae, which generally remain aseptate. Members of this group of fungi reproduce both by asexual and sexual mechanisms. *Achlya* is one of the best-studied fungi with respect to the hormonal mechanisms that are involved in the regulation of its sexual reproduction; many of these being undoubtedly surface-mediated phenomena. The involvement of diffusible hormones that control the sexual reproduction of *Achlya* species has been elegantly demonstrated by Raper (see review 1952). Among *Achlya* species four different strains are found: (1) pure male strains; (2) predominantly male strains with a latent capacity for producing oogonia (female sex organs); (3) pure female strains, and (4) predominantly female strains with a latent capacity for producing antheridia (male sex organs). None of the four types form sexual organs when grown alone. However, when grown in contact with, i.e. mated with, any of the other three types, each strain will form sexual organs with functional gametes and fertilization will take place. The series of morphological steps seen during sex organ formation and prior to fertilization are described in Fig. 6.4. When a male and a female hypha approach each other, the formation of antheridial hyphae are seen on the male. These hyphae are quite distinct from the vegetative hyphae in size and morphology. As the antheridial hyphae grow towards the female hyphae, oogonial initials develop on the female hyphae. Antheridial hyphae grow towards the oogonial initial and upon reaching it they become appressed to the oogonial wall, and a transverse wall is then developed, forming a terminal multinucleate antheridium.

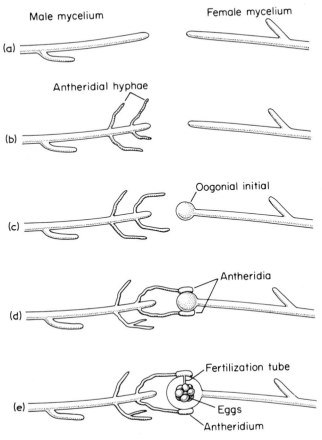

Fig. 6.4 Stages in sexual reproduction of *Achlya*. (a) Approach of male and female mycelia. (b) Induction of antheridial hyphae on male mycelium. (c) Induction of oogonial initial on female mycelium and attraction of antheridial hyphae to the oogonial initial. (d) Attraction of antheridial hyphae to the oogonial initial and delimination of antheridia. (e) Maturation of oogonium, differentiation of eggs and initiation of fertilization.

A cross wall is formed at the base of each oogonial initial and, within the oogonium thus formed, several eggs begin to differentiate. Fertilization tubes originating in the antheridia penetrate the oogonial wall and reach the eggs. The antheridial nuclei migrate from the antheridia to the eggs through the fertilization tubes; one nucleus enters each egg, the nuclei fuse and form a diploid zygote.

The proof that antheridial hyphae grow to developing oogonia in response to chemical signals from the oogonia, and that several other hormones are involved in the integration of sexual reproduction in *Achlya bisexualis* and *A. ambisexualis* was provided by Raper (1939, 1940). From his experiments, Raper concluded that the initiation of the sexual process was the result of the secretion of one or more chemical compounds by female hyphae which caused the development of antheridial hyphae on the vegetative male mycelium (hormone A complex). The antheridial hyphae then secreted hormone B, which induced the formation of oogonial initials on the female hyphae. The oogonial initials were then postulated to secrete hormone C which directed the growth of the antheridial hyphae to the oogonial initials, and was responsible for the delimitation of antheridia at the tips of the antheridial hyphae. The final chemical (hormone D) was secreted by the antheridia and caused the formation of oogonia by the oogonial initials and the differentiation of eggs within the oogonia. The presence of the different hormones and their sequential production was shown by the isolation of male and female plants at different stages with cellophane membranes, and the diffusion of the hormones through the membranes with the subsequent expression of the different specific morphological events. Further confirmation was obtained from the results of other ingenious experiments.

More recently, Barksdale (1963a,b) has found that hormone A not only induces the antheridial hyphae but is also responsible for their chemotrophic growth to the oogonial initials, a function attributed by Raper to hormone C. Polystyrene particles that had absorbed hormone A could attract the antheridial hyphae. When such hormone-treated particles were spread on a cellophane membrane placed over a male strain, they induced the formation of the antheridial branches in the male hyphae. In addition, cross walls were formed in the antheridial hyphae, delimiting antheridia, a function of Raper's hormone C. Hormone A thus seems to be responsible for the following functions: (1) induction of antheridial hyphae, (2) directional growth of the antheridial hyphae to the oogonial initials, (3) stimulation of production of hormone B by the male hyphae, and (4) delimitation of antheridia.

Hormone A, renamed antheridiol because it brings about the formation of branches on which antheridia are delimited, has been extracted from female hyphae, purified, and its structure determined. It has also been chemically synthesized (Arsenault *et al.*, 1968; Edwards *et al.*, 1969; McMorris and Seshadri, 1971; Edwards *et al.*, 1972; McMorris *et al.*, 1972). Antheridiol (hormone A) is a C−29 steroid (Fig. 6.5). It is effective in producing antheridial branches in certain male strains of *Achlya* in concentrations as low as 5−10 pg ml^{-1} (Barksdale *et al.*, 1974). The structural and stereochemical requirements for its activity are very specific. A large number of different steroids (53) including several isomers of antheridiol and related steroids were assayed for their ability to induce antheridial branches in a male strain of *Achlya* (Barksdale *et al.*, 1974). From these studies it appears that the stereochemistry at C−22 and C−23 in antheridiol is very important. The three C−22, C−23 stereoisomers of antheridiol all had less than 1/1000 the activity of antheridiol. The 7-keto group seems to be relatively unimportant since antheridiol was only 20 times as active as its 7-deoxy analog. A free hydroxyl at C−3 is not essential for full activity. Oxidation of the 22-hydroxyl causes a sharp fall in activity.

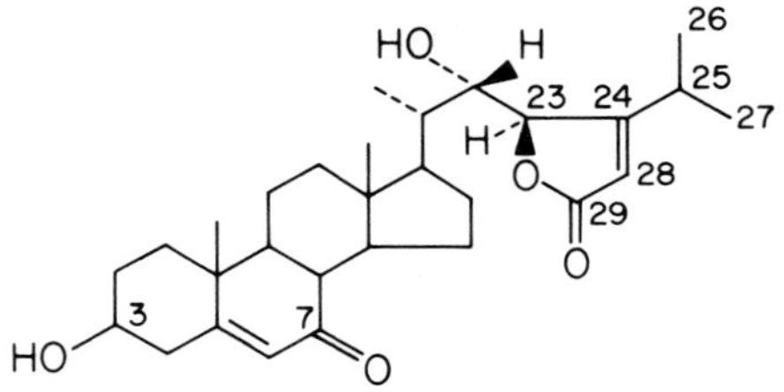

Fig. 6.5 Structure of antheridiol.

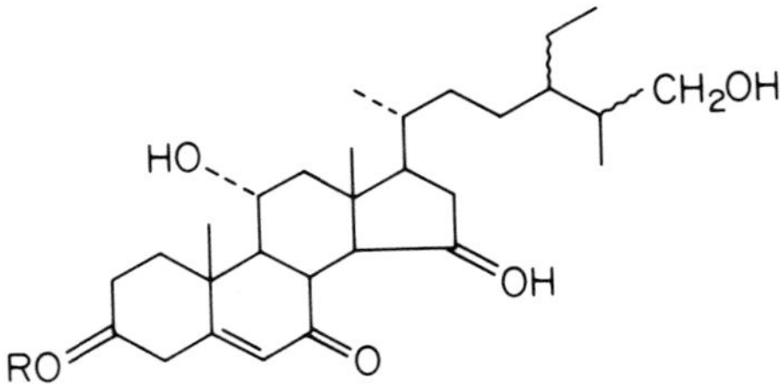

Oogoniol-1,   R = (CH$_3$)$_2$CHC = O

Oogoniol-2,   R = CH$_3$CH$_2$C = O

Fig. 6.6 Structures of the oogoniols.

A large number of mammalian steroid hormones and other steroids were inactive in the bioassay, i.e. the induction of antheridial hyphae.

More recently, compounds that have hormone B activity have been isolated and their structure determined (Fig. 6.6) (Barksdale and Lasure, 1974; McMorris *et al.*, 1975). (Hormone B, it will be recalled, is produced by antheridial branches after their stimulation by antheridiol and acts on the female causing the formation of oogonial initials). These compounds were isolated from extracts of a hermaphroditic strain of *A. heterosexualis,* which secretes hormone B without prior stimulation by exogenous antheridiol.

Compounds 1 and 2 (Fig. 6.6) which have been named oogoniol-1 and oogoniol-2, showed similar activity in biological tests for hormone B. The lowest concentration at which activity was observed was 620 and 460 ng ml^{-1} respectively. McMorris *et al.* (1975) have commented that sexual reproduction in *Achlya* seems to closely parallel sexual reproduction in mammals, antheridiol and the oogoniols being plant counterparts to mammalian androgens and estrogens.

There have been several studies aimed at elucidating the mechanism of action of antheridiol. Male *Achlya* strains seem to remove antheridiol added to the culture medium, and it cannot be extracted back from the hyphae (Barksdale, 1963a). The rate of uptake and the quantity of antheridiol removed from the medium roughly parallels the capability of the different strains to produce antheridial initials. Strains that are 'strong males' take up antheridiol more readily than 'weak male' strains. The fate of antheridiol once it is taken up by the male has not yet been studied.

The induction of male sexual organs by male cultures on the addition of antheridiol requires both transcription and translation. Inhibition of either of these processes eliminates the response (Kane *et al.*, 1973; Horowitz and Russell, 1974). The addition of antheridiol is also accompanied by increased rates of synthesis of ribosomal RNA, poly (A) containing RNA and protein (Silver and Horgen, 1974; Timberlake, 1976). In addition there is a temporal separation between the synthesis of rRNA and that of mRNA and protein (Silver and Horgen, 1974; Horgen *et al.*, 1975). A sharp rise in cellulase activity has been reported at the time antheridial primordia are initiated (Thomas and Mullins, 1967, 1969). Inhibitors of either transcription or translation inhibit the release of cellulase and the production of antheridial primordia (Kane *et al.*, 1973). Cellulose is a major component of the cell wall of *Achlya* and it has been proposed that a prerequisite for the formation of antheridial hyphae is a localized softening of the hyphal wall caused by cellulase. These weak spots are presumed to be the sites of antheridial primordia which grow out because of the turgor pressure of the cell (Mullins and Ellis, 1974). Processes of vesiculation and secretion are considered to provide a mechanism for concentration of cellulase at the sites of initiation of antheridial primordia, since freeze-etch studies of hormone-treated hyphae show aggregates of vesicles found associated with areas of wall thinning (Mullins and Ellis, 1974).

A protein with a molecular weight of 69 000 is induced 1 h after addition of antheridiol to a male strain of *A. ambisexualis* (Groner *et al.*, 1976). When *Achlya* chromatin is incubated with antheridiol and the cytosol from a male strain, there is an increase in the RNA synthetic capacity of the chromatin (Horgen, 1977). No stimulation of chromatin transcription was obtained when cytosol or antheridiol alone, or a mixture of hormone with cytosol from a female strain were added. Optimal hormone— cytosol stimulation of *in vitro* transcription required a temperature-dependent incubation of the steroid—cytosol complex and high ionic strength (0.05—0.12 M KCl) (Horgen, 1977). Several of the effects of antheridiol that have been studied thus seem to show a similarity in its mode of action to that of steroid hormones in animal systems.

Fucosterol-[3-^{3}H] when fed to a male strain of *A. ambisexualis* is converted to the oogoniols only when stimulated by the addition of antheridiol (McMorris and White, 1977). In the absence of antheridiol, labeled fucosterol added to the male strain was gradually taken up over a period of several hours. If antheridiol was added 2 h after the fucosterol, it required a further hour before oogoniol could be detected in the culture liquid. The enzymes which catalyze the conversion of fucosterol to oogoniol are presumably induced during this period. Protein synthesis is involved since cycloheximide completely inhibits the production of oogoniols (McMorris and White, 1977). Fucosterol, the major sterol of *Achlya,* is also a precursor of antheridiol (Popplestone and Unrau, 1974).

6.2.3 *Mucor* and related fungi

In *Mucor mucedo* (Blakeslee, 1904), when two sexually compatible hyphae grow
into close proximity with each other, special protruberances called copulation
branches or zygophores are produced. When the zygophores meet, a swollen outgrowth
the progametangium, develops on each zygophore at the point of contact. Plus (male)
and minus (female) progametangia remain attached to each other while they continue
to enlarge. At the apex of each progametangium a wall is formed delimiting a multinucleate gametangium. The two gametangia subsequently fuse to form the zygote
(Fig. 6.7). Zygophores of compatible strains are mutually attracted to each other.

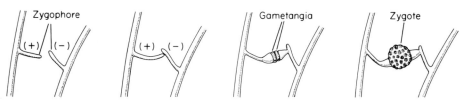

Fig. 6.7 *Mucor* — stages in the mating process.

The first experimental evidence for this chemotrophic growth of zygophores was
provided by Burgeff (1924) who named the phenomenon, zygotropism (see Machlis
and Rawitscher-Kunkel, 1967; and van den Ende and Stegwee, 1971, for review of
early work). There are thus two distinct events that occur, first the mutual induction
of zygophore formation by *plus* and *minus* mycelia and then the subsequent chemically directed growth of the two zygophores, to each other. Whether two different
molecules are involved in these two different processes is not yet known. The
substance(s) that induced the formation of zygophores was shown to be volatile and
to act through air (Burgeff, 1924; Hepden and Hawker, 1961). The details of the
hormonal control of the different steps of the sexual cycle were described by
Plempel and his associates (Plempel, 1957, 1960, 1963; Plempel and Dawid, 1961).

The trisporic acids (Fig. 6.8) have been shown to be responsible for the induction
of zygophores (van den Ende, 1967, 1968; Austin *et al.*, 1969; Reschke, 1969;
van den Ende *et al.*, 1970). It was known quite early (Burgeff, 1924) that zygophores
became yellow, and this was later shown to be caused by β-carotene. The study of
this relationship between carotene production and sexuality was responsible for the
trisporic acids being structurally characterized. Prieto *et al.* (1964) found that traces
of an acidic fraction obtained from a chloroform extract of a mixed culture of
Blakeslea trispora significantly increased the yield of β-carotene by the individual
strains. This acidic fraction was shown to consist of three substances named trisporic
acids A, B and C, with A constituting 1–2% of the mixture, B, 15% and C about 80%
(Caglioti *et al.*, 1967; Cainelli *et al.*, 1967). Trisporic acids B and C were shown to be
identical to the factors responsible for the induction of zygophores in *M. mucedo*
(van den Ende, 1967, 1968). These results were confirmed (Austin *et al.*, 1969;

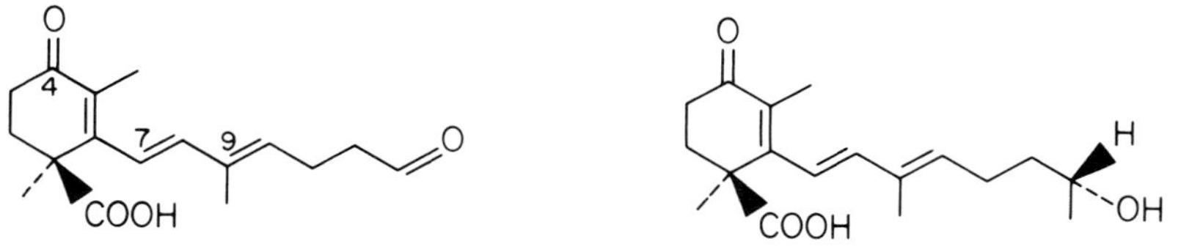

Fig. 6.8 Structures of trisporic acids.

Reschke, 1969; van den Ende *et al.,* 1970). An unexpected conclusion of this work is the apparent lack of mating-type specificity, since trisporic acids can induce zygophore formation in both mating types of several species of the Mucorales (van den Ende, 1968; Gooday, 1968; Bu'Lock *et al.,* 1972). The trisporic acids are moreover, not produced by single strains of the organisms, but only by mated cultures. These observations raise intriguing questions concerning the control of trisporic acid synthesis. How does one explain the fact that both plus and minus cultures produce trisporic acids only after they are mixed? Trisporic acid synthesis does not require physical contact since it occurs when the two mating types are separated by a membrane filter (van den Ende, 1968; van den Ende *et al.,* 1970). Moreover, both mating types contribute equally to trisporic acid production (van den Ende *et al.,* 1972), and inhibitors of protein and RNA synthesis inhibit de novo trisporic acid synthesis (Gooday, 1972; van den Ende and Stegwee, 1971). Control of trisporic acid synthesis thus seems to require that each mating type produce an inducer that has the ability to cause the necessary enzyme biosynthesis in the complementary mating type and the ability to respond to the inducer from the opposite mating type. Sutter and associates (Sutter, 1970, Sutter *et al.,* 1973, 1974) found that specific compounds were secreted by *plus* and *minus* mycelia. These were precursors of trisporic acids and they could be converted by the mating partner into trisporic acid. Only *plus* cultures produced 4-hydroxymethyl-trisporates, while trisporins and trisporols were found only in extracts of minus cultures (Bu'Lock *et al.,* 1974; Nieuwenhuis and van den Ende, 1975). The 4-hydroxymethyl-trisporates can be converted to trisporic acids by *minus* strains only, and the trisporins by *plus* strains only (Nieuwenhuis and van den Ende, 1975). Sex specificity is thus exhibited both in the production of precursors and in their conversion to trisporic acids. In unmated cultures, the production of these intermediates is very low; however, trisporic acids strongly stimulate their production. This stimulation is inhibited by RNA and protein synthesis inhibitors. Trisporic acids once formed in mated cultures, can further stimulate their own synthesis (Werkman and van den Ende, 1973). "Trisporic acid synthesis is therefore envisaged as the result of the combination of two incomplete but complementary pathways, which partially exhibit strong sex specificity" (Nieuwenhuis and van den Ende, 1975).

There is very little information concerning the mechanisms by which trisporic

acids cause the development of zygophores. Werkman (1976) has reported that a
NADP-dependent dehydrogenase and an esterase appear to be highly specific for the
minus mating type of *M. mucedo* and the synthesis of these enzymes is stimulated by
trisporic acids. The dehydrogenase was concentrated in the *minus* zygophores. In the
homothallic *Zygorhynchus moelleri* the copulating main branch which has a *minus*
character appears to be the major site of dehydrogenase activity.

As mentioned earlier, zygophores of opposite mating type tend to grow towards
one another. Volatile substances produced by the zygophores cause a positive tropic
response in the opposite partner (Banbury, 1954; Plempel, 1960, 1962; Plempel and
Dawid, 1961). Whether trisporic acid precursors are responsible for the tropism remains
to be determined (Mesland *et al.*, 1974).

6.3 CHEMOTAXIS IN BROWN ALGAE

There is a wide variety of ways in which the male and female sex cells of algae contact
each other and achieve fertilization. Only certain of the brown algae will be discussed
in this review (for details of sexual processes in other algae, see Machlis and Rawitscher-
Kunkel, 1967; Wiese, 1969; van den Ende, 1976). The brown algae are primarily
marine organisms. Many of them are common sea-weeds seen on the Atlantic coast
and in other cold waters. The brown algae multiply by various vegetative means.
Under certain specific environmental conditions the plants become reproductive and
produce male and female gametangia. In certain species such as *Ectocarpus* both the
gametes are motile and of the same size i.e., they are isogamous. In other species
such as *Cutleria* the female gametes are much larger than the male gametes (30 times
larger in volume) (anisogamous), although both are motile. In species such as *Fucus*
the female gamete is an egg which is large (20 000 times the volume of the sperm)
and immotile and is produced in small numbers in an oogonium, while the male
gametes are motile, and produced in very large numbers (Jaenicke, 1977). The
motile gametes are biflagellate with the two flagella of unequal length and laterally
inserted, the longer flagellum projecting forward and the shorter projecting backward;
with the opposite being true for the male gametes of *Fucus* (Smith, 1955).

When male and female gametes of *Ectocarpus* which are initially both motile and
morphologically alike, are mixed, one gamete type (female) settles down attaching
itself by its longer flagellum to the substrate. Only after becoming immotile does the
female gamete secrete a chemical compound that chemotactically attracts the male
gametes in clusters to it (Berthold, 1881; Hartman, 1934, as quoted by Machlis, 1972).
In the formation of such clusters, each male gamete attaches itself to the body of the
female gamete by the tip of its longer flagellum. Once fusion of one male gamete
with the female gamete begins, the flagella of the other males become detached and
the fusing zygote is no longer able to attract other male gametes. The chemotactic
agent is thus released by the female gamete for only a short interval; that between
attachment to the substratum and the beginning of fusion. The chemotactic agent

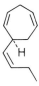

Fig. 6.9 Structure of ectocarpene.

is volatile and has been shown to be a hydrocarbon with three non-conjugated *cis* double bonds and a seven carbon ring (Müller *et al.,* 1971; Jaenicke *et al.,* 1971). It was later given the trivial name ectocarpene (Fig. 6.9).

When male gametes of *Ectocarpus* are labeled with 1', 2'-[^{3}H]-ectocarpene and the distribution of the label in the gametes then studied by radioautography, most of the radioactivity is first found over the long flagellum. At later times the cells are also labeled. These results have been interpreted to mean that the receptor proteins for ectocarpene are located in the flagellum, and the main body of the cell is where metabolism or storage of the degradation products of ectocarpene occurs (Jaenicke, 1977). This would seem to indicate that the mechanisms of perception and response to the chemotactic compound reside in the flagellum. The response of male gametes to ectocarpene is very rapid beginning within less than a minute from the time the hormone is added (Müller, 1976). Various analogues and derivatives of ectocarpene have been synthesized. Of all the compounds tested ectocarpene is the most active; a threshold concentration of 10^{-8} M for activity in the bioassay used, being determined. Several compounds with long hydrophobic alkyl substituents appeared to act as competitive inhibitors of ectocarpene (Jaenicke, 1977).

The sperm-attracting chemicals of *Cutleria multifida* and *Fucus serratus* have also been chemically characterized. The active substance from *Cutleria* has been identified as *trans*-4-vinyl-5-(*cis*-1'-butenyl) cyclopentane (Fig. 6.10) and has been given the name multifidene (Jaenicke *et al.,* 1974); that from *Fucus* is the conjugated hydrocarbon 1, 3-*trans*, 5-*cis*-octatriene (Fig. 6.10) renamed fucoserraten (Müller and Jaenicke, 1973; Jaenicke and Seferiadis, 1975).

Three compounds can be recovered by gas-chromatographic analysis of the volatile products secreted by female gametes of *Cutleria*: — multifidene, aucantene, and ectocarpene in a ratio of about 10:4:1 (Jaenicke *et al.,* 1974; Müller, 1974). Male gametes of *Cutleria* are most sensitive to multifidene. They also respond to ectocarpene and aucantene, although 10- and 30-fold higher concentrations, respectively, of these two compounds are required for the response to be seen (Müller, 1976).

Cook *et al.* (1948) and Cook and Elvidge (1951) obtained several volatile fractions from suspensions of eggs of *Fucus serratus* and *F. vesiculosus* that attracted the sperms. They also showed that many common hydrocarbons, including *n*-hexane, could attract the sperms in their bioassay. This relative non-specificity has been confirmed by Müller and Seferiadis (1977), who have shown that several derivatives

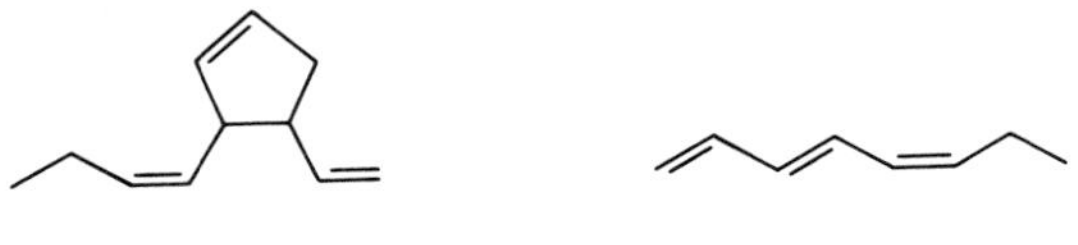

Multifidene   Fucoserratene

Fig. 6.10 Structures of multifidene and fucoserratene.

of fucoserratene and ectocarpene are active although at much higher concentrations than the natural compound. A concentration of *n*-hexane 3100 times that of fucoserratene was required for activity, indicating that *n*-hexane is not likely to be a natural attractant (Müller and Seferiadis, 1977). The sperms of *F. serratus* and *F. vesiculosus* respond equally well to fucoserratene, indicating no species specificity of the attractant. Unlike *Ectocarpus*, the chemotactic substance in *Fucus* is liberated by eggs still contained in oogonia and its production continues for 3–4 days in unfertilized eggs (Cook and Elvidge, 1951).

Although no information is currently available about the nature of the receptors on the sperm that respond to the tactic substances, nor the mechanisms by which the motility is directed, the brown algae seem to be ideal objects for such studies. Many derivatives of the active compounds have already been synthesized, and, in one case at least, that with ectocarpene, labeled material is available. Preliminary work indicates that the receptors might be located in the flagella (Jaenicke, 1977). It should thus be possible to isolate surface receptor molecules and to study the processes involved in the perception and response to the hormones.

6.4 CHEMOTAXIS OF MOSS, LIVERWORT AND FERN SPERMS

Mosses, liverworts and ferns, although quite different groups of plants, all bear their eggs at the bottom of an archegonium (Fig. 6.11). An archegonium is a female structure found in either the female or hermaphroditic haploid plants of these plant groups. When a mature archegonium is exposed to water the apical neck cells separate, followed by the breakdown and extrusion of the neck canal cells, forming a canal through which the sperm swim to the egg. The sperm in all these groups of plants are motile and the release of the sperm and fertilization only occur in the presence of water. The sperm of liverworts and mosses are biflagellate while those of ferns are multiflagellate.

Hanstein (1865–1866) and Strasburger (1868, 1869–1870) were the first investigators to report chemotactic movement of the sperm into the archegonial canal and down it to the egg. Pfeffer (1884) confirmed these observations for several different fern species and in addition described the chemotactic responses of sperm to the archegonia of several liverworts and moss species. Using an assay method that consisted of partially filling a capillary tube sealed at one end with a test

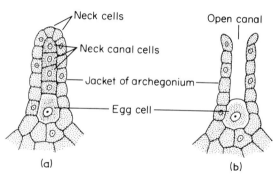

Fig. 6.11 Diagrammatic longitudinal section through an immature (a) and mature (b) archegonium showing its structure. The sperm swim down the canal to the egg.

solution and introducing the open end into a suspension of sperm, Pfeffer (1884) demonstrated that certain fern sperm very rapidly clustered around the tip, if the tube contained 0.1% sodium malate. Pfeffer thought that the receptive spot on the egg was the source of the attractant, presumably malate, although he did not demonstrate the presence of malate in the secretions from the archegonia. He tested the sperm of other plants to various compounds and found the sperm of several mosses to be attracted by sucrose (0.001 to 0.1%) but nothing else. The sperms of the spike moss, *Selaginella* were also attracted to malate. These results were confirmed and extended by several other workers (see Machlis and Rawitscher-Kunkel, 1967) and can be summarized as follows:

(1) the sperms of the plants under discussion are attracted to their archegonia and, in addition, to certain organic substances, all of which are common metabolites or plant products;

(2) some of the sperms respond to a variety of ions and organic substances;

(3) chemotactically active substances for liverworts were shown to be proteins; for mosses, sucrose; malate and maleate but not fumarate for ferns, malate and fumarate for the quillwort *Isoetes*; malate for the horsetails and citrate for the club mosses.

Unfortunately, to this day, we do not know whether the organic acids are indeed the native chemotactic attractants because no one has yet isolated and identified a chemotactic substance from archegonia or even determined whether archegonia contain a high enough concentration of the organic acids to exert a chemotactic effect.

Very few studies have been addressed to an explanation of how the directional information in the chemical concentration gradient of a chemotactic substance is used by a motile cell in its precise orientation to the gradient. Brokaw in a series of papers has attempted to do this (Brokaw, 1957, 1958a,b, 1974). Sperm of the bracken fern *Pteridium aquilinum* respond to the partially ionized form of malic acid, bimalate ion and also to calcium ions (Brokaw, 1957, 1958a, 1974). In addition, they also exhibit a response to voltage gradients (Brokaw, 1958b). Both calcium and bimalate ions are required for the chemotactic response and for the response to voltage gradients (Brokaw, 1974). Sperm that swim up a bimalate concentration gradient show a decrease in the radius of their helical paths; if they accidentally swim down the concentration gradient their paths show an unusually large helix-radius which becomes small when they turn around and swim back towards the source of the chemotactic mixture (Brokaw, 1974). These observations indicate that fern sperm can direct their movement relative to a gradient of bimalate and calcium ions, and Brokaw has suggested that the basis for the change in movement could be an alteration in the bending pattern of the flagella. Brokaw (1974) has proposed a 'coupled diffusion' hypothesis for chemoreception. This hypothesis postulates a membrane carrier which can only circulate freely in the membrane if it binds both bimalate and calcium ions. If a step increase in bimalate ion is applied to the outside of this membrane in the presence of calcium ions there will be an influx of bimalate and calcium ions until the internal bimalate concentration reaches a new equilibrium. There will also be an increase in the internal calcium concentration and this may cause a flagellar response. If the sperms have a mechanism which actively transports calcium ions out of the cell, the response to a bimalate concentration step will be a pulse of internal calcium ion concentration. This mechanism can thus account for a time differentiation of a chemical signal, so that the cell can respond to the rate of increase or decrease of external bimalate or calcium ions. This time differentiation could provide the sperm with a mechanism for sensing the directional information in a concentration gradient of the chemotactic substance(s). The hypothesis also explains the coupling of sensitivity to bimalate ions to a general mediator of intracellular events, calcium ions. The 'coupled diffusion' hypothesis seems reasonable and is one of the very few proposed mechanisms to explain oriented movement to a chemical gradient. Experimental proof, however, is needed to document it.

6.5 RECOGNITION EVENTS AND CHEMOTROPISM IN THE REPRODUCTION OF FLOWERING PLANTS

The egg located in the haploid embryo sac of flowering plants is embedded in a mass of diploid tissue in the ovule of the pistil. The pistil is the female organ of the plant, and consists of a stigma, style and ovary in which the ovules are borne. When a pollen grain (male gametophyte) which, depending on the plant species, may contain two or three haploid nuclei, is deposited on the stigma of a compatible pistil, it begins to germinate. The pollen grain germinates by extrusion of a tube, the pollen tube, through a germ pore in the grain. The pollen tube grows in between the cells of the stigma and down into the style. The two sperm cells are carried through the style in the pollen tube. Most pollen tubes grow very rapidly, some achieving rates greater than 35 mm h^{-1}. Styles can be extremely variable in length. In some species the style is practically non-existent, whereas in others, for example, corn, it may attain a length of about 50 cm. An outstanding feature of the organization of the pistil is that the stigma is connected with the interior of the ovary by a tissue, the transmitting tissue (Esau, 1977), consisting of cells that are secretory. Styles may be hollow, solid, or a combination of the two. In hollow styles, e.g. lily, the transmitting tissue lines the stylar canal. In most angiosperms the styles are solid. The transmitting tissue is present, nevertheless, usually in the form of strands of considerably elongated cells. Tranmitting tissue occurs on the placenta within the ovary and, in some species, on parts of the ovule as well (Esau, 1953). In solid styles the pollen tube usually passes through the transmitting tissues by intercellular growth. Upon reaching the ovarian cavity, the pollen tube follows the transmitting tissue lining the ovary wall and eventually comes in contact with an ovule. The ovary may contain from one to several hundred ovules depending on the species, attached to various parts of the lining of the ovary wall. The tube enters the ovule in a manner specific for each species. In most plants it enters through the micropyle. The tube penetrates the wall of the embryo sac, bursts open, discharges its contents and fertilization occurs. The pollen tube thus functions as a vehicle to transport the two sperm cells down the style and to the embryo sac. For a more detailed description of the events preceding fertilization in flowering plants, see Jensen (1972).

Whether a male gamete of a particular genotype will enter the embryo sac to effect fertilization is determined by interactions between the pollen grain and the receptive surface of the stigma or between the pollen tube and the transmitting tissue of the style. During pollination some pollen grains from foreign species are usually deposited on the stigma. These pollen grains normally tend to be rejected. In addition, most flowering plants exhibit some degree of self-incompatibility, i.e. rejection of pollen of identical genotype and the acceptance of that from another genotype of the same species (Brewbaker, 1957; Heslop-Harrison, 1975a). This recognition and rejection of self-pollen by the cells of the stigma and style is a fascinating area of study of flowering plant reproduction that has in the past few years yielded significant new information and advances in our understanding of incompatibility. The pollen tube, as described earlier, grows through the style and enters the embryo sac in a very specific manner. The evidence that the directional growth of pollen tubes is chemically controlled will also be considered.

6.5.1 Incompatibility

Incompatibility refers to the partial or complete incapacity of otherwise normal pollen to effect fertilization with certain genotypic combinations of pollen and pistil. Both interspecific and intraspecific incompatibility systems are known. This discussion will, however, be limited to intraspecific or self-incompatibility systems. Self-incompatibility, together with other mechanisms ensures a greater amount of outcrossing in a population. The phenomenon is widespread among flowering plants

(Brewbaker, 1957). An ideal incompatibility system would be one in which only the incompatible pollen grains were discriminated against, without a concomitant large-scale destruction or inactivation of the pistil tissues. If such a large-scale inactivation of female tissue were to occur, there would be no possibility of fertilization when compatible pollen was deposited on the stigma. This is how incompatibility systems operate in nature where the interactions between pollen and the female part of the flower are restricted to individual pollen grains or tubes and a single or a few cells of the stigma or style, leaving the bulk of the female tissue undamaged for pollination with compatible pollen (Heslop-Harrison, 1975b). In addition, in many plants, if there are no compatible pollinations, incompatibility becomes leaky when the pistil has aged a few days, and otherwise incompatible pollen tubes can grow down the style and effect fertilization (Ascher and Peloquin, 1966) — apparently it is better to have some seeds formed even if they are selfed, rather than none!

There are two major types of incompatibility systems: sporophytic and gametophytic. Sporophytic refers to the fact that genetic evidence indicates that pollen behavior is determined by the diploid male parental genotype, i.e. the sporophyte, interacting with the diploid female sporophyte. In other words, the effective gene products in the pollen grain that interact with the stigma must have been synthesized by diploid sporophytic cells, i.e. either in the pollen mother cells prior to meiosis or alternatively later in pollen development by the diploid cells surrounding the pollen and the transfer of these materials to the pollen grains during the terminal stages of their maturation. In gametophytic incompatibility the effective gene products in the pollen have been synthesized by the haploid genotype after meiosis and these interact with complementary material synthesized by the diploid pistil tissue. The incompatibility can express itself as an inhibition of pollen germination or early tube growth, while the tubes are still on the stigma, or during the growth of the pollen tube through the style. In such cases the growth rate of the pollen tubes is slow and growth may stop before the tubes reach the ovary. In addition, the inhibited tubes may show morphological aberrations of various sorts, such as branching, swelling of the tube tips, thickening of the cell walls, etc. For a more detailed treatment of the classification and genetics of incompatibility systems in flowering plants, see Lewis (1976) and de Nettancourt (1977).

The operation of a self-incompatibility system requires that the pistil be able to recognize self and non-self pollen. Such a recognition between cells is normally considered more typical of animal than of plant cells. It is clear, however, that the cell wall does not necessarily create a barrier to the operation of recognition molecules on the surfaces of plant cells. The interaction of a pollen grain with the pistil begins at the moment that the pollen grain is deposited on the stigma. The incompatibility-related inhibition of growth of the pollen tube may, however, take place at various sites in the pistil. A brief description of the receptive surfaces of the stigma and pollen grain might be of help in following the further discussion. There is a wide variation in stigmas both with respect to the morphology of the receptive cells and the amount of stigma secretions. There are two main types of stigmas:

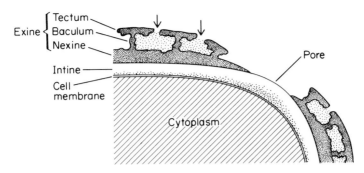

Fig. 6.12 Diagrammatic representation of the pollen grain wall. The arrows indicate the sites of deposition of sporophytically synthesized materials.

'dry' stigmas which do not have large amounts of fluid surface secretion at maturity and 'wet' stigmas in which there is a copious surface secretion. In the 'dry' stigmas of the Gramineae (grasses) the receptive cells are elongated and often pointed, while in those of many Cruciferae and Compositae the stigma is made up of elongated but rounded papillae (a papilla is a protruding epidermal cell). In the 'wet' stigmas of many Rosaceae the receptive surface has short papillae, while in those of the Solanaceae and Liliaceae the surface cells are non-papillate (Heslop-Harrison 1975a). The surface cells of 'dry' stigmas have a discontinuous cuticle which covers the cell wall. Overlying the cuticle of the papillae is a thin hydrated proteinaceous layer or pellicle, which is secreted by the papillae through the discontinuities in the cuticle (Heslop-Harrison *et al.,* 1975). In 'wet' stigmas the cuticle in the mature state is usually detached and disrupted (Konar and Linskens, 1966; Heslop-Harrison, 1975a). In plants with 'dry' stigmas the pollen tube after germination enters through the cuticle and makes its way through the wall of the papilla before entering the style where it then grows between cells of the transmitting tissue (Christ, 1959; Kroh, 1964; Dickinson and Lewis, 1973a). The cuticle in 'dry' stigmas could thus form a barrier to the penetration of pollen tubes.

Pollen grains when mature have thick walls of several layers often with elaborate and beautiful surface patterns. Depending on the species, one or more regions of the pollen grain might lack the thick walls. These regions are known as pores or apertures, and are the regions on the grain where a germ tube emerges on germination of the pollen grain. As seen under the electron microscope, angiosperm pollen walls consist of several layers of chemically different materials that have been given different names (Fig. 6.12). There are differences in various pollens between the relative thickness of the various layers, presence or absence of one or other layer or sublayer, types of morphological detail on the surface, etc. The exine is composed of a substance called sporopollenin, which is a unique polymer characterized by a high stability to anaerobic biological and chemical attack. Sporopollenins are highly unsaturated compounds, contain C-methyl and hydroxyl groups, and after oxidation give a mixture of simple dicarboxylic acids (C_2 to C_6) as the major products. They are co-polymers of carotenoids and carotenoid esters with oxygen (Brooks and Shaw, 1971). The intine contains pectinaceous material, cellulose and proteins. The pollen walls of all species of flowering plants thus far examined contain proteins that are rapidly released when the pollen grains are moistened (Tsinger and Petrovskaya-Baranova, 1961; Knox and Heslop-Harrison, 1969, 1971a, 1971b, 1971c; Knox *et al.*, 1970; Knox, 1971; Hubscher and Eisen, 1972; Howlett *et al.*, 1973). These proteins are localized at two sites in the wall, in the inner cellulosic intine layer, especially at the germinal apertures, and in the spaces and cavities of the exine. Several of the wall proteins are enzymes, principally hydrolytic enzymes (Knox and Heslop-Harrison, 1969, 1970), although only a part of the total wall protein appears to be enzymic. By cytochemical methods several hydrolytic enzymes; acid phosphatase, ribonuclease, esterase, amylase, and protease were demonstrated to be present in the walls of fifty different angiosperm pollens (Knox and Heslop-Harrison, 1970). In all cases enzyme activity was associated principally with the intine, with activity concentrated in or around the intine near a pore. Light and electron microscope studies seem to indicate that the enzymes are incorporated into the intine during the early period of wall growth following the release of the spores from the meiotic tetrads (Knox, 1971; Knox and Heslop-Harrison, 1971a). The proteins occur in strands, ribbons, or leaflets, encased in the polysaccharide matrix of the intine, and are produced by the male gametophyte and incorporated into the wall during its growth. At maturity the outer wall of the pollen grain, the exine, shows a distinct stratification (Fig. 6.12). Quite commonly a columnar layer is found, formed of numerous radially directed rods, the bacula, which rise from the nexine. This layer may be roofed over or the rods may stand free. If roofed over, the roof-wall is interrupted by perforations which allow movement of materials to or from the outside of the grains to the space between the columns. The structural features of the exine are thus well-adapted to receive and hold externally derived materials (Heslop-Harrison, 1975b). The proteins in the cavities of the exine are sporophytic in origin being transferred into the wall during the terminal stages of pollen development. They are derived from membrane-bound cisternae, released from the tapetum during its dissolution (Dickinson and Lewis, 1973b; Heslop-Harrison *et al.*, 1973). The tapetum is a sporophytic tissue that surrounds the developing pollen grains in the anther and which possibly has a nurse function (Mascarenhas, 1975). In summary, the pollen wall at maturity contains proteinaceous materials derived from both the haploid gametophyte and the parental diploid sporophyte.

When a mature pollen grain which is fairly dehydrated is deposited on a stigma or some other moist surface, the pollen grain hydrates and the exine-held proteins are released very rapidly through the pores in the wall, the release beginning with 30 s of hydration. The intine-held proteins tend to be released later (within about 5 min) (Heslop-Harrison *et al.*, 1973). These rapidly released materials have been shown to be both proteins and glycoproteins of molecular weights in the range 10 000—40 000(Howlett *et al.*, 1975; Knox *et al.*, 1975). In the sporophytic incompatible system exemplified by *Brassica* (Cruciferae), hydration of the pollen grain and emission of pollen wall proteins is completed within 5 min of deposition on the stigma. In a compatible cross, the pollen grain begins to germinate within 3–10 min and the pollen tube penetrates the cuticle in 10–30 min. In an incompatible pollination, each stigma papilla in contact with a pollen grain reacts by the deposition of callose, a β–1, 3-glucose polymer, within the papilla in the region of contact with the pollen grain or tip of the pollen tube. This callose deposition is not seen in compatible crosses (Heslop-Harrison, 1975a). This callose 'rejection reaction' in the stigma papillae seems to be a characteristic of the sporophytic incompatibility system and has provided a rapid assay for the incompatibility response (Dickinson and Lewis, 1973a; Knox, 1973). In *Iberis,* the callose response was induced when gel cubes into which pollen exine proteins from incompatible pollen had diffused, were placed on the stigma (Heslop-Harrison *et al.,* 1974). No response was obtained in similar experiments with compatible pollen. That the materials responsible for the rejection reaction were derived from a sporophyte tissue, the tapetum, was shown by dissecting out the tapetum just before the onset of its dissolution and applying it to the stigma of a flower from the same plant. A strong rejection reaction was obtained. Evidence from preliminary fractionation suggests that the active fractions are proteins or glycoproteins of molecular weights between 10 000–40 000 (Heslop-Harrison *et al.,* 1974; Heslop-Harrison, 1975a). Following the 'rejection reaction' in the stigma papilla, there is a deposition of callose within the pollen tube and grain with a concomitant inhibition of further growth of the pollen tube (Heslop-Harrison, 1975a).

Since the pollen wall proteins are first deposited on the pellicle of the stigma papillae, the pellicle proteins must form the receptor site(s) for the sporophytic pollen wall proteins and it is these proteins that must be involved in the recognitions of pollen and stigma. The consequence of binding of proteins of pollen and stigma seems to be the transmission of stimuli that trigger the rejection responses in stigma and pollen.

In plants with 'dry' stigmas, a successful pollination requires that the pollen tube penetrate the cuticle of the stigma papilla early in its growth. Christ (1959) suggested that incompatible pollen could fail to penetrate the stigma cuticle if a pollen-contributed cutinase was either inhibited, or if the activation of a cutinase precursor in the pollen were to be prevented in such a cross. Recent evidence appears to support the presence of a cutinase precursor in the pollen which is activated by some component of the stigma pellicle. Intine proteins do not digest cuticles of the style and stigma except in the region of the papilla surface pellicle and, if the proteinaceous pellicle is removed enzymatically, the capacity of the pollen tube to penetrate the cuticle is lost (Heslop-Harrison, 1975a; Heslop-Harrison and Heslop-Harrison, 1975). In the self-compatible system of *Gladiolus,* concanavalin A binds to the stigma surface and when the receptor sites for con A are occupied the pollen tube penetration of the papillar cuticle is prevented (Knox *et al.,* 1976). There are at least four glycoproteins with molecular weights between 43 000–93 000 in the stigma surface pellicle that bind to concanavalin A (Knox *et al.,* 1976) and that could possibly be involved in the recognition process (Clarke *et al.,* 1977). The above evidence suggests that in incompatibility systems such as those in the Cruciferae, the binding of specific recognition factors on the surfaces of the pollen grain and the stigma papilla deter- mine the success or failure of a mating. The details of how this recognition is achieved still remain a mystery.

For additional information concerning the other incompatibility systems in flowering plants the reader is referred to several articles in the volume edited by Duckett and Racey (1975).

6.5.2 Pollen-tube chemotropism

As seen earlier, the pollen tube of flowering plants grows in a manner characteristic for each species through the stylar tissue, enters the micropyle of an ovule and then discharges from its tip two non-motile sperm cells in the immediate vicinity of an egg. Is the growth of the pollen tube chemically directed, or is the anatomy of the pistil tissues such that just by elongating it will automatically arrive at the micropyle? From the discussion that follows it will be seen that both chemotropism and pistil structure are probably involved. Additional information about other aspects of pollen tube chemotropism will be found in the following reviews: Mascarenhas and Machlis, 1962a; Rosen, 1971, 1975; Mascarenhas, 1973. There has been little experimental work of any significance on chemotropism during the last few years that has substantially added to our understanding of the phenomenon.

Molisch (1889) was the first to demonstrate that pistil tissues contained some substance or substances that could control the direction of growth of pollen tubes. When styles of *Narcissus tazetta* (daffodil) were placed on a sugar gelatin drop, pollen tubes growing in the vicinity were strongly attracted towards the stigma and cut surface of the style. This sort of an assay procedure has been called a 'surface test' because the pollen, ovules, or other test materials are placed on the surface of the agar medium. Since Molisch, several other workers have demonstrated this type of chemotropism in a wide variety of plants. About 50% of plants tested have shown chemotropism of pollen tubes to pistil tissues (Mascarenhas and Machlis, 1962a). Pollens from many plants respond chemotropically to vegetative and pistil tissues from related and unrelated plant species (see review by Mascarenhas and Machlis, 1962a). Hence the chemotropic factor(s) seems to be widely dispersed among plants and/or there are several factors to which pollen tubes can react chemotropically. The chemotropic factor has been characterized as being of small molecular size, although it is associated with material of high molecular weight from which it can be partly dissociated by polar solvents (Tsao, 1949; Miki, 1954, 1955; Linck and Blaydes, 1960; Rosen, 1961; Mascarenhas and Machlis, 1962b). Several early reports in the literature claimed chemotropic activity for specific compounds and crude preparations such as compressed yeast, sucrose, glucose, fructose, lactose, egg albumin, diastase and sodium malate, although more recent work has failed to confirm these results (see review in Mascarenhas and Machlis, 1962a). Simple amino acid and amine mixtures coupled with sugars have also been reported to be responsible for the chemotropic attraction of pollen tubes of *Oenothera* and *Narcissus* (Schildknecht and Benoni, 1963a,b). However, neither lily pollen (Rosen, 1964) nor snapdragon pollen (Mascarenhas and Machlis, 1962b) react chemotropically towards amino acid mixtures or sugars. In the snapdragon (*Antirrhinum*) the calcium ion is the, or one of the, natural chemotropic factors for the pollen (Mascarenhas and Machlis, 1962c, 1964). The chemotropic activity of calcium for snapdragon pollen has been confirmed with two different assays by Rosen (1964) who also found that ashed snapdragon pistils were chemotropically active. An analysis of snapdragon pistil tissues showed an overall gradient of total calcium amounting to a four-fold increase in concentration between the upper third of the style and that in the ovules and placenta (Mascarenhas and Machlis, 1964). The calcium would have to be present in an ionic or soluble form if it were to be effective in directing the pollen tube to the ovule. The concentration of ionic calcium was found to be fairly low and almost constant throughout the length of the style, being slightly higher in the stigma and increasing in the region of the ovary, with the placenta and inside of the ovary wall containing the highest concentration of ionic calcium (Mascarenhas, 1966). The transmitting tissue and surrounding parenchyma cells in the style had a lower concentration of soluble calcium than that in the ovule and stigma. The cells of the ovule were relatively low in calcium and a higher concentration of soluble calcium was not found in the region of the micropyle and embryo sac. This anatomical distribution of calcium would not be expected if a continuously increasing calcium gradient was important in directing pollen tubes from the stigma to the ovule and one might accordingly expect some other factor besides calcium to be involved in directing the pollen tube to the micropyle.

The calcium ion exerts a pronounced stimulating effect on both pollen germination and tube growth of a large number of plant species (Brink, 1924; Brewbaker and Kwack, 1963). The chemotropic substance(s) from pistil tissues is known to have a growth-stimulating effect on pollen tubes, in addition to a tropic effect (Knowlton, 1922; Beck and Joly, 1941).

Although calcium might be the principal chemotropic agent for snapdragon pollen tubes, it has no effect on pollen tube growth in lily (Rosen, 1964) and corn (Cook and Walden, 1967) or on chemotropism of lily (Rosen, 1964). A very similar distribution of ionic calcium to that found in snapdragon is also seen in the pistil of *Oenothera* (Glenk *et al.,* 1971) and in this study it was concluded that calcium could not play a role in the chemotropism of pollen tubes, although it did have a promotive effect on germination and tube growth. A similar conclusion was reached by Kwack (1969) for *Clivia* and *Crinum* pollen tubes. As can be seen from the preceding discussion, there is no unanimity of opinion concerning the chemical identity of the chemotropic substance(s) in the plants studied. I have attempted to bring some meaning to all these apparently conflicting observations in proposing a hypothesis that might explain chemotropism (Mascarenhas, 1973).

How does a tropic factor effect a change in the direction of growth of a pollen tube?

Is it necessary to have a continuously increasing gradient of the chemotropic substance from the stigma to the micropyle of the ovule? Any discussion of the mechanism of action of tropic factors has to include a consideration of the special nature of growth of pollen tubes. Pollen tubes grow exclusively at their tips by the fusion of polysaccharide-containing vesicles derived from either Golgi bodies or endoplasmic reticulum (Dashek and Rosen, 1966). For a tube growing straight, the growth zone at the tip is perpendicular to the long axis of the tube. For the tip to change its direction of growth, all that is required is a small shift in the angle made by the center of the growth zone with respect to the rest of the tube. This would presumably occur in response to a chemotropic factor impinging on the tip of the tube in a directionally localized manner. There may be a concentration gradient at this point. The gradient, if any, need be effective over only a very small distance. Once the direction of growth was changed and the tube tip was now in a uniformly distributed field of the tropic substance, the tube would continue to grow straight, no concentration gradient being necessary. Any component contributing directly to the growth at the tip region could theoretically be the agent that would cause such a change in direction, i.e. be a tropic factor. One might accordingly expect those factors required for normal metabolism of the pollen tube or for the synthesis of wall precursor material behind the tip to contribute only to the growth of the tube. However, those factors responsible for the assembly of the various components of the tube wall at the growth zone would, in addition to being growth factors, also be chemotropic agents. The pollen tube depends for part of its nutrition and growth requirements on the pistil tissue through which it grows. There is evidence for the movement of sugars, amino acids, etc. from the pistil tissue into the pollen tube (Linskens and Esser, 1959; Kroh *et al.,* 1970). Thus it is possible that for one or more of the requirements for tip growth, the pollen tube is dependent on the pistil tissue and the missing component(s) would be the chemotropic factor(s).

If this hypothesis is correct, there would be no necessity for a continuously increasing concentration gradient of the tropic substance in the pistil along the pathway of the pollen tubes from the stigma to the embryo sac. It would only be necessary for the tropic factor to be present in the tissues through which the pollen tubes grew in a concentration greater than a certain threshold value. Only in the region where a sharp change in direction occurred, such as, for example, from the placenta to the ovule and from the sides of the ovule into the micropyle, would a very restricted gradient of the chemotropic substance be of use. If this reasoning is correct, one would not expect a continuously increasing gradient of calcium ions in the snapdragon pistil, or for that matter of any other chemotropically active substance in other plants, to be present in the pistil along the pathway of the pollen tube. One might also expect differences in the nature of the chemotropic factors in different plant species. Iwanami (1959) has carried out some very elegant experiments with lily style and stigma sections. Pollen was added to the basal or apical ends or in the centers of these sections and the direction of growth of the pollen tubes followed. His experiments indicated fairly conclusively that there was no gradient of chemotropic factor(s) from the stigma to the ovule in lily pistils.

The identification of chemotropic compounds in several additional species of plants and a better understanding of the biochemistry of pollen tube tip growth is necessary before the validity of the hypothesis can be determined.

REFERENCES

Arsenault, G.P., Biemann, K., Barksdale, A.W. and McMorris, T.C. (1968), The structure of antheridiol, a sex hormone in *Achlya bisexualis. J. Am. Chem. Soc.,* **90**, 5635−5636.

Ascher, P.D. and Peloquin, S.J. (1966), Effect of floral aging on the growth of compatible and incompatible pollen tubes in *Lilium longiflorum. Am. J. Bot.,* **53**, 99−102.

Austin, D.J., Bu'Lock, J.D. and Gooday, G.W. (1969), Trisporic acids: sexual hormones from *Mucor mucedo* and *Blakeslea trispora. Nature,* **223**, 1178−1179.

Banbury, G.H. (1954), Processes controlling zygophore formation and zygotropism in *Mucor mucedo* Brefeld. *Nature,* **173**, 499−500.

Barksdale, A.W. (1963a), The uptake of exogenous hormone A by certain strains of *Achlya. Mycologia,* **55**, 164−171.

Barksdale, A.W. (1963b), The role of hormone A during sexual conjugation in *Achlya ambisexualis. Mycologia,* **55**, 627−632.

Barksdale, A.W. and Lasure, L.L. (1974), Production of hormone B by *Achlya heterosexualis. Appl. Microbiol.,* **28**, 544−546.

Barksdale, A.W., McMorris, T.C., Seshadri, R. and Arunachalam, T. (1974), Response of *Achlya ambisexualis* E 87 to the hormone antheridiol and certain other steroids. *J. gen. Microbiol.,* **82**, 295−299.

Beck, W.A. and Joly, R.A. (1941), Some growth phenomena in cultured pollen tubes. *Trans. Am. Micros. Soc.,* **60**, 149−162.

Berthold, G. (1881), Die geschlechtliche Fortpflanzung der eigentlichen Phaeosporen. *Mitth. Zod. Stat. Neapel,* **2**, 401−413.

Blakeslee, A.F. (1904), Sexual reproduction in the *Mucorineae. Proc. natn. Acad. Sci. U.S.A.,* **40**, 205−319.

Blondel, B. and Turian, G. (1960), Relation between basophilia and fine structure of the cytoplasm in the fungus *Allomyces macrogynus* Em. *J. Biophys. Biochem. Cytol.,* **7**, 127−134.

Brewbaker, J.L. (1957), Pollen cytology and self-incompatibility systems in plants. *J. Hered.,* **48**, 271−277.

Brewbaker, J.L. and Kwack, B.H. (1963), The essential role of calcium ion in pollen germination and pollen tube growth. *Am. J. Bot.,* **50**, 859−865.

Brink, R.A. (1924), The physiology of pollen. IV. Chemotropism: effects on growth of grouping grains; formation and function of callose plugs; summary and conclusions. *Am. J. Bot.,* **11**, 417−436.

Brokaw, C.J. (1957), 'Electro-chemical' orientation of bracken spermatozoids. *Nature,* **179**, 525.

Brokaw, C.J. (1958a), Chemotaxis of bracken spermatozoids. The role of bimalate ions. *J. exp. Biol.,* **35**, 192−196.

Brokaw, C.J. (1958b), Chemotaxis of bracken spermatozoids. Implications of electrochemical orientation. *J. exp. Biol.,* **35,** 197–212.

Brokaw, C.J. (1974), Calcium and flagellar response during the chemotaxis of bracken
spermatozoids. *J. Cell Physiol.,* **83,** 151–158.

Brooks, J. and Shaw, G. (1971), Recent developments in the chemistry, biochemistry,
geochemistry, and post-tetrad ontogeny of sporopollenins derived from pollen
and spore exines. In: *Pollen Development and Physiology.* (Heslop-Harrison, J.,
ed.), Butterworths, London, pp. 99–114.

Bruce, S.A. and Mascarenhas, J.P. (1977), Gene activity during zygote germination
and early sporophyte germling development in the aquatic fungus, *Allomyces
macrogynus. Exp. Mycol.,* **1,** 194–210.

Bu'Lock, J.D. (1976), Hormones in fungi. In: *The Filamentous Fungi.* (Smith, J.E. and
Berry, D.R., eds), Vol. 2, pp. 345–368, John Wiley, New York.

Bu'Lock, J.D., Drake, D. and Winstanley, D.J. (1972), Specificity and transformations
of the trisporic acid series of fungal sex hormones. *Phytochemistry,* **11,**
2011–2018.

Bu'Lock, J.D., Winskill, N. and Jones, B.E. (1974), Structures of the mating type-
specific prohormones of Mucorales. *Chem. Comm.,* 708–709.

Burgeff, H. (1924), Untersuchungen über Sexualität und Parasitismus bei Mucorineen.
Botanische Abhandlungen (Goebel, K., ed.), **4,** 1–135.

Butler, E.J. (1911), On *Allomyces,* a new aquatic fungus. *Ann. Bot.,* **25,** 1023–1035.

Caglioti, L., Cainelli, G., Camerino, B., Mondelli, R., Prieto, A., Quilico, A.,
Salvatori, T. and Selva, A. (1967), The structure of trisporic acid–C acid.
Tetrahedron, Suppl., **7,** 175–187.

Cainelli, G., Grasselli, P. and Selva, A. (1967), Struttura dell'acido trisporico B.
Chimica e l'industria (Milano) **49,** 628–629.

Carlile, M.J. and Machlis, L. (1965), A comparative study of the chemotaxis of the
motile phases of *Allomyces. Am. J. Bot.,* **52,** 484–486.

Christ, B. (1959), Entwicklungshichtliche und physiologische Untersuchungen über
die Selbsterilität von *Cardamine pratensis* L. *Z. Bot.,* **47,** 88–112.

Clarke, A.E., Harrison, S., Knox, R.B., Raff, J., Smith, P. and Marchalonis, J.J. (1977),
Common antigens and male-female recognition in plants. *Nature,* **265,**
161–163.

Cook, A.H. and Elvidge, J.A. (1951), Fertilization in the Fucaceae: investigations
on the nature of the chemotactic substance produced by eggs of *Fucus serratus*
and *F. vesiculosus, Proc. R. Soc. Ser. B.,* **138,** 97–114.

Cook, A.H., Elvidge, J.A. and Heilbron, I. (1948), Fertilization including chemotactic
phenomena in the Fucaceae. *Proc. R. Soc. Ser. B.,* **135,** 293–301.

Cook, F.S. and Walden, D.B. (1967), The male gametophyte of *Zea mays L. II.* The
influence of temperature and calcium on pollen germination and tube growth.
Can. J. Bot., **45,** 605–613.

Dashek, W.V. and Rosen, W.G. (1966), Electron microscopical localization of
chemical components in the growth zone of lily pollen tubes. *Protoplasma,* **61,**
192–204.

de Nettancourt, D. (1977), *Incompatibility in Angiosperms.* Springer-Verlag,
New York, Berlin.

Dickinson, H.G. and Lewis, D. (1973a), Cytochemical and ultrastructural differences
between intraspecific compatible and incompatible pollinations in *Raphanus.
Proc. R. Soc. Lond. Ser. B.,* **183,** 21–38.

Dickinson, H.G. and Lewis, D. (1973b), The formation of the tryphine coating the pollen grains of *Raphanus* and its properties relating to the self-incompatibility system. *Proc. R. Soc. Lond. Ser. B.,* **184**, 149−165.

Duckett, J.G. and Racey, P.A. (eds) (1975), *The Biology of the Male Gamete.* Academic Press, London.

Edwards, J.A., Mills, J.S., Sundeen, J. and Fried, J.H. (1969), The synthesis of the fungal sex hormone antheridiol. *J. Am. Chem. Soc.,* **91**, 1248−1249.

Edwards, J.A., Sundeen, J., Salmond, W., Iwadare, T. and Fried, J.H. (1972), A new synthetic route to the fungal sex hormone antheridiol and the determination of its absolute stereochemistry. *Tetrahedron Letters,* **9**, 791−794.

Emerson, R. (1941), An experimental study of the life cycles and taxonomy of *Allomyces. Lloydia,* **4**, 77−144.

Emerson, R. and Wilson, C.M. (1954), Interspecific hybrids and the cytogenetics and cytotaxonomy of *Euallomyces. Mycologia,* **56**, 393−434.

Esau, K. (1953), *Plant Anatomy.* John Wiley, New York.

Esau, K. (1977), *Anatomy of Seed Plants.* John Wiley, New York.

Glenk, H.O., Wagner, W. and Schimmer, O. (1971), Can Ca^{2+} ions act as a chemotropic factor in *Oenothera* fertilization? In: *Pollen: Development and Physiology,* Heslop-Harrison, J. ed)., Butterworths, London, pp. 255−261.

Gooday, G.W. (1968), Hormonal control of sexual reproduction in *Mucor mucedo. New Phytol.,* **67**, 815−821.

Gooday, G.W. (1972), Fungal sex hormones. *Biochem. J.,* **127**, 2P−3P. .

Gooday, G.W. (1975), Chemotaxis and chemotropism in fungi and algae. In: *Primitive Sensory and Communication Systems.* Carlile, M.J. ed), pp. 155−204, Academic Press, London, New York.

Groner, B., Hynes, N., Sippel, A.E. and Schutz, G. (1976), Induction of specific proteins in hyphae of *Achlya ambisexualis* by the steroid hormone antheridiol. *Nature,* **261**, 599−601.

Hanstein, J. (1865−1866), *Jahrb. Wiss. Botan.,* **4**, 197 (as quoted by Machlis and Rawitscher-Kunkel, 1967).

Hartmann, M. (1934), Untersuchungen über die Sexualität von *Ectocarpus siliculosus. Arch. Protistenk.,* **83**, 110−153.

Hatch, W.R. (1938), Conjugation and zygote germination in *Allomyces arbuscula. Ann. Bot. N.S.,* **2**, 583−614.

Hepden, P.M. and Hawker, L.E. (1961), A volatile substance controlling early stages of zygospore formation in *Rhizopus sexualis. J. gen. Microbiol.,* **24**, 155−164.

Heslop-Harrison, J. (1975a), Male gametophyte selection and the pollen-stigma interaction. In: *Gamete Competition in Plants and Animals.* (Mulcahy, D.L. ed.), North-Holland, Amsterdam, pp. 177−190.

Heslop-Harrison, J. (1975b), Incompatibility and the pollen-stigma interaction. *Ann. Rev. Plant. Physiol.,* **26**, 403−425.

Heslop-Harrison, J. and Heslop-Harrison, Y. (1975), Enzymic removal of the proteinaceous pellicle of the stigma papilla prevents pollen tube entry in the Caryophyllaceae. *Ann. Bot.,* **39**, 163−165.

Heslop-Harrison, J., Heslop-Harrison, Y. and Barber, J. (1975), The stigma surface in incompatibility responses. *Proc. R. Soc. Lond. Ser. B.,* **188**, 287−297.

Heslop-Harrison, J., Heslop-Harrison, Y., Knox, R.B. and Howlett, B. (1973), Pollen wall proteins: gametophytic and sporophytic fractions in the pollen walls of the Malvaceae. *Ann. Bot.,* **37**, 403—412.

Heslop-Harrison, J., Knox, R.B. and Heslop-Harrison, Y. (1974), Pollen wall proteins: exine held fraction associated with the incompatibility response in Cruciferae. *Theoret. Appl. Genet.,* **44**, 133—137.

Horenstein, E.A. and Cantino, E.C. (1969), Fungi. In: *Fertilization.* (Metz, C.B. and Monroy, A., eds), Vol. 2, pp. 95—133, Academic Press, New York and London.

Horgen, P.A. (1977), Cytosol—hormone stimulation of transcription in the aquatic fungus *Achlya ambisexualis. Biochem. biophys. Res. Comm.,* **75**, 1022—1028.

Horgen, P.A., Smith, R., Silver, J.C. and Craig, G. (1975), Hormonal stimulation of ribosomal RNA synthesis in *Achlya ambisexualis. Can. J. Biochem.,* **53**, 1341—1345.

Horowitz, D.K. and Russell, P.J. (1974), Hormone-induced differentiation of antheridial branches in *Achlya ambisexualis:* dependence on ribonucleic acid synthesis. *Can. J. Microbiol.,* **20**, 977—980.

Howlett, B.J., Knox, R.B. and Heslop-Harrison, J. (1973), Pollen wall proteins: release of the allergen antigen ε from intine and exine sites in pollen grains of ragweed and cosmos. *J. Cell Sci.,* **13**, 603—619.

Howlett, B.J., Knox, R.B., Paxton, J.D. and Heslop-Harrison, J. (1975), Pollen-wall proteins: physiochemical characterization and role in self-incompatibility in *Cosmos bipinnatus. Proc. R. Soc. Lond. Ser. B.,* **188**, 167—182.

Hubscher, T. and Eisen, A.H. (1972), Localization of ragweed antigens in the intact ragweed pollen grain. *Int. Arch. Allergy Appl. Immunol.,* **42**, 466—473.

Iwanami, Y. (1959), Physiological studies of pollen. *J. Yokohama Municipal Univ.,* **116**, [C—34, Biol—13], 1—137.

Jaenicke, L. (1977), Sex hormones of brown algae. *Naturwissenschaften,* **64**, 69—75.

Jaenicke, L., Akintobi, T. and Müller, D.G. (1971), Synthesis of the sex attractant of *Ectocarpus siliculosus. Angew. Chem., Int. edn.,* **10**, 492—493.

Jaenicke, L., Müller, D.J. and Moore, R.E. (1974), Multifidene and aucantene, C_{11} hydrocarbons in the male-attracting essential oil from the gynogametes of *Cutleria multifida* (Smith) Grev. (Phaeophyta). *J. Am. Chem. Soc.,* **96**, 3324—3325.

Jaenicke, L. and Seferiadis, K. (1975), Die Stereochemie von Fucoserraten, dem Gameten-Lockstoff der Braunalga *Fucus serratus* L. *Chem. Ber.,* **108**, 225—232.

Jensen, W.A. (1972), The embryo sac and fertilization in angiosperms. Univ. of Hawaii, H.L. Lyon, Arboretum Lecture No. 3, 1—31.

Kane, B.E., Reiskind, J.B. and Mullins, J.T. (1973), Hormonal control of sexual morphogenesis in *Achlya*: dependence on protein and ribonucleic acid synthesis. *Science,* **180**, 1192—1193.

Knowlton, H.E. (1922), Studies in pollen, with special reference to longevity. *Cornell Univ. Agri. Expt. Sta. Mem.,* **52**, 746—793.

Knox, R.B. (1971), Pollen wall proteins: localization, enzymic and antigenic activity during development in gladiolus (Iridaceae). *J. Cell Sci.,* **9**, 209—237.

Knox, R.B. (1973), Pollen wall proteins: pollen stigma interactions in ragweed and cosmos (Compositae). *J. Cell Sci.,* **12**, 421–443.

Knox, R.B., Clarke, A., Harrison, S., Smith, P. and Manchalonis, J.J. (1976), Cell recognition in plants: determinants of the stigma surface and their pollen interactions. *Proc. natn. Acad. Sci. U.S.A.,* **73**, 2788–2792.

Knox, R.B. and Heslop-Harrison, J. (1969), Cytochemical localization of enzymes in the wall of the pollen grain. *Nature,* **223**, 92–94.

Knox, R.B. and Heslop-Harrison, J. (1970), Pollen wall proteins: localization and enzymic activity. *J. Cell Sci.,* **6**, 1–27.

Knox, R.B. and Heslop-Harrison, J. (1971a), Pollen wall proteins: electron microscopic localization of acid phosphatase in the intine of *Crocus vernus. J. Cell Sci.,* **8**, 727–733.

Knox, R.B. and Heslop-Harrison, J. (1971b), Pollen wall proteins: The fate of intine-held antigens on the stigma in compatible and incompatible pollinations of *Phalaris tuberosa. J. Cell Sci.,* **9**, 239–251.

Knox, R.B. and Heslop-Harrison, J. (1971c), Pollen wall proteins: localization of antigenic and allergenic proteins in the pollen grain walls of *Ambrosia* spp. (ragweeds). *Cytobios,* **4**, 49–54.

Knox, R.B., Heslop-Harrison, J. and Heslop-Harrison, Y. (1975), Pollen-wall proteins: localization and characterization of gametophytic and sporophytic fractions. In: *Biology of the Male Gamete,* (Duckett, J.G. and Racey, P.A., eds), Academic Press, London, pp. 177–187.

Knox, R.B., Heslop-Harrison, J. and Reed, C. (1970), Localization of antigens associated with the pollen grain wall by immunofluorescence. *Nature,* **225**, 1066–1068.

Konar, R.N. and Linskens, H.F. (1966), The morphology and anatomy of the stigma of *Petunia hybrida. Planta,* **71**, 356–371.

Kroh, M. (1964), An electron microscopic study of the behavior of *Cruciferae* pollen after pollination. In: *Pollen Physiology and Fertilization,* (Linskens, H.F., ed.), North-Holland, Amsterdam, pp. 221–224.

Kroh, M., Miki-Hirosige, H., Rosen, W.G. and Loewus, F. (1970), Incorporation of label into pollen tube walls from myoinositol-labeled *Lilium longiflorum* pistils. Plant Physiol., **45**, 92–94.

Kwack, B. (1969), Chemotropic growth of *Clivia* and *Crinum* pollen towards pistils as influenced by calcium action. *Korean J. Hort. Sci.,* **6**, 81–84.

Lewis, D. (1976), Incompatibility in flowering plants. In: *Receptors and Recognition.* Ser. A., Vol. 2 (Cuatrecasas, P. and Greaves, M.F., eds), Chapman and Hall, London, pp. 165–198.

Linck, A.J. and Blaydes, G.W. (1960), Demonstration of the chemotropism of pollen tubes *in vitro* in four plant species. *Ohio J. Sci.,* **60**, 274–278.

Linskens, H.F. and Esser, K. (1959), Stoffaufnahme der Pollenschläuche aus dem Leitgewebe des griffels. *Proc. Kon. Ned. Akad. Wetensch.,* Amsterdam C62:150.

Lovett, J.S. (1963), Chemical and physical characterization of 'nuclear caps' isolated from *Blastocladiella* zoospores. *J. Bact.,* **85**, 1235–1246.

Machlis, L. (1958a), Evidence for a sexual hormone in *Allomyces. Physiol. Plant.,* **11**, 181–192.

Machlis, L. (1958b), A procedure for the purification of sirenin. *Nature,* **181,** 1790–1791.

Machlis, L. (1958c), A study of sirenin, the chemotactic sexual hormone from the watermold *Allomyces. Physiol. Plant.,* **11,** 845–854.

Machlis, L. (1969a), Zoospore chemotaxis in the watermold *Allomyces. Physiol. Plant,* **22,** 126–139.

Machlis, L. (1969b), Fertilization induced chemotaxis in the zygotes of the watermold *Allomyces. Physiol. Plant,* **22,** 392–400.

Machlis, L. (1972), The coming of age of sex hormones in plants. *Mycologia,* **64,** 235–247.

Machlis, L. (1973a), The chemotactic activity of various sirenins and analogues and the uptake of sirenin by the sperm of *Allomyces.* Plant Physiol., **52:** 527–530.

Machlis, L. (1973b), Factors affecting the stability and accuracy of the bioassay for the sperm attractant sirenin. *Plant Physiol.,* **52,** 524–526.

Machlis, L., Nutting, W.H. and Rapoport, H. (1968), The stucture of sirenin. *J. Am. Chem. Soc.,* **90,** 1674–1676.

Machlis, L. and Rawitscher-Kunkel, E. (1967), Mechanisms of gametic approach in plants. In: *Fertilization,* (Metz, C.B. and Monroy, A., eds), Vol. **1,** pp. 117–161, Academic Press, New York.

Machlis, L., Nutting, W.H., Williams, W.H. and Rapoport, H. (1966), Production, isolation, and characterization of sirenin. *Biochemistry,* **5,** 2147–2152.

Mascarenhas, J.P. (1966), The distribution of ionic calcium in the tissues of the gynoecium of *Antirrhinum majus. Protoplasma,* **62,** 53–58.

Mascarenhas, J.P. (1973), Pollen tube chemotropism. In: *Behavior of Microorganisms.* (Perez-Miravete, A., coord.), Plenum Press, London, New York, pp. 62–69.

Mascarenhas, J.P. (1975), The biochemistry of angiosperm pollen development. *Bot. Rev.,* **41,** 259–305.

Macarenhas, J.P. and Machlis, L. (1962a), The hormonal control of the directional growth of pollen tubes. *Vitamins and Hormones.* **20,** 347–372.

Mascarenhas, J.P. and Machlis, L. (1962b), The pollen tube chemotropic factor from *Antirrhinum majus*: bioassay, extraction, and partial purification. *Am. J. Bot.,* **49,** 482–489.

Mascarenhas, J.P. and Machlis, L. (1962c), Chemotropic response of *Antirrhinum majus* pollen to calcium. *Nature,* **196,** 292–293.

Mascarenhas, J.P. and Machlis, L. (1964), Chemotropic response of the pollen of *Antirrhinum majus* to calcium. *Plant Physiol.,* **39,** 70–77.

McMorris, T.C., Arunachalam, T. and Seshadri, R. (1972), A practical synthesis of antheridiol. *Tetrahedron Letters,* **26,** 2673–2676.

McMorris, T.C. and Seshadri, R. (1971), Synthetic studies on antheridiol. *Chem. Comm.,* **24,** 1646.

McMorris, T.C., Seshadri, R., Weihe, G.R., Arsenault, G.P. and Barksdale, A.W. (1975), Structures of oogoniol −1, −2, and −3, steroidol sex hormones of the water mold, *Achlya. J. Am. Chem. Soc.,* **97,** 2544–2545.

McMorris, T.S. and White, R.H. (1977), Biosynthesis of the oogoniols, steroidol sex hormones of *Achlya*: The role of fucosterol. *Phytochemistry,* **16,** 359–362.

Mesland, D.A.M., Huisman, J.G. and van den Ende, H. (1974), Volatile sexual hormones in *Mucor mucedo. J. gen. Microbiol.,* **80**, 111–117.

Miki, H. (1954), A study of tropism of pollen tubes to the pistil. I. Tropism in *Lilium. Bot. Mag. Tokyo,* **67**, 143–147.

Miki, H. (1955), A study of tropism of pollen tubes to pistils II. Tropism in *Camellia sinensis. Bot. Mag. Tokyo,* **68**, 293–298.

Molisch, H. (1889), Über die Ursachen der Wachstumsrichtungen bei Pollenschläuchen. *Sitz. Math. Naturw. Kl. Akad. Wiss., Wien* (Anz. Akad. Wissensch.) Wien **28**, 11–13.

Müller, D.G. (1974), Sexual reproduction and isolation of a sex attractant in *Cutleria multifida* (Smith) Grev. (Phaeophyta) *Biochem. Physiol. Pflanzen,* (BPP), **165**, 212–215.

Müller, D.G. (1976), Quantitative evaluation of sexual chemotaxis in two marine brown algae. *Z. Pflanzenphysiol.,* **80**, 120–130.

Müller, D.G. and Jaenicke, L. (1973), Fucoserraten, the female sex attractant of *Fucus serratus* L. (Phaeophyta). *FEBS Letters,* **30**, 137–139.

Müller, D.G., Jaenicke, L., Donike, M. and Akintobi, T. (1971), Sex attractant in a brown alga: chemical structure. *Science,* **171**, 815–817.

Müller, D.G. and Seferiadis, K. (1977), Specificity of sexual chemotaxis in *Fucus serratus* and *Fucus vesiculosus* (Phaeophyceae) *Z. Pflanzenphysiol.,* **84**, 85–94.

Mullins, T.J. and Ellis, E.A. (1974), Sexual morphogenesis in *Achlya*: ultrastructural basis for the hormonal induction of antheridial hyphae. *Proc. natn. Acad. Sci. U.S.A.,* **71**, 1347–1350.

Nieuwenhuis, M. and van den Ende, H. (1975), Sex specificity of hormone synthesis in *Mucor mucedo. Arch. Microbiol.,* **102**, 167–169.

Pfeffer, W. (1884), Locomotorische Richtungsbewegungen durch chemischen Reize. *Untersuch. Botan. Inst.,* Tubingen, **1**, 364–482.

Plattner, J.J., Bhalerao, U.T. and Rapoport, H. (1969), Synthesis of *dl*-sirenin. *J. Am. Chem. Soc.,* **91**, 4933.

Plattner, J.J. and Rapoport, H. (1971), The synthesis of *d*- and *l*-sirenin and their absolute configurations. *J. Am. Chem. Soc.,* **93**, 1758–1761.

Plempel, M. (1957), Die Sexualstoffe der Mucoraceae. *Arch. Microbiol.,* **26**, 151–174.

Plempel, M. (1960), Die zygotropische Reaktion bei Mucorineen. I. *Planta,* **55**, 254–258.

Plempel, M. (1962), Die zygotropische Reaktion bei Mucorineen. III. *Planta,* **58**, 509–520.

Plempel, M. (1963), Die chemischen Grundlagen der Sexualreaktion bei Zygomyceten. *Planta,* **59**, 492–508.

Plempel, M. and Dawid, W. (1961), Die zygotropische Reaktion bei Mucorineen. II. *Planta,* **56**, 438–446.

Pommerville, J. (1977), Chemotaxis of *Allomyces gametes. Exp. Cell Res.,* **109**, 43–51.

Pommerville, J. and Fuller, M.S. (1976), The cytology of the gamete and fertilization of *Allomyces macrogynus. Arch. Microbiol.,* **109**, 21–30.

Popplestone, C.R. and Unrau, A.M. (1974), Studies on the biosynthesis of antheridiol. *Can. J. Chem.,* **52**, 462–468.

Prieto, A., Spalla, C., Bianchi, M. and Biffi, G. (1964), Biosynthesis of β-carotene by strains of Choanephoraceae. *Comm. 2nd Int. Fermentation Symp.,* London, p. 38.

Raper, J.R. (1939), Sexual hormones in *Achlya.* I. Indicative evidence for a hormonal coordinating mechanism. *Am. J. Bot.,* **26**, 639–650.

Raper, J.R. (1940), Sexual hormones in *Achlya.* II. Distance reactions, conclusive evidence for a hormonal coordinating mechanism. *Am. J. Bot.,* **27**, 162–173.

Raper, J.R. (1952), Chemical regulation of sexual processes in the thallophytes. *Bot. Rev.,* **18**, 447–545.

Reschke, T. (1969), Die Gamone aus *Blakeslea trispora.* Zur Struktur der Sexualstoffe aus Mucoraceae. I. *Tetrahedron Letters,* **39**, 3435–3439.

Rosen, W.G. (1961), Studies on pollen tube chemotropism. *Am. J. Bot.,* **48**, 889–895.

Rosen, W.G. (1964), Chemotropism and fine structure of pollen tubes. In: *Pollen Physiology and Fertilization.* (Linskens, H.F. ed), North-Holland, Amsterdam, pp. 159–166.

Rosen, W.G. (1971), Pistil-pollen interactions in *Lilium.* In: *Pollen: Development and Physiology.* (Heslop-Harrison, J. ed), Butterworths, London, pp. 239–254.

Rosen, W.G. (1975), Pollen/pistil interactions. In: *The Biology of the Male Gamete.* (Duckett, J.G. and Racey, P.A., eds), Academic Press, London, pp. 153–164.

Schildknecht, H. and Benoni, H. (1963a), Über die Chemie der Anziehung von Oenotheren. *Z. Naturforsch.,* **18b**, 45–54.

Schildknecht, H. and Benoni, H. (1963b), Versuche zur Aufklärung des Pollenschlauch-Chemotropismus von Narcissen. *Z. Naturforsch.,* **18b**, 656–661.

Silver, J.C. and Horgen, P.A. (1974), Hormonal regulation of presumptive mRNA in the fungus *Achlya ambisexualis. Nature,* **294**, 252–254.

Smith, G.M. (1955), *Cryptogamic Botany.* Vol. 1. *Algae and Fungi.* McGraw-Hill Book, C., New York.

Strasburger, E. (1868), *Bot. Ztg.,* **26**, 822 (as quoted by Machlis and Rawitscher-Kunkel, 1967).

Strasburger, E. (1869–1870), *Jahrb. Wiss. Botan.,* **7**, 390 (as quoted by Machlis and Rawitscher-Kunkel, 1967).

Sutter, R.P. (1970), Trisporic acid synthesis in *Blakeslea trispora. Science,* **168**, 1590–1592.

Sutter, R.P., Capage, D.A., Harrison, T.L. and Keen, W.A. (1973), Trisporic acid biosynthesis in separate plus and minus cultures of *Blakeslea trispora:* identification by *Mucor* assay of two mating type-specific components. *J. Bact.,* **114**, 1074–1082.

Sutter, R.P., Harrison, T.L. and Galasko, G. (1974), Trisporic acid biosynthesis in *Blakeslea trispora* via mating type-specific precursors. *J. biol. Chem.,* **249**, 2282–2284.

Thomas, D. des S. and Mullins, J.T. (1967), Role of enzymatic wall-softening in plant morphogenesis: hormonal induction in *Achlya. Science,* **156**,84–85.

Thomas, D. des S. and Mullins, J.T. (1969), Cellulase induction and wall extension in the water mold *Achlya ambisexualis. Physiol. Plant,* **22**, 347–353.

Timberlake, W.E. (1976), Alterations in RNA and protein synthesis associated with steroid hormone-induced sexual morphogenesis in the water mold *Achlya. Dev. Biol.,* **51**, 202–214.

Tsao, T. (1949), A study of chemotropism of pollen tubes *in vitro*. *Plant Physiol.,* **24**, 494—504.

Tsinger, N.V. and Petrovskaya-Baranova, T.P. (1961), The pollen grain wall — a living physiologically active structure. *Doklady Akad. Nauk. SSSR,* **138**, 466—469.

Turian, C. (1955), Sur la nature ribonucleique du corps para nucleaire et ses relations avec la differenciation du sexe chez *Allomyces javanicus. C. R. Acad. Sci. Ser. D.,* **240**, 2344—2349.

van den Ende, H. (1967), Sexual factor of the Mucorales. *Nature,* **215**, 211—212.

van den Ende, H. (1968), Relationship between sexuality and carotene synthesis in *Blakeslea trispora. J. Bact.,* **96**, 1298—1303.

van den Ende, H. (1976), *Sexual Interactions in Plants.* Academic Press, New York.

van den Ende, H. and Stegwee, D. (1971), Physiology of sex in Mucorales. *Bot. Rev.,* **37**, 22—36.

van den Ende, H., Wiechmann, A.H.C.A., Reyngoud, D.J. and Hendriks, T. (1970), Hormonal interactions in *Mucor mucedo* and *Blakeslea trispora. J. Bact.,* **101**, 423—428.

van den Ende, H., Werkman, B.A. and van den Briel, M.L. (1972), Trisporic acid synthesis in mated cultures of the fungus *Blakeslea trispora. Arch. Mikrobiol.,* **86**, 175—184.

Werkman, B.A. (1976), Localization and partial characterization of a sex-specific enzyme in homothallic and heterothallic Mucorales. *Arch. Microbiol.,* **109**, 209—213.

Werkman, B.A. and van den Ende, H. (1973), Trisporic acid synthesis in *Blakeslea trispora*. Interaction between *plus* and *minus* mating types. *Arch. Mikrobiol.,* **90**, 365—374.

Wiese, L. (1969), Algae. In: *Fertilization.* (Metz, C.B. and Monroy, A., eds), Vol. 2, pp. 135—188, Academic Press, New York and London.

7 Insect Pheromones

ERNST KRAMER

Taxis and Behavior
(*Receptors and Recognition,* Series B, Volume 5)
Edited by G.L. Hazelbauer
Published in 1978 by Chapman and Hall, 11 New Fetter Lane, London EC4P 4EE
© Chapman and Hall

'Chemical substances secreted to the outside by an individual and received by a second individual of the same species, in which they release a specific reaction', is the definition of pheromones as given by Karlson and Butenandt (1959), who also proposed the name 'pheromone'. The similarity between pheromones and hormones — the latter acting in a comparable manner but within a single individual — was already seen in 1932 by Bethe who called these chemicals 'ectohormones'. Although this name seems to be good because it is self-explanatory the prefix ecto- partly contradicts the meaning of hormone since hormones by definition are produced by endocrine glands.

Surprisingly, hormones were given a collective name long before the pheromones— the name hormones goes back to Bayliss and Starling (1912) — though the existence of pheromones has been well known since at least the end of the 19th century. At this time there were many reports by lepidopterists who observed that male butter-flies and moths are attracted by the scent of females. One observation of Riese published by Noll (1869) may be cited here. 'Riese, who lived in the midst of the older part of the town in a narrow, crowded lane, placed a crippled female of *Lasiocampa prunei* outside the window together with some caterpillar boxes. He enjoyed watching the exposed female, surrounded by fluttering males, which were a welcome booty for the collector. In this case the chances of the sexes meeting was rather low, the female being sequestered within the town and this species being extremely rare in that region. If the animals in this case were guided by their smell — and what else is imaginable — what should we be more astonished about, the male's delicacy of sense or the immense divisibility of matter emanating from the female?'

For a long time, lepidopterists have used traps baited with females to attract and catch conspecific males. The efficacy of this method is not reduced when the females are hidden such that visual cues are excluded. This led to the conclusion that the attraction is based on chemical emanations. Furthermore it was known that these emanations differ between species since only males of the same species were lured. Dubois (1896) proposed using this fact to crossbreed closely related species which, under normal conditions, will not mate, by deceiving the males with females scented with the secretions of conspecifics. Breeders of silk worms also knew about the chemical attractiveness of the females: they surmised that the odour emanates from a paired organ which 'calling' females extrude from their abdomen. In addition there is a striking dimorphism in the structure of the antennae in many species of lepidoptera. Those of the males appear better developed for the perception of odours. Hence at the end of the 19th century, all the points included in the

1932 definition of ectohormones were known. Nevertheless, little attention was given to this kind of communication system.

In fact, at that time, the investigation of such a phenomenon seemed to be hopeless. On the one hand there were reports in which the distance over which some butterflies lured their males was claimed to be in the order of kilometres, though a human nose could not smell anything even when close to the female gland. It was obvious that almost infinitesimal dilution of these substances can alert males, and moreover, will suffice to guide them to the source. On the other hand, the state of art of chemistry before the late 1950's was such that chemical analysis required quantities far too great to be practicable for the analysis of insect scents.

Three circumstances then led to an explosive increase of efforts and knowledge in this field. The first was the refinement of analytical methods in chemistry especially the development of gas chromatography and mass spectrometry. These reduced the quantities needed for an analysis to the order of micrograms. As a consequence, in 1959, the first pheromone was identified by Butenandt. The extract of some hundred thousand silk moth (*Bombyx mori*) glands were needed for the analysis. The substance was found to be (E)-10, (Z)-12-hexadecadien-1-ol, and it was given the name bombykol. The identification was soon followed by a synthesis of the compound. From that time, the silk moth became a favourite 'guinea pig' in pheromone research.

Like the first, the second development which promoted pheromone research was an advance in methodology. Several electrophysiologists succeeded in recording receptor potentials from olfactory sensilla on insect antennae (Roys, 1954; Schneider, 1955; Boistel *et al.*, 1956). Stimulating isolated silk moth antennae with an extract of female glands, Schneider and Hecker (1956) obtained nerve impulses as well as summed potentials. The latter they called 'EAG' (electroantennogram) in analogy to EKG, EEG and EMG.

The third circumstance is of more complex character and is connected to the growing environmental consciousness. Worldwide, people were becoming concerned about the unrestricted and thoughtless application of pesticides, which not only endanger human health but disturb the balance of ecological systems by their non-specificity of effect. Pheromones, which in the meantime had been found in a great number of pest insects, offered a new means of control. It appeared possible to attack pest insects specifically either by luring the males into traps baited with the appropriate pheromone or confusing their orienting system by application of an excessive amount of pheromone over the region to be protected.

Within the past twenty years a great number of pheromones have been chemically identified. A comprehensive list has been recently compiled by Inscoe and Beroza (1976). Pheromone receptors must be very sensitive since single molecules suffice to evoke a response (Kaissling and Priesner, 1970). This sensitivity is combined with a similarly high specificity; even very closely related compounds are often orders of magnitude less effective. Availability of pure pheromone allows an estimation of the rate of emmission from female glands. This in combination with data on the receptor thresholds has made possible calculations of the distances over which pheromones may be effective (Bossert and Wilson, 1963). Investigations of the mechanisms by which the animals are guided when orienting to a pheromone source have also been facilitated by using pure pheromones.

On the molecular level progress in pheromone research has been less impressive. Little is known about how a pheromone is recognized by the 'acceptor' on the receptor membrane or how the pheromone—acceptor interaction results in a change in membrane conductivity. In this regard there are some promising hypotheses but as yet no convincing biochemical results.

Compared to the original optimism, practical results in pest control are somewhat disappointing. An effective way to control a pest insect solely by the application of pheromones has not yet been found. However, pheromones have proved to be a useful tool in monitoring population densities, so that application of pesticides can be reduced to cases of serious infestation.

Up to this point we have dealt exclusively with sex pheromones — also called sex attractants — but there are others just as important and widespread. Ants and termites mark their trails with trail pheromones or alert their nest mates in case of danger with alarm pheromones. Cockroaches, bedbugs and other insects secrete aggregation pheromones. Honeybees invite their hive mates to follow by fanning backward an airstream laden with a special odour. The architecture of termite hills seems to be determined to a great extent by the flow and diffusion of pheromones. One phero- mone can have multiple functions. For example the pheromone of the honeybee queen attracts drones during the nuptial flight, keeps together swarming bees and inhibits development of the rudimentary ovaries in worker bees.

Pheromones, however, are not restricted to insects. Many mammals mark their territories with the secretion of a special gland or actively scent their trails in order to signal their presence to conspecifics. Males are sexually excited by the urine or vaginal secretions of estrous females. The reproduction of mice is controlled by several 'primer pheromones'. Unlike releaser pheromones, which elicit more or less innate behavioural responses, primer pheromones act on the endocrine system of the receiver changing their physiological state over longer spans of time.

Though there are numerous observations indicating the important role of phero- mones in vertebrates, knowledge has not progressed to a state comparable to that in arthropods. Mammalian pheromones generally seem to consist of a rather complex bouquet of commonplace substances. Behavioural responses are much less stereotyped than in insect and therefore much more difficult to classify and quantify. The olfactory epithelium is not as easily accessible to microelectrodes as the superficial sensilla of arthropods, and receptor cells of different specificities are not morpholo- gically distinguishable.

The above shows the variety of problems in the field of pheromone research. A comprehensive review would not be within the scope of this book. In the following sections only a few aspects will be presented in more detail. For further information the reader is referred to reviews recently written or edited by Priesner (1973), Birch (1974) and Shorey and McKelvey (1977).

7.2 SPECIAL FEATURES OF CHEMICAL COMMUNICATION

7.2.1 Physical properties of pheromones

The molecular weights of pheromones chemically identified lie in the range between 74 and ca. 300. Most of them belong to classes with a rather simple structure such as aliphatic hydrocarbons without any functional group (e.g. undecan, an alarm pheromone of several formicid ants) (Bergström and Löfquist, 1968, 1970; Dumpert, 1972), alcohols, esters, aldehydes, ketones and acids. The carrier of these functional groups is aliphatic, either saturated or unsaturated, or aromatic. More exotic substances have also been found e.g. epoxides (Bierl *et al.,* 1970), pyrrolizidone (Meinwald *et al.,* 1969), dichlorphenol (Berger, 1972).

The boiling points range between 150 and 250°C, hence the vapour pressure under normal conditions is between 9 and 0.2 mbar. However, there are some exceptions to this rule. Many alarm pheromones have boiling points as low as 100°C (hexenal, formic acid, dimethysulfide). Due to their high volatility they spread rapidly and only last a short time. Such a correlation may exist for trail pheromones as well, in this case between the need for persistance and pheromone volatility, but too few of these substances have been chemically identified. Pheromones which act over greater distances commonly have boiling points between 200 and 250°C.

Whenever thorough chemical analyses of pheromones have been carried out, it has been shown that mixtures of at least two components are produced, rather than single substances. Commonly the different components are all active as pheromones, but there are cases in which some are not perceived by the pheromone receiver. In those cases the boiling point of the inactive substances is rather high; thus these components probably serve to reduce the emission rate of the behaviourally active substance(s). Also not yet understood is the function of so-called 'pheromone particles' as occur in some danaid butterflies. Their sex pheromone danaidone is produced by males and acts as a aphrodisiac. Danaidone is carried by a fine powder which the male dusts over the female during the courtship flight (Schneider *et al.,* 1975).

Though many pheromones have one or more double-bonded oxygen atoms they are relatively stable. There is no evidence that the substances decompose during the aerial phase such that the active area would be markedly reduced by this kind of loss. A significant reduction can result from adsorption to surfaces. This can be demonstrated dramatically by passing an airstream leaden with bombykol through a small cotton pad. Such treated air is almost free of the pheromone and no longer arouses males.

7.2.2 The propagation of chemical signals

In visual and acoustical communication systems the linear propagation of waves allows location of the signal source over considerable distances by rather simple structures guiding the signal to the receptors. This is not true for communication systems using diffusing chemicals as a signal. Evaporating or dissolving molecules have a considerable velocity and would move away from the source linearly if no other molecules hindered their way. But in fluids and gases of normal pressure a released molecule collides with other molecules and changes direction billions of times per second and thus has a mean free path shorter than a micron. The original direction of the molecule is lost almost immediately and the net velocity of the molecule is very small compared to the instantaneous velocity. Hence chemical communication by release of a substance in still air or water can work only over distances of centimeters or over long time periods. The limits of molecular diffusion are easily overcome by small movements of the medium which are the rule in nature. Therefore, in most cases propagation of the signal is determined predominantly by flow of the medium. Since this flow is of a very complex nature under normal conditions it is not possible to direct transmission to a certain destination nor to prevent the concentration from being modulated by irregularities in flow. This almost precludes the use of intentional modulations of the signal intensity in order to increase the flow of information (Bossert, 1968).

Undisturbed molecular diffusion will occur only in small, completely enclosed compartments and there only in the absence of small spatial differences of temperature which would produce convection streams.

If a chemical is released in moving air or water its distribution depends on the degree of turbulence in the medium. In laminar streams, which are rather exceptional in nature and occur only in very slowly streaming media, the resulting odour plumes are very narrow. The plumes widen only as a result of molecular diffusion; hence the concentration decreases with distance from the central axis following a Gaussian function. However, the body of an animal exposing an endocrine gland in the stream will destroy the laminar flow. The resulting eddies then disturb the even distribution at the very beginning of the plume. Though these eddies fade out while travelling down the stream the discontinuities do not. Hence at any point downwind from the source the odour concentration fluctuates around a mean value. In turbulent streams, spreading of the odour depends on the size and frequency of eddies which in turn depend on the structure and number of obstacles upwind as well as on the speed of flow, (Aylor, 1976). Recent field experiments indicate active spaces in the 100 m range for the cabbage looper (Sower *et al.*, 1971) and the tobacco cutworm (Nakamura and Kawasaki, 1977).

7.3 THE RECEIVER SYSTEM

7.3.1 Morphology

Like all olfactory receptor cells the pheromone receptors are primary sense cells responsible for both the perception and transfer of information to the central nervous system by their own axons. All experimental results and the morphology indicate that the dendritic process of the sense cell is the receptive area.

In insects the dendrite lies in a thin-walled structure of the cuticule and communicates with ambient air or water by means of pores penetrating the cuticule. The gap between the dendritic membrane and the cuticule is filled with the dendritic liquor. The dendrite itself is divided into two parts by a ciliary structure. This ciliary structure, the 'neck' is closely related to those in motor cilia. In both cases, they are based on the structure of a centriole. The characteristic element of centrioles is a circle of nine doublets of filaments around an axis of two additional filaments. Within the neck of olfactory cells in insects, however, this set of filaments is incomplete in that the cental axis is missing. Nevertheless, the outer segement with the neck can be viewed as a modified motor cilium in which the receptive area (the outer segment) corresponds to the shaft of a motor cilium. The outer segment is free of mitochondria. The only cell structures found in this region are vesicles and numerous microtubules. The length of the outer segment reaches 500 μm in Sphingids. The outer segment may or may not be branched.

Cell soma, axon and the proximal part of the dendrite do not significantly differ from other sensory cells. The nucleus is always large with respect to the size of the cell. The perikarion contains a normal set of cell organelles. Mitochondria are often accumulated in the proximal part of the dendrite. The axons are very thin (about 0.2 μm) and do not fuse or contact others by synapses in the periphery.

Unlike those of vertebrates the arthropod's olfactory cells are grouped within sensilla of varying architecture. Despite these variations in shape the underlying structure of the sensilla is always the same. Commonly a group consists of two to several tens of sensory cells surrounded by three auxiliary cells, which form an inner (thecogen), middle (trichogen) and outer (tormogen) sheath (Schmidt and Gnatzy, 1971; Steinbrecht and Müller, 1976). Besides the morphogenetic function of secreting the cuticular structures of the sensillum they are assumed to contribute to the generation of electric membrane potentials. This assumption is supported by the presence of gap junctions which electrically interconnect the auxiliary cells and by the strongly folded distal membranes of the trichogen and tormogen cells which are adjacent to the sensillum liquor (Thurm, 1969). (Fig. 7.1).

The sensilla of insects have been classified according to the form of the auxilliary structures of the cuticula. Sensilla of sensory modalities other than olfaction look very similar and are found intermingled with the olfactory sensilla. It is therefore hazardous to deduce the modality from form alone. However, a common feature of olfactory sensilla seems to be the presence of pores in the cuticule (for exceptions see Ernst and Altner, 1977). Tiny tubules connect these pores with the dendrite (Steinbrecht, 1973; Meinecke, 1975). Pores have been seen in sensilla trichodea, s. basiconica, s. coeloconica and s. placodea. The first are characterized by very long hairs. S. basiconica have shorter hairs, whereas in s. placodea the hair is reduced to a pore plate either lying in the same plane as the surrounding cuticula or forming the bottom of a depression of varying depth. Sensilla coeloconica have a hair within a pit.

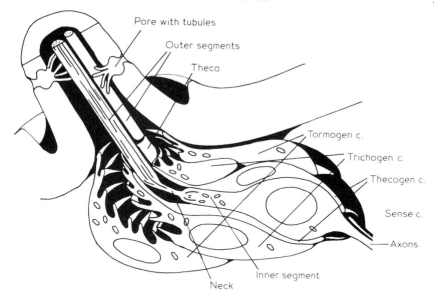

Fig. 7.1 Schema of a sensillum trichodeum illustrating characteristic elements of insect pheromone receptors (after Steinbrecht; Schmidt and Gnatzy).

Most olfactory sensilla are found on the antennae. Their total number on one antenna can sum up to severals tens of thousands, commonly of more than one olfactory type (silk moth: Steinbrecht, 1970; cockchafer: Meinecke, 1975; honeybee: Esslen and Kaissling, 1976).

The sensitivity of olfactory organs is determined largely by their ability to filter out molecules from the carrier medium. This can be achieved by either increasing the surface area of single receptors (long free-standing hairs) or by increasing the number of receptors. This demand is often incompatible with the other functions of the antennae. In the honeybee for example many kinds of odours and several pheromones play an important role, but the antennae are not notably large nor do they bear long haired sensilla trichodea. S. placodea (pore plates) which are found in great numbers on the bee's antennae obviously are better protected against mechanical damage when the antennae serve largely as mechanical feelers.

The highest degree of specialization for the perception of pheromones is found in the antennae of several lepidopteran species. In these the activity of the male imago is reduced to searching for and mating with females. The antenna of the saturnid moth *Antheraea,* for example, has a profile area of about 1 cm². A stem with two rows of sidebranches form a structure like a feather the plane of which is exposed to the airstream. Each sidebranch in turn has two rows of sensilla trichodea with extremly long hairs (Fig. 7.2). The hairs are spaced such that their 'diffusion spaces' (the volume out of which molecules are caught by diffusion and adsorption) overlap. The

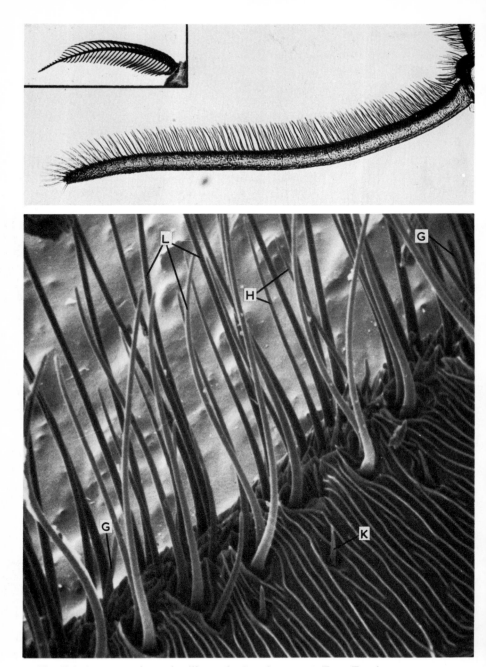

Fig. 7.2 Antenna of a male silk moth, *Bombyx mori*. Top: Total antenna.
Middle: Side branch with sensilla trichodea. Bottom: Detail from a side branch
showing long-haired sensilla trichodea. Shorter hairs belong to sensilla
coeloconica. (From Steinbrecht, 1973, courtesy of Springer Verlag, Hamburg).

whole antenna comprises a sieve which can collect most of the pheromone molecules from a penetrating airstream, as has been shown in quantitative experiments with the smaller but similarly built antenna of the silk moth *Bombyx mori* (Adam and Delbrück, 1968; Kaissling, 1971).

7.3.2 Methods of study

The only way of investigating the physiological properties of olfactory receptor cells is by recording of their response electrophysiologically. The first advances were in recording summed responses of numerous receptor cells in olfactory epithelia (Ottoson, 1956) and whole insect antennae (Roys, 1954; Schneider, 1955). One electrode was placed somewhere in a neutral part of the experimental animal's body, the second either in the olfactory epithelium or in the tip of the antenna. The time course of potentials obtained by this method is about the same as that of the applied stimulus. The origin of both the electro-olfatogram (EOG) and the electro-antennogram (EAG) is not fully understood. The most plausible explanation is that the ionic current flowing through the depolarized dendritic membrane induces compensating currents within the surrounding medium. These currents act like numerous batteries. Depending on their mutual positions these batteries are either connected in parallel or in series. This method is not adequate for the study of single receptor cells. It can only give information as to whether the olfactory organ as a whole is responsive to the applied test substance. Nevertheless, in insects having highly specialized antennae for the perception of pheromones this procedure is still an excellent tool. Priesner *et al.* (1975, 1977) predicted the chemical constitution of pheromone components in numerous noctuid and tortricid moth species by using the EAG method.

Measuring thresholds, specificity, dynamic properties, noise levels, adaptation and other characteristics of olfactory receptors requires recording from single units. By placing the electrode close to the somata of a sensillum basiconicum on the antenna of the carrion beetle Boeckh (1962) obtained the first data on single receptor types. This method allows for the recording of both slow receptor potentials and action potentials (spikes). It proved applicable in many insects and led especially to the elucidation of the specificity of a number of receptors (Lacher, 1964, 1967; Vareschi, 1971; Kaissling and Priesner, 1970; Kafka, 1970; Dumpert, 1972; Sass, 1976).

A further improvement in the technique of extracellular recording from sensilla trichodea was made by Kaissling (1974). The tip of the trichodeum is cut off and the recording capillary slipped over the hair. With this arrangement of electrodes a better insulation from the electrical activities of neighbouring sensilla is achieved. The technique is also applicable with rather short hairs (DenOtter, 1977). Nevertheless, it is still difficult to discriminate between the activities of more than two receptor cells belonging to the same sensillum. Intracellular recordings would solve many problems but due especially to the minuteness of the receptor cells intracellular recordings have been obtained only in a few accidental cases.

Though the amount of substances needed for modern microanalytical methods are unimaginably small, concentrations employed in pheromone communication are even smaller and in most cases cannot be directly monitored by these methods. Hence the pheromone concentration in experiments can be evaluated only by indirect methods. Usually, the airstream used for stimulation is passed over a piece of filter paper, glass or metal impregnated with a known quantity of the pheromone. The number of molecules emitted by this source can be calculated by using radioactively labelled pheromones (Boeckh, 1967; Kaissling and Priesner, 1970).

7.3.3 The specificity of receptor cells

Theoretically, there are two ways of recognizing olfactory signals. One uses receptor cells tuned such that they respond to one and only one chemical compound. A response of these receptors signals the presence of the compound without the need for further processing. A special receptor cell would be required for each biologically relevant odour. Olfactory organs organized exclusively according to this principle would be 'blind' for all odours for which there was no specific receptor cell. Since the number of volatile organic compounds is almost unlimited a 'general olfactory sense' can not be established in this way. However, because of their 'narrow bandwidth' such receptor cells can be enormously sensitive. Highly specialized receptors, therefore, appear especially well suited for the detection of pheromones.

The second way of recognizing olfactory signals is based on receptor cells which are sensitive to a wide 'spectrum' of substances. (One must be aware that the use of the term spectrum in this context differs from its usual meaning where it implies some order based upon the magnitude of one variable. As long as we do not know what physical parameter is 'read' by the receptor this term should be avoided.) Given a set of receptor cells having multiple, low specificities, each chemical compound to which at least two different cells respond produces a unique pattern of excitation. This pattern can be discriminated from others by a suitable process in the central nervous system. Olfactory systems organized according to this principle are able to sense and discriminate odours to which they are not specially adapted. The lower the specificity the more the receptors are affected by noise, i.e. excited by irrelevant odours, hence their sensitivity can not be as high as in the specialized type. Schneider *et al.* (1964) coined the term 'specialist' for the receptor type mentioned first and 'generalist' for the latter. However a clear separation between these two classes is not possible. All receptors lie somewhere between these extremes; neither specialists nor generalists in the strict sense are known.

The bombykol receptor on the silk moth's antenna comes very close to an ideal specialist. Minute changes in the structure of bombykol (E)-10, (Z)-12-hexadecadien-1-ol), such as an interchange of the *cis-* and *trans-* positions reduce the efficacy of the substance by a factor of 100 or more (Schneider *et al.,* 1967) (Fig. 7.3). The pheromone of the summerfruit moth *Adoxophyes orana* consists of a mixture (9:1) of (Z)-9-, and (Z)-11-tetradecen-1-ol-acetate (TDA). DenOtter (1977) using single cell

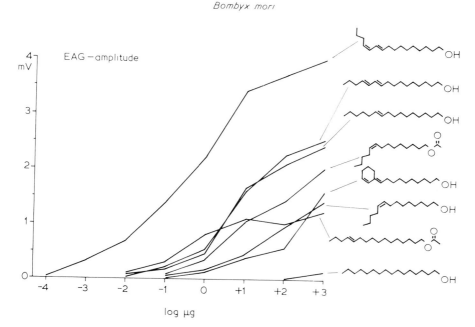

Bombyx mori

Fig. 7.3 EAG responses from the antenna of a male silk moth to bombykol and seven analogues (redrawn from Kaissling, 1974).

recordings found two receptors on the female antenna, one more sensitive to (Z)-9-TDA, the other to (Z)-11-TDA. In both cells the corresponding *trans* configurations ((E)-9-TDA, (E)-11-TDA, respectively), were at least one order of magnitude less effective. Single cell recordings from the pheromone receptor of the pine weevil *Hylobius abietis* also indicate a very high specificity (Mustaparta, 1975).

An extensive study on the problem of specificity was carried out by Priesner *et al.* (1974, 1977). The EAGs of some twenty species of Noctuidae, Tortricidae and Cochylidae, chosen because of their closely related pheromones (mainly alkenyl acetates) were recorded in response to both the corresponding pheromones and to each of several hundred analogues. These analogues were synthesized such as to vary systematically one parameter of structure, e.g. chain length, position of double bonds, number of double bonds etc. The response spectra obtained by this method come close to the above-mentioned correct meaning of this term. However, since these data were obtained by the EAG method it is not absolutely sure that the spectra belong to single receptor cells. Nevertheless, these results give not only a general survey of the specificity but also allow one to theorize about the nature of interactions between the pheromone and the acceptors on the dendritic membrane. These results are compatible with the current assumption that odour molecules are

Bombyx mori

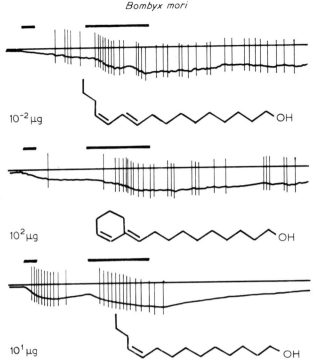

Fig. 7.4 Patterning of action potentials and slow potentials of the bombykol receptor when stimulated with bombykol (top), cyclobombykol (middle) and (Z)-10-tetradecadecen-1-ol (bottom). Odour sources were pieces of filter paper laden with substances in amounts as given in the figure. Bars indicate stimulus duration (100 and 500 ms, respectively) (redrawn from Kaissling, 1974).

reversibly and non-covalently bound to an acceptor molecule. This binding leads to a conformation change in the acceptor molecule as a result of which the flow of ions through the membrane is locally enhanced. Two features of the odour molecule are prerequisite to this binding. (a) Their steric dimensions may not hinder access to the binding site. (b) The spatial pattern of functional groups must correspond to that of the binding sites in the acceptor molecule. Since the energy of binding in this model is low and within the order of thermal fluctuations the binding can also occur with molecules not fitting exactly. In highly specialized receptors three or four different specific regions of interaction within a single binding site would be sufficient to explain the relative efficacies of pheromone analogues (Kafka and Neuwirth, 1974). A variant of this concept is discussed by Kaissling (1974) who observed that the time courses of receptor potentials elicited by either the pheromone or its analogues

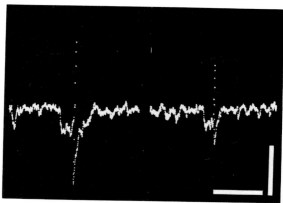

Fig. 7.5 Averaged action potentials of bombykol receptors. The action potentials lie within a depression of the slow receptor potential ('bumps'). Bumps are thought to reflect brief openings of ion channels which might be caused by single pheromone molecules (courtesy of K.E. Kaissling).

differ. Slow potentials of single bombykol receptors show a rather fluctuating time course when stimulated with a weak bombykol concentration, correspondingly the action potentials show a very irregular time pattern. (E)-10-tetradecen-1-ol, when applied in a 1000-fold greater concentration, elicits about the same receptor potential amplitude and spike number, but the potential is smooth and the spikes are spaced rather regularly. The response to cyclobombykol, however, resembles that to bombykol though the required concentration is 10 000-fold greater (Fig. 7.4). This phenomenon can be explained by assuming that the opening of an ion channel is not stereotyped, i.e. the width of the opening or its duration depends on the molecular structure of the releasing molecule. Kaissling proposes a two step mechanism of binding and activation. In the first step, the molecules is attached to the acceptor by, for instance, two binding points while, in the second, the acceptor is deformed by the attraction of a third binding point which allows ions to penetrate the membrane (Fig. 7.5). A high percentage of molecules of substances which cause a smooth receptor potential would then be attached to the acceptor, but these would not completely open the ion channel or would only do so for a short time; whereas irregular potentials are produced by chemicals which cause a wide or (and) longer-lasting opening. According to this concept, bombykol and cyclobombykol would differ in their probability of being bound in the first step of the mechanism.

Although in insects many pheromone receptors have been found which can be classified as specialists this does not imply that pheromone receptors in general are of this type. Vareschi (1971) showed that 9-oxo-(Z)-2-decanoic acid (a pheromone of the honeybee queen) excites a receptor cell on the worker antenna which is somewhat generalist. In parallel behavioural experiments, Vareschi (1971) also showed, that bees can easily be trained to extend the proboscis in response to the pheromone. Apparently, in honeybees, the above-mentioned possibility of direct behaviour release by an exclusive pheromone receptor is not verified. This obviously and generally holds true in vertebrates. No evidence has been found that there are receptors solely for the perception of pheromones in this class of animals. We must assume that the recognition of pheromone signals in vertebrates is performed in the same way as in general olfaction.

7.3.4 The sensitivity of pheromone receptors

The few experimental data on absolute response thresholds for odourous substances in both arthropods and vertebrates indicate that behavioural threshold concentrations for substances perceived by generalists cannot be far below a concentration of some million molecules per ml of air. This corresponds to a concentration of the order of 1 in 10^{14}. Thresholds lie between 10^8 and 10^{11} molecules ml^{-1}. Insects with specialized pheromone receptors, however, have a behavioural threshold a few orders of magnitude lower. Kaissling and Priesner (1970) could show that the pheromone receptor of the silk moth has reached the theoretical limit. This receptor requires only one molecule of bombykol on the dentritic membrane to fire a spike. Since this receptor produces spontaneous spikes intermittently, about 320 of the 50 000 receptors must be impinged by a molecule per second to overcome this noise. The bombyx antennae can filter out these 320 molecules from air which contains 600 molecules/ml and which flows with a speed of 60 cm s^{-1} around the antennae. This concentration corresponds to only one milligram of bombykol evenly distributed in 100 km^3 of air.

Such a high degree of sensitivity is not restricted to the silk moth. Although Kaissling's method has not been applied to other species, other experiments indicate sensitivities which come close to that of the silk moth. *Adoxophyes* for example responds to sources containing 10^{-6} μg of its pheromone (DenOtter, 1977). From Priesner's data one can also conclude that, in the numerous species he studied, the sensitivity must be close to the theoretical limit. In all species he tested, 1 ng of the most efficient substance produced an EAG response well above a limit of confidence. One nanogram of bombykol is sufficient to evoke a significant EAG amplitude in the silk moth.

7.3.5 Dynamic properties

Pheromone receptors of insects respond to stimuli of rectangular time course with a latency period followed by an increase of the receptor potential to a transient maximum and then a decrease to a plateau maintained for the remainder of the stimulus duration. The end of the stimulus is followed by a slow decline in the potential. The latency as well as the rise time are functions of the applied concentration. With high concentrations only a few milliseconds elapse before the onset of the receptor potential. In a few more milliseconds the response reaches its maximum. With very weak stimuli, delay and rise time both increase up to values of several hundred ms. The fall time is less affected by the stimulus strength and is fairly constant over a large range of concentrations. In general, the fall time is longer than the rise time. For the silk moth's bombykol receptor, the half time of the EAG decline is about 400 ms. However, after the application of very high concentration this time increases remarkably (Kaissling, 1972). This effect may be due to integrating properties of the antennal surface where the molecules accumulate by adsorption. Not all molecules diffuse immediately onto the dendritic membrane, many still arrive after the end of the stimulus, drawing out the response. Kasang (1971) could show that the *Bombyx* antenna contains enzymes which decompose bombykol. Nevertheless, there must be an additional process which inactivates errant pheromone molecules since this enzymatic process seems too slow for the observed fall times. The spiking frequency of the receptors follows approximately the time course of the slow receptor potential. Nevertheless, action potentials are predominantly found in those part of the slow potential where its differential quotient is negative. As in other olfactory cells the maximal rate of action potentials is not very high (ca 200 s^{-1}).

No studies have yet been carried out to determine whether there are responses to small variations in the concentration. Besides the interest in these properties from a fundamental point of view these data are required for a discussion of the mechanisms by which the animals are guided to the source.

The dynamic range of receptors so far measured covers about five decades of concentration (Kaissling, 1969, 1971; Kaissling and Priesner, 1970; DenOtter, 1977). In EAGs this range appears to be even wider which is probably due to receptors having different sensitivities.

7.3.6 Chemical mixtures as pheromones

The number of organic compounds which theoretically could serve as pheromones is almost unlimited. From this point of view, therefore, pheromone systems based on single compounds would function without the danger of interspecific interference. Nevertheless, such systems seem to be exceptional. Even in moths where the receptors are extremely well tuned to the pheromones at least two substances are normally found. In *Bombyx* as well a second compound was recently detected; it is the aldehyde of bombykol (bombykal; Kaissling, in preparation).

Three different possibilities are conceivable to explain this phenomenon. However, it seems dangerous to look for a general explanation. One possibility is that each component belongs to a different pheromone system and thus releases a different behavioural response. These responses may or may not exclude one another. Mixtures of such pheromones therefore, may show different effects depending on which behavioural element or result thereof (wing beating, approach to a source, mating etc.) is examined by the experimenter. Under such experimental conditions a pheromone could appear to be an inhibitor. Bombykal, the second compound produced by the female silk moth's glands, is released in amounts much smaller than bombykol. If its proportion is artificially increased, greater and greater bombykol concentrations are needed to arouse males. With a 10:1 ratio (bombykal to bombykol) the response is completely suppressed. In the silk moth as in all cases in which single receptor recordings have been obtained, special receptors of equal sensitivity for each component have been found. Are we dealing in the case of bombykal with a pheromone which controls a behavioural element not yet detected?

The second possibility is based on the idea that mixtures are a means of enhancing the number of possible chemical codes without a similar increase in chemical substances and receptor types. Since each component would have its special receptor, theoretically it would be possible to discriminate between differing mixtures by evaluating the ratio of excitation among these receptor types. This possibility is probably not applicable in the silk moth since as yet no differences in the behavioural response to pure bombykol and female extracts have been observed. The ratios of mixtures are often as high as 9:1. The sensitivity of the receptor type for the less concentrated component, however, is not correspondingly higher. Thus the active space (the area from which males are attracted) would be determined by the component having the lowest concentration. A 9:1 ratio in this case would reduce the active space to one third of that which could be achieved with one substance alone.

Evolution could also favour mixtures of substances. Pheromone systems with only one chemical compound and highly specialized receptors are very inflexible with respect to the development of new species. Transmitters and receivers must undergo parallel mutation lest pheromone communication be disrupted. Indeed, the biological relationships of species are also reflected by the degree of chemical relationship of their pheromones and mixtures thereof.

7.4 MECHANISMS OF GUIDANCE

Despite numerous efforts, we are far from understanding the strategies insects apply in searching for a pheromone source. As already pointed out odours under natural conditions do not spread in a predictable manner; hence a method of measuring differences in concentration and simply moving up the gradient is hardly applicable.

Locomotory responses to chemical signals are commonly divided into two categories. Those in which the animal responds to the stimulus by changing speed or direction without these changes being directed with respect to the source are called 'chemokinesis'. Kineases are subdivided in ortho- and klinokinesis. In orthokinesis, the speed of locomotion is modified by the stimulus whereas in klinokinesis, the direction is changed. Responses directed to the source are called 'chemotaxes'. If this directed response is a result of a comparison between two spaced sensors e.g. left and right antenna, this is termed tropotaxis. If this comparison is made by a single sensor which samples at different times and different loci it is called klinotaxis (Kühn, 1919; Dethier *et al.,* 1969; Fraenkel and Gunn, 1961).

In practice this classification brings about many difficulties. It does not include all possible strategies for orientation even using only a single sensory modality. Real orientation systems, however, are rarely based on only a single modality. In experiments, even a discrimination between chemokinesis and chemotaxis turns out to be problematical. If, for example, the experimenter observes in single turns of an animal no apparent relation to the position of the source, but the animal consistently comes closer to it after a longer series of turns, then the overall movement is certainly directed. Thus each of the turns is also directed though with a very high average error. How can this behaviour be classified in terms of kinesis and taxis? There is no room to discuss this problem at length here. The difficulties which arise when using these terms are also pointed out in the critical article on this subject by Kennedy (1977).

Some systems of chemical orientation do not call for an orientation response at all (marking of territories, alarm pheromones). Some do not demand an ability of the receiver to find the maximal concentration (trail pheromones). In still others a distinct absolute value of concentration is probably of the greatest importance (pheromones controlling the structure of termite hills).

Quantitative experiments on mechanisms of orientation to pheromones so far have mainly dealt with trail following in ants and termites and with orientation of moths in windborne pheromone plumes.

Like many other ants, *Lasius fuliginosus* marks the path home from a food source by continuously touching the ground with the tip of the abdomen thereby depositing a pheromone from the rectal ampulla. Conspecific individuals are able to follow these paths and thus are guided to the food source. The pheromone in this species is a mixture of fatty acids the main component being hexanoic acid (Huwyler *et al.,* 1975). Hangartner (1967, 1969) studied the behaviour of *Lasius fuliginosus* when following an artificial trail of extracts from rectal ampullae laid on filter paper. Intact ants placed on a straight, narrow line of this extract followed it precisely with only slight oscillations in their path (Fig. 7.6a1). The behaviour suggested the presence of an chemotropotactic mechanism of guidance, i.e. the ant keeps a position in which both antennae are equally stimulated by turning towards the side of the more strongly excited antenna. Such a mechanism depending on feedback tends to oscillate under these conditions causing the wiggly line of motion. Further support for this came from experiments with two closely adjacent, parallel trails. The concentration of one trail decreased stepwise along its course. At the very beginning where both trails were equally concentrated, the ant's path lay between these two trails. A 10% reduction in one trail was sufficient to cause about 30% of the ants to switch over to the more strongly concentrated trail. It is difficult to explain these results by any mechanism other than chemo-tropotaxis. Ants with one antenna removed showed a pronounced turning tendency towards the intact side when exposed to a homogeneous trail pheromone distribution (Fig. 7.6a2). This is further support for a tropotactic orientation mechanism. Nevertheless, these animals were still capable of following a trail. Even ants with antennae fixed in a crossed position inducing laterally inverted inputs had not completely lost this ability (Fig. 7.6a3). The paths of unilaterally amputated ants, however, resembled a series of arcs like a garland, whereas the course

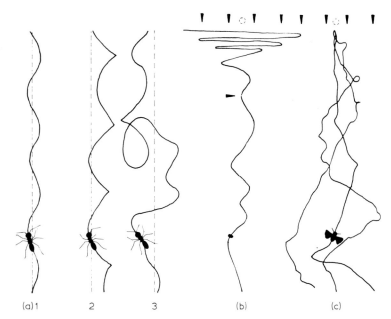

Fig. 7.6(a) Paths of *Lasius fuliginosus* following a straight line impregnated with the trail pheromone, 1, intact animal. 2, Left antenna amputated. 3, Antennae fixed in a crossed position (after Hangartner, 1967).

(b) Flight path of male *Cadra cautella* flying in a wind tunnel towards a point source of the sex pheromone. When the source is suddenly removed (horizontal arrowhead) the angle of the moth's flight with respect to the wind increases to almost 90 degrees (after Kennedy and Marsh, 1974).

(c) Three paths of male *Bombyx mori* walking in a zigzag course upwind in a pheromone plume (Kramer, 1975).

of those with crossed antennae was rather irregular and convoluted. Hangartner therefore claims that *Lasius fuliginosus* can also orient chemo-klinotactically as do honeybees (Martin, 1964).

From a cybernetic point of view, tropotaxis is relatively well-defined and under-standable. This is not true in the case of klinotaxis. Numerous suitable algorithms to evaluate the direction of a gradient by successive measurements with only one sensor are conceivable. Which of these algorithms ants apply when orienting klinotactically is not yet known.

Trail following in termites is obviously also based on a combination of tropo- and klinotaxis (Kaib, in preparation). Tropotaxis seems to prevail along narrow paths deposited by one or few animals. These trails have steep gradients of concentration as required for this type of response, whereas in wider trails with flatter and less regular gradients klinotaxis predominates.

There is no evidence that pheromone trails are polarized. For the most part visual cues seem to determine the correct direction of walking (Leuthold *et al.*, 1976).

American cockroaches (*Periplaneta americana*) have two pheromones, a sex pheromone secreted by the female and an aggregation pheromone to which immatures and adults of both sexes are attracted. These insects also orient by both chemo-tropotaxis and chemo-klinotaxis (Rust *et al.*, 1976). But in addition, the sex phero-mone releases a positive anemotaxis (orientation with respect to the direction of wind). This response is widespread in insects orienting to point sources of odour over long distances. In airborne odour plumes, the gradients along the longitudinal axes are much smaller than in the transverse axes. Anemotaxis therefore, is a good means of polarizing the aerial trail. Chemo-klinotaxis (−kinesis?) polarized in such manner is obviously the basis of long-range orientation in Lepidoptera. Nevertheless, because of the vague term klinotaxis this statement does not mean much. What can be observed in many species is a zigzag upwind flight. But one can only speculate as to which events cause the changes in course. Has the insect detected a difference between the actual excitation and that a few moments before? Has the ambient concentration fallen below an internal (fixed or variable) reference value? Or is the change of course induced by the more frequent fluctuations in concentration in the marginal parts of the plume as Wright (1958) surmised?

Male silk moths (*Bombyx mori*) when exposed to an airstream homogeneously laden with bombykol walk upwind keeping a distinct angle of about 30 to 50 degrees to the wind (silk moths are unable to fly). The sign of this angle intermittently changes. The resulting path resembles the course of a sailing boat tacking upwind (Fig. 7.6c). Changes of sign can also be released by sudden drops of the pheromone concentration (Kramer, 1975 and Kramer in preparation). Gypsy moths (*Lymantria dispar*) with clipped wings show a similar behaviour (Kafka personal communication). These results coincide with the zigzag flights observed in field and wind tunnel experiments. However, the results obtained from walking insects may not be applic-able to flying insects, especially since detection of wind in flight can no longer be achieved by mechanoreceptors, which then only measure the speed of flight relative to the air. In flying insects wind can only be detected visually with respect to the ground. Kennedy and Marsh (1974) recorded the flight of three moth species (*Plodia interpunctella, Anagasta kühniella, Cadra cautella*) in a wind tunnel when orienting to sources of the corresponding sex attractants. This wind tunnel was equipped with a movable carpet of either black stripes or dots. With a stationary ground pattern the moths flew upwind approaching the source in a moderately zigzag course. When the ground was moved in the downwind direction the moths reduced their airspeed such as to keep the ground speed constant. With respect to the observers reference system the zigzag pattern of path appeared compressed. When the pheromone source was suddenly removed the angle of the moth to the wind increased to almost 90°. Its sign in this case changed from plus to minus with increasing intervals. The resulting 'castings' appear to be a good means of recovering a lost contact with the odour plume (Fig. 7.6b). The experiments demonstrate that flying insects can orient with respect to the wind by visual cues. Furthermore, a chemically released 'optomotor anemotaxis' in combination with a suitable strategy of locomotion is a sufficient means to find a point source of odour without chemotaxis in the strict sense. This does not imply, however, that chemotaxis is not involved in the process of orienting as a whole. The cabbage looper *Trichoplusia ni* can chemotactically follow an artificial terrestrial trail (Shorey and Farkas, 1973). Male silk moths respond chemo-tropotactically to concentration differences smaller than 10%. Temporal changes of concentration as low as 1% s^{-1} are also perceived by this animal if this decrease lasts for at least 5 seconds. It is not clear to what extent, if at all, these capabilities contribute to orientation over long distances. Probably their role is restricted to the final phase of approach.

REFERENCES

Adam, G. and Delbrück, M. (1968), Reduction of dimensionality in biological diffusion processes. In: *Structural Chemistry and Molecular Biology*, (Rich, A. and Davidson, N. eds), Freeman Co., San Francisco, London.

Altner, H. (1977), Insektensensillen: Bau- und Funktionsprinzipien. *Verh. Dtsch. Zool. Ges.* **70**, 139−153.

Aylor, D.E. (1976), Physics and insect pheromones. Frontiers of plant science. *Connecticut Agric. Exp. Station. VSDA.*, **28**, 4−7.

Bayliss, W.M. and Starling, E.H. (1912), The mechanism of pancreatic secretion. *J. Physiol.*, **28**, 29.

Berger, R.S. (1972), 2, 6-Dichlorphenol, sex pheromone of the lone star tick. *Science*, **177**, 704−705.

Bergström, G. and Löfquist, J. (1968), Odor similarities between the slave-keeping ants *Formica sanguinea* and *Polyergus rufenscens* and their slaves *Formica fusca* and *Formica rufibarbis*. *J. Insect Physiol.* **14**, 995−1011.

Bergström, G. and Löfquist, J. (1970), Chemical basis of odour communication in four species of *Lasius* ants. *J. Insect Physiol.*, **16**, 2353−2357.

Bethe, A. (1932), Vernachlässigte Hormone. *Naturwissenschaft* **20**, 177−183.

Bierl, B.A., Beroza, M. and Collier, C.W. (1970), Potent sex attractant of the gypsy moth: its isolation, identification and synthesis. *Science*, **170**, 87−89.

Birch, M.C. (1974), Pheromones. In: *Frontiers of Biology*, Vol. **32**, North Holland Publishing Co., Amsterdam, London.

Boeckh, J. (1962), Elektrophysiologische Untersuchungen an einzelnen Geruchsrezeptoren auf den Antennen des Totengräbers (*Necrophorus, Coleoptera*). *Z. vergl. Physiol.*, **46**, 212−248.

Boeckh, J. (1967), Reaktionsschwelle, Arbeitsbereich und Spezifität eines Geruchsrezeptors auf der Heuschreckenantenne. *Z. vergl. Physiol.*, **55**, 378−406.

Boistel, J., Lecomte, J. and Coraboeuf, F. (1956), Quelques aspects de l'étude électrophysiologique des récepteurs sensoriels des antennes d'Hymenoptères. *Insects sociaux*, **3**, 25−31.

Bossert, W.H. (1968), Temporal patterning in olfactory communication. *J. theoret. Biol.*, **18**, 157−170.

Butenandt, A., Beckmann, R., Stamm, D. and Hecker, E. (1959), Über den Sexual-Lockstoff des Seidenspinners *Bombyx mori*. Reindarstellung und Konstitution. *Z. Naturforsch.,* **14b**, 1283−1284.

DenOtter, C.J. (1977), Single sensillum responses in the male moth *Adoxophyes orana* (F.v.R.) to female sex pheromone components and their geometrical isomers. *J. comp. Physiol.,* **121**, 205−222.

Dethier, V.G. Browne, L.B. and Smith, C.N. (1960), The designation of chemicals in terms of the response they elicit from insects. *J. econ. Ent.,* **53**, 134−136.

Dubois, R. (1895), Sur le rôle de l'olifaction dans les phenomènes d'accouplement chez les papillons. *Assn. France pour l'Avancement des Sciences.* **24**, Sess. 293−294.

Dumpert, K. (1972), Alarmstoffrezeptoren auf der Antenne von *Lasius fuliginosus* (Latr.) (*Hymenoptera, Formicidae*). *Z. vergl. Physiol.,* **76**, 403−425.

Esslen, J. and Kaissling, K-E. (1976), Zahl und Verteilung antennaler Sensillen bei der Honigbiene (*Apis mellifera* L.). *Zoomorphologie,* **83**, 227−251.

Fraenkel, G.S. and Gunn, D.L. (1940), The orientation of animals. Kineses, taxes and compass reactions. Oxford University Press, New York, Oxford.

Hangartner, W. (1967), Spezifität und Inaktivierung des Spurpheromones von *Lasius fuliginosus* Latr. und Orientierung der Arbeiterinnen im Duftfeld. *Z. vergl. Physiol.,* **57**, 103−136.

Hangartner, W. (1969), Orientierung von *Lasius fuliginosus* Latr. an einer Gabelung der Geruchsspur. *Insects Sociaux,* **16**, 155−160.

Huwyler, S., Grob, K. and Viscontini, M. (1975), The trail pheromone of the ant, *Lasius fuliginosus:* Identification of six components. *J. Insect Physiol.,* **21**, 299−304.

Insco, M.N. and Beroza, M. (1976), Insect behavior chemicals active in field trials. ACS Symposon Series. (Beroza, M. ed.), Washington D.C.

Kafka, W.A. (1970), Analyse der molekularen Wechselwirkung bei der Erregung einzelner Riechzellen. (Elektrophysiologie einzelner Rezeptorzellen auf der Antenne von *Locusta migratoria*.) *Z. vergl. Physiol.,* **70**, 105−143.

Kafka, W.A. and Neuwirth, J. (1975), A model of pheromone molecule-acceptor interaction. *Z. Naturforsch.,* **30c**, 278−282.

Kaissling, K-E. (1969), Kinetics of olfactory receptor potentials. Olfaction and Taste III. (Pfaffmann, C. ed.), pp. 52−70, Rockefeller University Press, New York.

Kaissling, K.E. (1971), Handbook of sensory physiology. Vol. IV. (Beidler, L.M. ed.), Springer Verlag, Berlin.

Kaissling, K.E. (1972), Kinetic studies of transduction in olfactory receptors of *Bombyx mori*. Olfaction and Taste IV. (Schneider, D. ed.), pp. 207−213, Wissenschaftliche Stuttgart. *Verlagsgesellschaft.*

Kaissling, K.E. (1974a), Sensorische Transduktion bei Riechzellen von Insekten. *Verh. Dtsch. Zool. Ges.,* **67**, 1−11.

Kaissling, K.E. (1974b), Topical stimulation of the outer dendrites of single olfactory cells in saturnid moth. *Abst. 1st Congr. Europ. Chemoreception Research Org., Paris.* p. 26.

Kaissling, K.E. and Priesner, E. (1970), Die Riechschwelle des Seidenspinners. *Naturwissenschaft* **57**, 23−28.

Kasang, G. (1971), Bombykol reception and metabolism on the antenna of the silk-moth *Bombyx mori*. Gustation and Olfaction. (Ohloff, G. and Thomas, A.F., eds), pp. 245–250, Academic Press, London, New York.

Kennedy, J.S. (1977), Chemical control of insect behaviour. (Shorey and McKelvey, eds), pp. 67–91, New York.

Kennedy, J.S. and Marsh, D. (1974), Pheromone-regulated anemotaxis in flying moths. *Science,* **184**, 999–1001.

Kramer, E. (1975), Orientation of the male silkmoth to the sex attractant bombykol. Olfaction and Taste V. (Denton, D.A. and Coghlan, J.P. eds), pp. 329–335, Academic Press, New York.

Kuhn, A. (1919), *Die Orientierung der Tiere im Raum.* Jena.

Lacher, V. (1964), Elektrophysiologische Untersuchungen an einzelnen Rezeptoren für Geruch, Kohlendioxyd, Luftfeuchtigkeit und Temperatur auf den Antennen der Arbeitsbiene und der Drohne (*Apis mellifica* L.). *Z. vergl. Physiol.,* **48**, 587–623.

Lacher, V. (1967), Elektrophysiologische Untersuchungen an einzelnen Geruchs-rezeptoren auf den Antennen weiblicher Moskitos (*Aedes aegypti* L.). *J. Insect Physiol.,* **13**, 1461–1470.

Leuthold, R.H., Bruinsma, O. and van Huis, A. (1976), Optical and pheromonal orientation and memory for homing distance in the harvester termite *Hodotermes mossambicus* (Hagn). *Behav. Ecol. Sociobiol.,* **1**, 127–139.

Martin, H. (1964), Zur Nahorientierung der Biene im Duftfeld, zugleich ein Nachweis für die Osmotropotaxis bei Insekten. *Z. vergl. Physiol.,* **48** , 481–533.

Meinecke, C.C. (1975), Riechsensillen und Systematik der *Lamellicornia (Insecta, Coleoptera)*. *Zoomorphologie,* **82**, 1–42.

Meinwald, J., Thompson, W.R., Eisner, T. and Owen, D.F. (1971), Pheromones. VII. African monarch: major components of the hairpencil secretion. *Tetrahedron Letters,* **38**, 3485–3488.

Mustaparta, H. (1975), Responses of single olfactory cells in the pine weevil *Hylobius abietis* L. (*Col.: Cucurlionidae*). *J. comp. Physiol.,* **97**, 271–290.

Nakamura, K. and Kawasaki, K. (1977), The active space of the *Spodoptera litura* (F.) sex pheromone and the pheromone component determining this space. *Appl. Ent. Zool.,* **12**, 162–177.

Noll, (1869), Feiner Geruch bei Schmetterlingen. *Zool. Garten* **10**, 254–255.

Ottoson, D. (1956), Analysis of the electric activity of the olfactory epithelium. *Acta physiol. Scand.,* **35**, Suppl. 122, 1–83.

Priesner, E. (1973), Artspezifität und Funktion einiger Insektenpheromone. *Fortschritte der Zoologie,* **22**, 49–135.

Priesner, E., Bestmann, H.J., Vostrowsky, O. and Rosel, P. (1977), Sensory efficacy of alkyl-branched pheromone analogues in noctuid and tortricid lepidoptera. *Z. Naturforsch,* **32c**, 979–991.

Priesner, E., Jacobson, M. and Bestmann, H.J. (1975), Structure relationships in noctuid sex pheromone reception *Z. Naturforsch.* **30c**, 283–293.

Roys, Ch. (1954), Olfactory nerve potentials a direct measure of chemoreception in insects. *Ann. New York Acad. Sci.,* **58**, 250–255.

Rust, M.K., Burk, T. and Bell, W. (1976), Pheromone-stimulated locomotory and orientation responses in the american cockroach. *Animal Behavior,* **24**, 52–67.

Sass, H. (1976), Zur nervösen Codierung von Geruchsreizen bei *Periplaneta americana*. *Z. comp. Physiol.*, **107**, 49−65.

Schmidt, K. and Gnatzy, W. (1971), Die Feinstruktur der Sinneshaare auf den Cerci von *Gryllus bimaculatus*. Deg. (*Saltoria, Gryllidae*). *Z. Zellforsch. mikrosk. Anat.*, **122**, 190−209.

Schneider, D. (1955), Mikroelektroden registrieren die elektrischen Impulse einzelner Sinnesnervenzellen der Schmetterlingsantenne. *Industrieelektronik, Hamburg*, **3**, 3−7.

Schneider, D., Block, B.C., Boeckh, J. and Priesner, E. (1967), Die Reaktion der männlichen Seidenspinner auf Bombykol und seine Isomeren: Elektro-antennogram und Verhalten. *Z. vergl. Physiol.*, **54**, 192−209.

Schneider, D., Boppre, M., Schneider, H., Thompson, W.R., Boriak, C.J., Petty, R.L. and Meinwald, J.A. (1975), A pheromone precursor and its uptake in the male *Danaus* butterflies. *J. comp. Physiol.*, **97**, 245−256.

Schneider, D. and Hecker, E. (1956), Zur Elektrophysiologie der Antenne des Seidenspinners *Bombyx mori* bei Reizung mit angereicherten Extrakten des Sexuallockstoffes. *Z. Naturforsch.*, **11b**, 121−124.

Schneider, D., Lacher, V. and Kaissling, K-E. (1964), Die Reaktionsweise und das Reaktionsspektrum von Riechzellen bei *Antheraea pernyi* (*Lepidoptera, Saturniidae*). *Z. vergl. Physiol.*, **48**, 632−662.

Shorey, H.H. and McKelvey, J.J. eds. (1977), Chemical control of insect behavior. John Wiley Sons, New York.

Shorey, H.H. and Farkas, S.R. (1973), Sex pheromone of Lepidoptera. 42. Terrestrial odor-trail following by pheromone-stimulated males of *Trichuplusia ni*. *Ann. ent. Soc. Am.*, **66**, 1213−1214.

Sower, L.L., Gaston, L.K. and Shorey, H.H. (1971), Sex pheromones of noctuid moths 26. Female release rate, male response thresholds and communication distance for *Trichuplusia ni*. *Ann. ent. Soc. Am.*, **63**, 1090−1092.

Steinbrecht. R.A. (1970), Zur Morphometrie der Antenne des Seidenspinners, *Bombyx mori* L. Zahl und Verteilung der Riechsensillen (Insecta, Lepidoptera). *Z. Morph. der Tiere*, **68**, 93−126.

Steinbrecht, R.A. (1973), Der Feinbau olfaktorischer Sensillen des Seidenspinners (*Insecta, Lepidoptera*). *Z. Zellforsch.*, **139**, 533−565.

Steinbrecht, R.A. and Muller, B. (1976), Fine structure of the antennal receptors of the bed bug, *Cimex lectularius* L. *Tissue and Cell*, **8**, 615−636.

Thurm, U. (1969), General organization of sensory receptors. *Estratto da Rendiconti della Scuola Intern. di Fisica 'E. Fermi'*, **43**, 44−68.

Vareschi, E. (1971), Duftunterscheidung bei der Honigbiene: Einzelzellableitungen und Verhaltensreaktionen. *Z. vergl. Physiol.*, **75**, 143−173.

Wright, R.H. (1958), The olfactory guidance of flying insects. *Can. Ent.*, **30**, 81−89.

8 Insect Chemoreception

KAI HANSEN

Acknowledgements

I thank Dr Helmut Wieczorek for valuable discussion and many critical comments on the manuscript and Dr Gerald L. Hazelbauer for his editorial revisions.

I thank Miss Christine Meier for drawing the figures carefully and Mr. Bill Colmers for linguistic corrections.

Taxis and Behavior
(*Receptors and Recognition*, Series B, Volume 5)
Edited by G.L. Hazelbauer
Published in 1978 by Chapman and Hall, 11 New Fetter Lane, London EC4P 4EE
© Chapman and Hall

8.1 INTRODUCTION

In insects, chemoreception plays an important role in the search for food, control of its choice and quality, oviposition and intraspecific communication by pheromones (for the latter topic see Kramer, this volume.) The responsible gustatory and olfactory organs are hairlike and show a rather simple organization. In many cases they contain only 1−5 receptor cells. It is possible to record the electrical response of single receptor cells upon stimulation by electrophysiological methods. It has been shown that each cell has a distinct and defined specificity for a certain group of structurally related substances. Most insects possess receptor cells specialized for primary nutrients, such as sugars, amino acids and water. In addition, several olfactory receptors are known to respond to food odors (green odors, carrion odors) and flower scents. The discovery of another group of receptors responsible for recognition of host plants was unexpected. These receptors are sensitive to mustard oil glycosides, alkaloids, steroids and other secondary plant substances. Haemophageous insects localize their hosts with CO_2 and lactic acid receptors and check blood for its nucleotide content.

The combination of diverse specificities, simple organisation and accessibility to electrophysiological techniques has made these organs favourable objects for studying basic processes of chemoreception.

In this report, new results and viewpoints on the physiology of insect chemo-sensory organs are discussed. The gustatory system is accentuated more than the olfactory one, beceause the latter is also discussed in the chapter 'pheromone reception' (Kramer, this volume). Emphasis is directed towards two main topics. The first problem is the understanding of the sequence of processes between arrival of stimulating molecules at the outside of the sense organ and occurrence of nerve impulses in the axon. This sequence may be outlined by the key words: conduction of stimulant molecules, transduction at the receptor membrane, generation of receptor potential and of spike frequency. Several unresolved questions are discussed in the light of results obtained for other, well-studied chemoreceptive systems as for example the acetylcholine receptor protein of the subsynaptic membrane.

The second problem is that of specificity. In contrast to the narrowly specific pheromone receptors (and synaptic transmitter receptor proteins) most receptors involved in food detection exhibit broad specificity patterns to numerous chemically related substances. This situation offers us the possibility of studying structure−activity relationships. Thus the recognition sites of the receptor proteins may be characterized with some precautions and limitations, under *in vivo* conditions. For reviews on general chemoreception see *Handbook of Sensory Physiology,* Vol. IV (Beidler 1971a, ed.); International Symposia on Olfaction and Taste I−VI

(Zottermann, 1963; Hayashi, 1967; Pfaffmann, 1969; Schneider, 1972; Denton and Coglan, 1975; Le Magnen and MacLeod, 1977; eds); Bardach, 1975; Benz, 1976; Moncrieff, 1967; Oakley and Benjamin, 1966; Poynder, 1974. For reviews on Insect chemoreception see Altner, 1977a,b; Boeckh, 1977; Boeckh *et al.,* 1965, 1976; Chapman, 1974; Dethier, 1976; Galun, 1977; Hodgson 1965, 1968, 1974; Kaissling, 1969–1977; Priesner, 1973; Schneider, 1971; Schneider and Steinbrecht, 1968; Schoonhoven, 1968, 1972, 1973; Slifer, 1970; Städler, 1977; Stürckow, 1970; Wolbarsht, 1965.

8.2 STRUCTURAL ORGANIZATION OF THE SENSORY ORGANS

8.2.1 General features and ontogeny

Insects possess small cuticular sensory organs, called sensilla. They respond to different kinds of stimuli such as chemical substances, mechanical forces, temperature or humidity. Because of several structural and ontogenetical similarities, the sensilla belong, together with epidermal glands, non-innervated hairs and the scales of the butterflies to the group of 'Kleinorgane' (Henke, 1953) or 'organules' (Lawrence, 1966). Being small cuticular organs, these organules represent multifunctional units, which cover the entire cuticle of insects in densities up to several thousand per square millimeter. Each organule develops from one epidermal mother cell. This divides a few times and its descendent cells differentiate into the complete organ (Table 8.1). It consists of a small and rather constant number of cells, which are arranged in a typical manner. After two divisions of the mother cell, three (named cells 1,2,3) of the four resulting cells surround one axial cell concentrically (4). A long ciliary process is typical of the axial cell. Cells 1 and 2 are the only cells of the sensillum capable of secreting cuticular protein like normal epidermal cells. But, in contrast to the latter, the cuticular products of cells 1 and 2 exhibit a genetically fixed, highly complex structure. Cell 1, the tormogen, or socket-forming cell, establishes the junction between the sensillum and the surrounding tegumentary cuticle. Cell 2, the trichogen or hairshaft-forming cell, is responsible for formation of the sensilla's stimulus-conducting structures: namely the pore-tubule systems of the olfactory hairs, and the distal openings of the taste hairs.

After having completed the cuticular parts, cells 1 and 2 modify themselves drastically (cf. Fig. 8.1a). They develop the extracellular lymph cavity II with its tightly folded membrane system. At this point the cells can hardly be distinguished from gland cells (Noirot and Quennedey, 1974). Cell 3, the inner sheath cell, forms a tube-like sheath around the dendrites. Thereby the small lymph cavity I is separated from the cavity II in gustatory sensilla. Cell 4 gives rise to the receptor cells by further divisions. It is present in gland organules too, but degenerates completely during further development (Sreng and Quennedey, 1976; Happ and Happ, 1977). In the sensilla, cell 4 reduces its ciliary process temporarily. The final form of the dendrite develops after hair formation (Ernst, 1972).

Table 8.1 Simplified cell lineage of a gustatory sensillum, modified after Lawrence (1966). For explanation see text.
M : epidermal mother cell. The lineage within the receptor cells is hypothetical

Cell types in the complete sensillum	Arrangement	Products of differentiation	Sensory function
tormogen cell		socket	electrogenic pump
trichogen cell	concentrically	hairshaft with pore or pore-systems	production of viscous fluid
inner sheath cell		dendritic sheath	isolation cavity I/II ?
receptor cells	central bundle	dendrites and axons	sugar cell / water cell
			anion cell / cation cell
			mechano-receptor cell

8.2.2 Special features of gustatory and olfactory sensilla

(a) *The fine structure*
In spite of their uniform ontogeny, the outer cuticular specializations show a very great variety of shapes. The fine structure of a gustatory sensillum is shown in Fig. 8.1a. Because most electrophysiological work on gustatory receptors is done with this fly hair, it is chosen as representative for the whole group. But considering the existing variety of shapes, it should not be designated as a 'typical' taste hair. In olfactory hairs, the arrangement of cells below the cuticle is rather similar to that of taste hairs. However, the dendritic sheath is perforated or reduced. Therefore, the lymph cavities are connected.

Striking differences exist in the stimulus-conducting structures of the hairshaft walls. Gustatory receptors are found only in the 'terminal pore sensilla'. Olfactory receptors are localized in 'wall pore sensilla'. The latter group is further subdivided into 'single-walled sensilla' with systems of pore tubules (Fig. 8.1c) and 'double-walled sensilla' with pore canals without tubules (Fig. 8.1d). The terms used here have recently been proposed by Altner (1977b).

The number of receptor cells per sensillum varies, but is constant for a certain hair type of a certain species. Most olfactory and gustatory hairs contain 1—10 receptor cells. In several large olfactory sensilla receptor cells are more numerous (locust: 20—50, cotton bug: 40—70, bee: 15—30) (Schneider and Steinbrecht, 1968; Hansen and Heumann, 1971; Gaffal and Bassemir, 1974). The receptor cells of each hair differ in their specificity. For example, one particular cell found in the taste hairs of flies, is stimulated specifically by sugars and amino acids, while others react to inorganic salts or water (see Section 8.4). For further literature on the fine structure of sensilla see Slifer, 1970 (review); Steinbrecht, 1973; Harbach and Larsen, 1976; Altner, 1977a (review); McIver and Siemicki, 1978.

(b) *Types and terminology of sensilla*
In the literature, a typology based on the outer shape of the sensilla is used for description and identification by light or scanning electron microscopy. The following types are currently recognized (see Schneider, 1964):

(1) Sensilla chaetica: sensory bristles with specialized socket regions;
(2) Sensilla trichodea: sensory hairs without sockets;
(3) Sensilla basiconica: sensory pegs or cones, without sockets, often hardly differing from sensilla trichodea;
(4) Sensilla coeloconica: pegs in pits;
(5) Sensilla placodea: sensory plates, reduced hairshaft.

It must be emphasized that neither the modality nor the specificity of a hair type can be predicted from its appearance under the light microscope. Nevertheless such typologies are helpful in performing electrophysiological investigations. It is a common experience that, for example, all sensilla basiconica type I on the antenna of the carrion beetle contain one and the same type of carrion receptor cells. For the complete identification of a certain receptor cell, the hair type, its exact location and the species must be stated. The value of a terminology based on the hair shapes is limited further

(a) by the existence of several fantastically styled forms (olfactory dorsal and predominantly gustatory terminal organ in fly larvae, Chu and Axtell, 1971; Chu-Wang and Axtell, 1972; antennal glandular-olfactory complex sensilla in collembola, Altner and Thies, 1973) and

(b) by the existence of different types with intermediate stages on one and the same antenna (olfactory sensilla of Lamellicornian beetles; Meinecke, 1975).

(c) *Distribution of chemosensitive sensilla*
Olfactory sensilla are found chiefly on the antennae, less on the palps or on the ovipositor. More widely distributed are gustatory sensilla (taste hairs, taste pores without hairshafts): on the outer mouth parts, within the pharynx, on the antennae, on the distal parts of the legs, especially on the lower side (the sole) and on the ovipositor.

8.3 HOW DOES A CHEMOSENSORY SENSILLUM WORK ?

8.3.1 How do stimulus molecules reach the receptor membrane?

(a) *Stimulus conduction in taste hairs*
The structure of the taste hair tip is shown in Fig. 8.3a. The dendritic outer segments, containing microtubuli, end less than 1 μm below the opening of canal I. The taste hair tips are covered by a small droplet of a so-called 'viscous fluid'. It can be observed in the light microscope at high magnification; in electron micrographs it is seen as a dense material (Morita and Takeda, 1957; Stürckow, 1967; Stürckow *et al.*, 1973; Hansen and Heumann, 1971). A solution of stimulating substances must first come into contact with the viscous fluid. The fluid may be responsible for the stimulating effects of solid crystals of sucrose and leaf-surface substances (Dethier, 1955; Bernays *et al.*, 1975, 1976). Stimulating substances reach the dendritic membranes by passive diffusion through the viscous fluid. As discussed later, the first stimulating molecules will reach the membrane within less than 2 ms. Within 50 ms, the concentration of stimulating molecules at the membrane should equal the applied concentration. There is no evidence that the viscous fluid has any influence on the specificity of the sensillum.

Mucopolysaccharides are responsible for the high viscocity of the viscous fluid (Bernays *et al.*, 1975). The fluid is probably produced by the membrane system of lymph cavity II, but the possibility of its originating from cavity I cannot be excluded.

(a)

(b)

(c)

(d)

Fig. 8.1 Schematic organization of insect chemosensory hairs. The cuticular parts are solid, the receptor cell is shaded.

(a) Longitudinal section through a taste hair from the leg of the fly *Phormia* (Hansen and Heumann, 1971; modified according to Altner, 1977a). The structure of the labellar hairs used preferentially for electrophysiological recording is quite similar (Larsen, 1962; Felt and Vande Berg, 1976). Here only one — instead of four — receptors is shown. The structures of the articulation-like socket region with the cuticular ring (CR) and the flexible membrane (FM) are simplified, the mechanoreceptor cell is omitted (for details see Gaffal *et al.*, 1975).

The main feature common to all taste hairs is the opening (O) at the tip of the hairshaft. Through this fluid-filled opening, stimulating molecules diffuse from the outside to the tip (T) of the dendritic outer segment (DD), where they interact with the membrane (transduction). The receptor cell is divided into the following segments:

(i) the receptor cell body (RCB) and the dendritic inner segment (PD). At the membrane of the latter, spike generation occurs;

(ii) the axon (AX) which passes to the central nervous system;

(iii) the dendritic outer segment (DD) which contains no organelles except microtubuli. The dendritic inner and outer segments are connected by a modified cilium (C) of $9 \times 2 + 0$ structure with two basal bodies and a ciliary root in the inner segment (for details see Gaffal and Bassemir, 1974). The receptor cell is concentrically surrounded by three (or four) sheath cells: 1. the inner sheath cell (SC) forming the dendritic sheath (DS); 2. the trichogen (TRC) and 3. the tormogen cell (TOC). The cell membranes of all cells are apically connected by intercellular junctions (J). A small lymph cavity (I) exists around the proximal parts of the dendritic outer segments. This cavity is connected with the labyrinth-like narrow invaginations (L) of the sheath cell as well as to the canal I (CI) of the hairshaft. Apical invaginations of the tormogen and trichogen cells form the lymph cavity II (LC II). Its wall is distinguished by a system of folded membranes (MS II). This cavity II opens into the canal II (C II) of the hairshaft. The canal is connected to the outside by tiny pores (TP). A complete separation of the two lymph cavities has been observed only in gustatory hairs; in olfactory hairs the dendritic sheath can be perforated or reduced.

(b) Cross-section through the hair shaft of sensilum a. In the canal I, four dendrities (DD) are visible, each of which belongs to one receptor cell.

(c) Cross-section through a single-walled olfactory hair (sensillum basiconicum of the carrion beetle containing a carrion-sensitive cell; Boeckh, 1962; Ernst, 1969). The hairshaft exhibits only one lumen filled up by ramified dendritic branches (DB) of one receptor cell. The cuticular wall is pierced by numerous olfactory pores associated with tubules on the inner side. The total number of pore systems is 15 000 per hair.

(d) Cross-section through a double-walled olfactory hair (sensillum coeloconicum of locust, containing green odor receptors; Boeckh, 1967; Steinbrecht, 1968; Kafka, 1970). The dendrites of three receptor cells are connected to the outside by long pore canals, which seem to be filled by a secretion product. Tubules are absent.

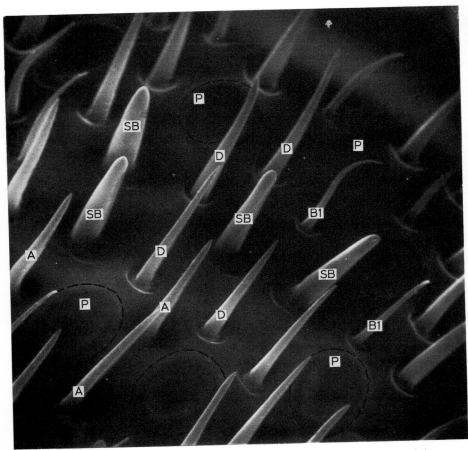

Fig. 8.2 Typical pattern of different types of sensilla on the antenna of the worker bee *Apis mellifera*. P: Sensilla placodea (= plate organs) containing 5—35 olfactory receptor cells, responding to several pheromones and flower scents. 75% of the antennal receptor cells fall into the plate organs (Vareschi, 1971); SB: Sensilla basiconica with many olfactory receptor cells of unknown specificity; B1: Sensilla trichodea type B1 with one mechanoreceptor cell; D: Sensilla trichodea type D, with gustatory receptors which mediate behavioral reaction to sugars; A: Sensilla trichodea type A, with olfactory receptors of unknown specificity.

Length of the sensillum trichodeum type D: 32 μm. Terminology according to Esslen and Kaissling (1976).

There are indications that passage of stimulating molecules to the receptor membrane can be blocked under some conditions. Taste hairs of the locust do not exhibit an electrophysiological response to stimulation immediately after feeding.

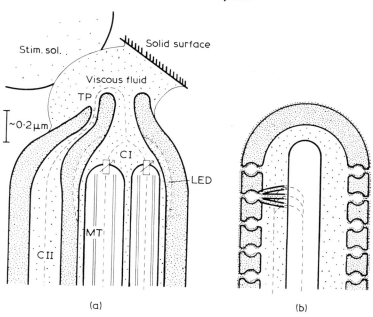

Fig. 8.3 Schematic representation of the site of chemosensory transduction.
(a) The taste hair tip, enlarged area of Fig. 8.1a. Transduction occurs at the apical membranes of the dendritic outer segment by binding of stimulus molecules to receptor proteins and by a subsequent change in membrane conductivity. The latter is symbolized as variable resistance in the receptor current path (broken line). C I, C II: canal I, II; LED: less electron-dense layer; MT: microtubules; TP: tiny pores.
(b) Olfactory hair of the single-walled type (cf. Fig. 8.1c). The pore system consists of the outer opening, an inner cavity and the tubules. Dotted lines mark the outer lipophilic layer. The broken line marks the path of the receptor current.

In that situation the transepithelial resistance of the taste hair population is about 30% higher than normal. The same effect is evoked in unfed animals by injection of hemolymph derived from fed locust, or by injection of extracts prepared from the corpora cardiaca. Therefore, hormonal factors seem to be involved in establishing this inactive state. Reactivation seems to occur only in the hungry locust. It may be that reactivation is the result of replenishing the viscous fluid used for food testing (Bernays *et al.*, 1972; Bernays and Chapman, 1972). Such effects have also been observed in flies (Stürckow, 1967; Stürckow *et al.*, 1973). However, the striking physiological effects have led to the less convincing suggestion that the terminal pores of the taste hairs may be opened and closed mechanically (Blaney *et al.*, 1971; Stürckow *et al.*, 1973; van der Wolk, 1977).

(c) *Stimulus conducting structures of the olfactory hairs*

Here (Fig. 8.3b), three physiologically relevant features of the single-walled hairs should be mentioned (for further details see Kramer, this volume; Kaissling, 1971; 1974, Steinbrecht, 1973):

(1) Odor molecules do not have to hit the outer openings of pore tubuli system directly. They can be adsorbed to the outer lipophilic cuticle layer of the hair and reach the pores by two-dimensional diffusion in this layer.

(2) During stimulation by an air stream containing odor molecules, more and more molecules are adsorbed to the cuticle layer. Within one second the concentration can reach values several orders of magnitude higher than the concentration in the airstream (Adam and Delbrück, 1968; Steinbrecht and Kasang, 1972; Kaissling, 1974; Mankin *et al.*, 1977). The efficiency of this concentration process should depend largely on the hydrophobicity of the odor molecules. Therefore the sensitivity of the hair seems to be determined not only by the binding properties of the receptor protein, but also to a considerable extent by the rate of this concentration process. In spite of a stimulus concentration which increases during stimulation, the receptor potential remains constant. Kaissling (1974) explains this effect by assuming a concentration-dependent 'early inactivation'.

(3) Stimulus molecules diffuse through pore material and tubuli directly to the dendritic membrane without leaving this hydrophobic medium.

8.3.2 Chemosensory transduction

(a) *General aspects*

Transduction is a phenomenon in which receptor membranes — in our case those of dendritic outer segments — increase conductivity in response to stimulating molecules. A detailed understanding of transduction in insect chemoreception awaits the isolation of receptor and channel proteins from the membranes of appropriate chemosensory cells. Until that is accomplished, a useful alternative is to look for analogies with the few membrane receptor systems that have been well characterized. It is fortunate that one of the best-known membrane receptors — the acetylcholine receptor (AChR) of the subsynaptic membranes of electric organs of fish — is a chemoreceptor. In this case, the identification of the purified protein as the AChR was based on correlations of binding of cholinergic agonists, antagonists and specific and irreversible blockers to the protein in the biochemical assays *in vitro* with effects of those compounds on electrophysiological activity *in vivo* (for literature see Changeux, 1972; Raftery *et al.*, 1974; Eldefrawi *et al.*, 1977). The following considerations of chemosensory transduction in insects are undertaken on the assumption that important analogies exist between AChR and the system of interest here.

Sites, receptor proteins

Kinetics considerations demonstrate that the number of identical sites for the stimulus molecules on chemosensitive membranes is large but limited (Beidler, 1971; Kaissling, 1971; Colquhoun, 1973). In the following discussion it will be assumed that the concentration dependence of conductivity or spike frequency reflects the fraction of sites occupied by stimulus molecules.

The chemical nature of insect chemoreceptor sites is not clear, but there are theoretical and experimental bases for assuming that most, if not all, are proteins. Binding of ligand to protein, based on configurationally complementary fitting, is the only class of interactions of biological molecules that could provide the variety of specificities and sensitivities that have been documented for chemoreception in insects. Receptors for some neurotransmitters and hormones have already been identified and isolated as protein molecules, and there is general agreement that receptor proteins are responsible for the recognition of neurotransmitters, several hormones and many other physiologically important ligands (Greaves, 1976).

However, in the field of gustatory and olfactory chemoreception only a few authors postulate a central role for proteins of the cell membrane in the process of recognition (for vertebrates: Price, 1974; for insects: Hansen, 1974; Norris, 1976; Kijima *et al.* 1977). Many others prefer the neutral terms 'receptor molecules' and 'acceptors' (Beidler, 1971b; Kaissling, 1974; Kafka and Neuwirth, 1975).

In some cases suggestions have been made that substances other than proteins could function as receptors. Phospholipids have been discussed as receptors for salt and bitter taste in vertebrates (for literature see Price and Desimonis, 1977). Another hypothesis suggests that bitter substances should act inside the receptor cells by decreasing cAMP level (Kurihara, 1972; Price, 1974).

Specificity

The specificity and sensitivity of a receptor cell is a direct function of the properties of the receptor proteins on its receptive membrane since other characteristics of the cell, as well as the subsequent electrical events are common to different types of receptor cells; moreover, the stimulus-conducting structures (pore-tubules system) and media (viscous fluid) do not exhibit any specificity.

Channel proteins

Recently, it has become more and more evident that ion channels are specialized regions of proteins (vertebrate rhodopsin (Montal, 1977), sodium channels of excitable membranes (Reed and Raftery, 1976), channels in the subsynaptic membrane). These channel proteins (pore proteins, ion-conductance modulators, ionophores) extend across the entire thickness of the membrane in a highly oriented manner (Korenbrot, 1977). The receptor site and the ion channel are on the same protein (Fig. 8.4C) in the case of rhodopsin (Montal, 1977), but apparently on different proteins in the case of the AChR-channel protein system (Eldefrawi *et al.*, 1977).

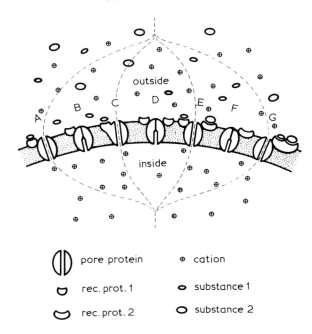

Fig. 8.4 Possible models of association between receptor proteins and channel- or pore-proteins in the chemosensitive membrane. The broken lines mark elementary receptor currents. For explanation see text.

In a simple model, the channel is closed in the resting state (Fig. 8.4B), but binding of a stimulus molecule to receptor protein triggers a temporary opening, resulting in an elementary current pulse (Fig. 8.4A). In the case of acetylcholine receptor, various agonists all induce similar open channel conductances in the subsynaptic membrane but differ in average open times induced and therefore in maximal depolarizations (Neher and Stevens, 1977). For insect chemosensory membranes, two or more receptor proteins have often been postulated (sugar receptor: Evans, 1963; Shimada *et al.*, 1974; Morita *et al.*, 1977; glycoside receptor: Wieczorek, 1976; deterrent receptors: see Section 8.4.2). In such a situation (a) each receptor protein might use its own channel protein (Fig. 8.4A and F), simultaneous stimulation of two receptor sites results in an additive response (Wieczorek, 1976); (b) different receptor proteins might use the same channel protein (Fig. 8.4E), the resulting response would be complex. Complex situations would also result if two or more receptor proteins had to be occupied before the channel opened (Morita and Shiraishi, 1968, Fig. 8.4D). For insect mechanoreceptors, the possibility of two types of channels lying interspersed in the dendritic membrane has been discussed (Thurm, 1974). Another relation between receptor and channel occurs in the *Limulus* photoreceptor and the bombykol receptor of the silk moth, where one quantum of light or one bombykol molecule, respectively, interacting with a single receptor molecule can open many channels simultaneously (Cone, 1973; Kaissling and Priesner, 1970).

Biochemical approaches in insects

Although no protein has been identified unequivocally as a receptor protein from chemosensitive sensilla, there is evidence that the so-called pyranose site of the sugar receptor may be identical with the substrate binding site of an α-glucosidase (Hansen, 1969; Morita, 1972; Section 8.4.1e). But it is not clear which of the more than ten glucosidases which have been detected in taste hair-rich segments, might act *in vivo* as a receptor protein. Naphthochinons are feeding inhibitors for the cockroach *Periplaneta* and proteins showing redox interactions with those compounds have been isolated from antennae; however, the type of sensilla involved is not yet clear (see Norris and Chu, 1974; Norris, 1976 for further literature).

(b) *The membrane area involved in transduction*

Fifty milliseconds after onset of stimulation of a taste hair the receptor current is half of its plateau value, and the spike frequency is maximal (Fig. 8.5). In this time period sucrose molecules diffuse a mean distance of 5 μm; only 1% of the molecules diffuses more than 3.5 times further than 5 μm. Remarkably stimulus molecules load only the tip of the dendrites. Therefore in the case of the largest labellar hairs of flies less than 2% of the length and surface of the dendrites serves for transduction. The absolute value of the membrane area, the conductance of which is altered during stimulation, appears to be in the range of 3 μm^2. The density of receptor channel protein complexes is not known in insect chemoreceptors. However, in all the analogous systems investigated, high densities have been observed by freeze etching techniques (subsynaptic membranes of the muscle end plate: $7.5 \times 10^3 \, \mu$m^{-2}, Peper *et al.*, 1974; olfactory cilia of vertebrates: $10^3 \, \mu$m^{-2}, Kerjaschki and Hörandner, 1976; Kerjaschki, 1977; disc membrane of rod outer segment: 20×10^3 rhodopsin molecules μm^{-2}, Bownds and Gaide-Hughin, 1970) in contrast with the low density of sodium channels (35–75 μm^{-2}) of axonal membranes (Ulbricht, 1974).

8.3.3 The electrical events

(a) *Receptor potential and spike frequency*

Changes in receptor membrane conductivity result in an ion current, which can be recorded as the first electrical signal after stimulation. These currents are superpositions of many elementary current pulses reflecting the transitory opening of pores. The driving force for these currents may be either potentials across the membrane, which are generated elesewhere, or diffusion potentials, which are based on differential ion concentrations across the membrane.

The sequence and time courses of electrical events are diagrammed in

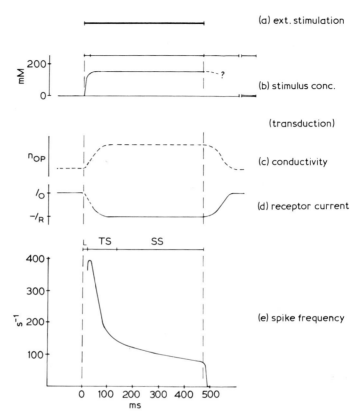

Fig. 8.5 The sequence and time course of processes during stimulation, shown schematically for the sugar cell of the fly. Electrode arrangement EA2-3 is used (see Fig. 8.7). The time scale of (e) is valid for the whole diagram.

(a) The black bar marks the interval of contact between the hair tip and the stimulating electrode containing 200 mM sugar solution.

(b) Within a few milliseconds, the sugar concentration at the membrane reaches a constant value equal to the applied one. After removal of the stimulating electrode, sugar remaining at the hair tip disappears in an unknown manner. Three minutes later the hair will give the same responses as before.

(c) The hypothesized time course of conductivity increase is drawn symmetrically to the receptor current (d). It has not been measurable in insect sensilla.

(d) Receptor current, shown schematically according to the receptor potential measurements of Morita, 1969. The onset (dotted line) is not exactly known.

(e) The spike frequency curve is calculated from the reciprocal distance between adjacent spikes. The first spike occurs after a latency (L) of a few

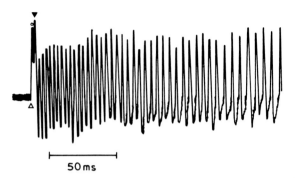

50 ms

Fig. 8.6 Spike response of the sugar receptor cell of a labellar taste hair from the fly *Phormia* upon stimulation by 1 M maltose. △ onset of stimulation, ○ contact artifact, ▼ first spike after a latency of 4 ms. Original record using the electrode arrangement EA 1 of Fig. 8.7. The spike amplitude is about 0.8 mV (Wieczorek and Dietz, unpublished observations).

Fig. 8.5c—e. Fig. 8.6 shows an original recording of a spike response. Fig. 8.7 indicates the various possible arrangements of recording electrodes.

Morita and Yamashita (1959) made the first measurements of receptor potentials during sugar and salt stimulation of labellar taste hairs of flies (Fig. 8.7, electrode arrangement (EA) 2). Later, Morita (1969) demonstrated, with an improved method (Fig. 8.7, EA 2 + 3), that for the sugar receptor

(1) the receptor potential reaches a constant amplitude after 100 ms (Fig. 8.5d, SS) called the steady state in analogy to enzyme reactions,

(2) receptor potential amplitude rises with increasing sugar concentration, and

(3) spike frequency is proportional to the steady-state amplitude of the receptor potential. The same relationship between receptor potential and spike frequency was obtained in insect mechanoreceptors by Thurm (1963). In the extremely sensitive bombykol receptors of the silk moth discrete potential fluctuations can be observed. They seem to be the quantal units of the receptor potential and are able to trigger single spikes (Kaissling, 1974; Kramer, this volume). Comparable small potentials are known as 'bumps' in invertebrate visual cells. They might reflect the synchronous opening of numerous ion channels elicited by single photons (Cone, 1973).

Fig. 8.5 (*continued*)
milliseconds. The high initial frequency of the transitional phase (TS) decreases rapidly to the rather constant values in the steady state (SS). A spontaneous discharge frequency has never been observed in the sugar receptors. At the end of stimulation, the spike frequency seems to disappear faster than the receptor current. In the olfactory receptors the electrical events c—e are the same as in taste hairs. The stimulation time course is, however, more complex; see Section 8.3.1 and Kaissling, 1974 (Fig. 6, p. 252).

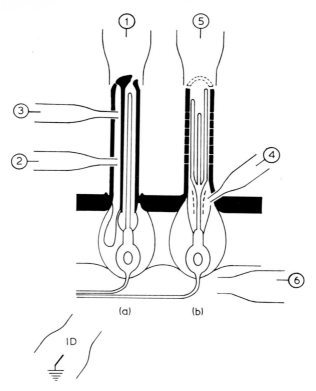

Fig. 8.7 Electrode arrangements (EA) used in electrophysiological recording techniques from taste (a) and olfactory (b) hairs. All electrodes lie extracellularily. EA 1 means that signals are recorded between electrode 1 and the indifferent electrode (ID), which lies in the hemolymph space. Spike series from up to three or four cells of one sensillum can be distinguished by their different amplitudes.

EA 1 The recording electrode 1 also contains the stimulating solution (Hodgson and Roeder, 1956) (see recording Fig. 8.6). Receptor potentials cannot be obtained.

EA 2 In the 'side wall recording technique' the hair is pierced laterally, capillary 1 is used for stimulation only (Morita and Yamashita, 1959). Thus the receptors can be studied before stimulation (spontaneous spike activity) and after the end of stimulation (rebound effects, off responses). A more advanced form is the recording between the electrodes 2 and 3 (EA 2–3) (Morita, 1969).

EA 4 For recording from olfactory cells (Boeckh, 1962, 1967).

EA 5 The tip of long olfactory hairs is cut off before electrode 5 is put over the hair (Kaissling, 1974). Stimulation of olfactory hairs is achieved by an airstream which contains the odor molecules (for quantitative aspects see Kafka, 1970).

EA6 Electroantennogram (EAG) technique. The electrode 6 and the indifferent electrode are inserted into the tip and base of an antenna. An integrated response is obtained (Schneider, 1957).

A more complex situation occurs during the rising phase of the receptor potential (Fig. 8.5d,e, TS). Here the rate of change of potential controls spike frequency, as also observed in olfactory sensilla by Boeckh (1962). Although the highest spike frequencies are obtained during these first 100 ms, and most behavioral responses are triggered during this interval, we do not sufficiently understand its kinetics. The latency between onset of stimulation and occurence of the first spike ranges from 1–40 ms at high stimulus concentrations (Fig. 8.5e). The shortest times are found for the salt receptors. Values of 5–10 ms for the sugar (Fig. 8.6) and water receptor and 40 ms for the glycoside receptor have been reported (Evans and Mellon, 1962; Brown and Hodgson, 1962; Rees, 1970b; Wieczorek, 1976). Comparably short latencies of 3 ms occur in olfactory hairs (green odor receptor of locust, Kafka, 1970; CO_2-receptors of the bee, Stange, 1974); longer latencies are observed in the bombykol receptor (Kaissling, 1976).

The conductance change induced by the stimulus is transformed into the receptor current by the movement of cations surrounding the dendrites (Morita, 1967). Since stimulating molecules diffuse so rapidly from the outside of the taste hair to the dendrites, it is unclear what prevents dilution of the ion concentration by diffusion in the opposite direction. If this dilution would actually occur it should result in a decrease of excitability of the receptors (Broyles and Hanson, 1976).

(b) *Mechanism of receptor potential formation*

Most authors (Morita, 1967, 1969; Wolbarsht, 1965; Boeckh, 1969; Maes, 1977; Morita *et al.,* 1977) have discussed the formation of receptor potentials in insect receptor cells in terms of a model adopted from the rather different mechanoreceptors of vertebrates. Of these, the Pacinian corpuscle is the best-studied (Loewenstein, 1971). It is a specialized end of an axon and is not part of an epithelium. In this system, the receptor potential is a diffusion potential, seen as a transitory decrease of resting potential during stimulation. It results from an increase of conductivity for all ions and depends on differential ion concentrations inside (K^+ high, Na^+ low) and outside the membrane (K^+ low, Na^+ high). In the light of new studies of mechanoreceptive sensilla of flies it is clear that the situation in insect sensilla is quite different (Thurm, 1974). Using different techniques, Küppers (1974) and Kaissling (unpublished observations) have demonstrated that the ionic milieu around the dendrites contains high potassium (130 or 300 mM) but low sodium concentrations in mechanoreceptive sensilla of flies or olfactory hairs of the silkmoth, respectively. Such a ionic composition is the same as that assumed to be inside the receptor cells and thus no diffusion potentials would exist.

Thurm's model makes the following radical change in the electrical analog circuit of the sensilla: The increased conductance controls a receptor current, the main voltage source of which is a transepithelial potential of 30–100 mV. The latter is generated in the membrane systems of the tormogen cell. There potassium is pumped by an electrogenic transport mechanism from the cell into lymph cavity II. Furthermore, this pump is responsible for the above mentioned high potassium content of the fluid around the dendrites (for details and further aspects see Thurm, 1970, 1974a,b). The recorded 'receptor potentials' correspond to receptor currents and represent the voltage drop across the resistance between electrodes 2 + 3 (Fig. 8.7). This altered interpretation does not influence Morita's result, that spike frequency is proportional to the relative amplitude of the receptor potential. Transepithelial potentials are well known in taste hairs (Wolbarsht, 1958), but they have never been adequately recorded and are normally nullified together with asymmetric potentials of the electrodes by the introduction of a compensatory potential.

The receptor current passes through the dendrite to control the spike generator which is located at the membrane of the dendritic inner segment. The localization of spike-initiating membrane areas is discussed by Tateda and Morita (1959); Wolbarsht and Hanson (1965) and Thurm (1974a). In olfactory hairs the outer current path is through the fluid surrounding the dendrites (Fig. 8.3b). In taste hairs with two canals, canal II is assumed to be the outer current path (Rees, 1967, 1968). However the connection of canal II to the dendritic tips in canal I is not clear. Tiny pores between canal II and the outside have been observed several times (Gaffal, 1973; van der Wolk, 1977). However, impedance measurements (Stürckow, 1971) and studies of ^{14}C-glucose diffusion into both canals of the hair (Hanamori, 1976) indicate that it is unlikely that the tiny pores of canal II provide the only functional current paths.

8.3.4 Receptor kinetics

The most distinctive features of a receptor cell are its specificity and sensitivity. Each parameter is adequately described by a concentration-response curve for each stimulating substance. These curves represent the basis of all kinetic considerations. A prerequisite for generating such curves is the possibility of making single cell recordings from a well-defined sensillum. Data from taste receptors are treated preferentially in this section because the kinetics are less complex than in olfactory receptors; for the latter see Kaissling (1969, 1971, 1975, 1976). In general, response is measured as the spike frequency in the steady state (Fig. 8.5e). In a direct plot, concentration-response curves are usually rectangular hyperbolas. Customarily the magnitude of response is plotted as a function of the logarithm of stimulus concentration, allowing a wide range of concentrations to be included. Then the curve is sigmoid and symmetrical about the inflection point. Examples of concentration-response curves for a sugar receptor cell are shown in Fig. 8.8. Each curve can be characterized by three parameters:

(1) The inflection point which represents the concentration of stimulating substance evoking half-maximal response. This point has been called the 'K_b value' (Morita, 1969; Kaissling, 1971, 1975), $a_{V/2}$(Hanamori *et al.*, 1972) or $1/K$ (Beidler, 1961, 1971b).

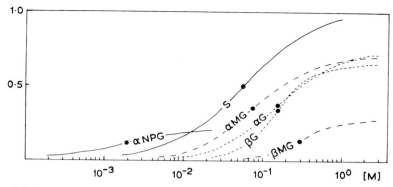

Fig. 8.8 Concentration-response curves of the sugar receptor cell from the largest labellar hairs of the fly *Boettcherisca*. The relative response of the receptor is plotted against the logarithmically scaled molar concentration of the stimulating sugars. The response is equal to the number of spikes during the steady state period from 150–350 ms after onset of stimulation; the maximal response for sucrose is set at unity. The K_b values are marked by filled circles. The K_b values and the Hill coefficients are listed in the columns 4 and 6 of Table 8.2.

Abbreviations: α-G: α-D-glucopyranose, β-G: β-D-glucopyranose, α-MG: methyl-α-glucoside, β-MG: methyl-β-glucoside, α-NPG: *p*-nitrophenyl-α-glucoside. (Modified after Hanamori *et al.*, 1972).

(2) The 'maximal response' (R_{max}) which is reached at high stimulus concentrations. It is often expressed as percentage of response to a reference substance.

(3) The slope of the curve at its inflection point which is expressed as the Hill coefficient (n_H) obtained from a separate Hill plot.

Concentration-response curves with a Hill coefficient of unity satisfy the Michaelis-Menten equation. Then K_b values formally correspond to but are not equal to the dissociation constant of the complex of stimulus molecule and receptor protein. As was first calculated by Morita (1969), for the case of a simple binding function, K_b values are always smaller than dissociation constants by a certain factor because of the non-linear relationship between receptor current and conductance change. This factor should be a site-specific constant, but, as can be derived from the more complex kinetic model discussed by Morita in the appendix of his paper, this assumption is valid only in cases of equal maximal responses, as for example in the case of the α-glucosidic disaccharides (see Table 8.2, column 5). Consequently, the ratios of K_b values of a certain site for several stimulating substances should directly reflect the ratios of the respective dissociation constants. For example, it can be deduced from the K_b values of Fig. 8.8 and column 4 (Table 8.2) for sucrose (24), maltose (27) and *p*-nitrophenyl-α-glucoside (45) that the ratios of the dissociation constants should be 1.0: 1.7: 0.03.

Table 8.2 Behavioral thresholds and electrophysiological data of the fly's sugar receptor cells for various sugars

1		2 50% acceptance threshold	3	4 K_b
1	ribose	0		
2	arabinose			
3	L-arabinose			
4	xylose			
5	L-xylose			
6	lyxose	0		
7	fucose		P	
8	L-fucose			
9	allose			
10	altrose	0		
11	glucose, equil. mix.			130
12	α-glucose		E	150
13	β-glucose		E	150
14	L-glucose		P	
15	mannose			~700
16	gulose	0		
17	idose	0		
18	galactose			80
(19	talose)			
20	ribulose	0		
21	fructose		P	75
22	L-sorbose			
23	tagatose	0	P	
24	sucrose Glcα1-2βFru			60
25	turanose Glcα1-3Fru			
26	palatinose Glcα1-6Fru		P	
27	maltose Glcα1-4Glc		P	100
28	isomaltose Glcα1-6Glc	+	W	
29	trehalose Glcα1-1Glc			
30	cellobiose Glcβ1-4Glc		P	

Column 2 scale (mM): 1000 — 100 — 10 (mM) — 1

5 R_{max}	6 n_H	7 p-MB	8 Mut.	9 site	10 hydr./inh.	11		
						1	ribose	
1.05		0.4		(F)	i+	2	arabinose	
0.70		< 0.2		P		3	L- arabinose	
		< 0.2		P	i+	4	xylose	
						5	L- xylose	
						6	lyxose	
0.90		0.9		F		7	fucose	
1.05		< 0.2		P		8	L- fucose	
0.33*						9	allose	
						10	altrose	
= 1.0	1.4	< 0.2	++	P	i+	11	glucose, equil. mix.	
1.0+	1.1					12	α- glucose	
0.9+	1.7					13	β- glucose	
0.90						14	L- glucose	
~ 0.3+		< 0.2		P		15	mannose	
						16	gulose	
						17	idose	
0.60	1.2	0.6		F		18	galactose	
						(19	talose)	
						20	ribulose	
0.85	1.2	1.0	–	F	i–	21	fructose	
		< 0.2		P	i+	22	L- sorbose	
						23	tagatose	
1.35	1.0	< 0.2	+	P	++	24	sucrose	Glcα1-3Fru
		< 0.2	+	P	++	25	turanose	Glcα1-3Fru
1.45		< 0.2	–	(P)	+	26	palatinose	Glcα1-6 Fru
1.35	1.0	< 0.2	+	P	++	27	maltose	Glcα1-4Glc
						28	isomaltose	Glcα1-6Glc
0.95		< 0.2	–	(P)	(++)	29	trehalose	Glcα1-1Glc
		< 0.2		P	–	30	cellobiose	Glcβ1-4Glc

Table 8.2 (*continued*) Behavioral thresholds and electrophysiological data of the fly's sugar receptor cells for various sugars

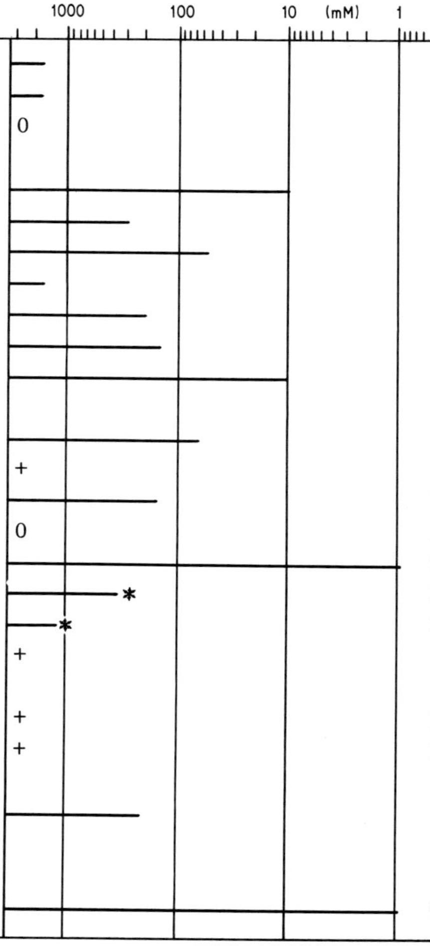

1		2 50% acceptance threshold	3	4 K_b
31	gentiobiose Glcβ1-6Glc	▬	P	
32	melibiose Galα1-6Glc	▬	P	
33	lactose Galβ1-4Glc	0		
34	maltotriose		P	
35	panose	▬▬	P	
36	melezitose	▬▬▬		
37	planteose	▬	P	
38	raffinose	▬▬		
39	gentianose	▬▬	P	
40	maltopentaose		P	
41	methyl-α-Glcp			73
42	ethyl-α-Glcp	+		100
43	methyl-β-Glcp		P	280
44	methyl-β-Fruf	0	J	
45	4-nitrophenyl-α-Glcp		P	2
46	4-nitrophenyl-β-Glcp	*	P	
47	4-nitrophenyl-α-Manp	*	P	
48	phenyl-α-Glcp	+		
49	sorbitol	+	E	
50	mannitol	+	E	
51	myo-inositol			
52	chiro-inositol			
53	L- phenylalanine		G	0.6

Column 1:1—8: aldopentoses, 9—19: aldohexoses, 20—23: ketoses, 24—29: α-glucosidic disaccharides, 30—33: other disaccharides, 34—39: trisaccharides of the following structures: 34: Glcα1-4Glcα1-4Glc, 35:Glcα1-6Glcα1-4Glc, 36: Glcα1-3Frufβ2-1αGl, 37: Glcα1-2βFruf6-1αGal, 38: Galα1-6Glcα1-2βFruf, 39: Glcβ1-6Glcα1-2βFruf, 40: Glcα1-(4Glcα1)$_3$-4Glc. 41—44: alkylglycosides, 45—48: arylglycosides.

5 R_{max}	6 n_H	7 p-MB	8 Mut.	9 site	10 hydr./inh.	11	
					−	31	gentiobiose Glcβ1-6Glc
					−	32	melibiose Galα1-6Glc
					−	33	lactose Galβ1-4Glc
						34	maltotriose
						35	panose
1.35		<0.2	+	P	+	36	melezitose
						37	planteose
		<0.2	−			38	raffinose
						39	gentianose
						40	maltopentaose
1.0+	1.1	++	P		+	41	methyl-α-Glcp
0.7+	1.1					42	ethyl-α-Glcp
0.4+	2.0				−	43	methyl-β-Glcp
0.0*						44	methyl-β-Fruf
1.25	1.0				++	45	4-nitrophenyl-α-Glcp
						46	4-nitrophenyl-β-Glcp
						47	4-nitrophenyl-α-Manp
1.05					+	48	phenyl-α-Glcp
						49	sorbitol
						50	mannitol
0.5*						51	myo-inositol
0.2*						52	chiro-inositol
0.3+		~0.8	F			53	L- phenylalanine

Column 1:49−50: sugar alcohols, 51−52: cyclitols, 53: amino acid. All compounds belong to the D-series if not stated otherwise. Column 2: The behavioral threshold values of the tarsal sugar receptors of the fly. Note the inverse logarithmic scale, in millimolar sugar concentrations. The bars represent the stimulation effectiveness ('sweetness'). The right end of each bar is equal to the behavioral threshold

The observation of different maximal responses for stimulating substances reacting at the same site indicates that the fractional occupancy of receptor protein molecules is not the sole determinant of conductance change. It might be that the complex between stimulus molecule and receptor protein exists in two states, only the second of which controls conductivity. If the ratio between the two states varied with the stimulus molecule, then different maximal responses would be produced (Morita, 1969; Kaissling, 1974).

Hill coefficients greater than one are generally considered as indications of positive co-operativity. In these cases the binding sites are not independent of each other. Binding of the first stimulus molecule at one site of a co-operative group of

Table 8.2 (*continued*)
(see text, Section 8.4.1b). Long bars correspond to a low threshold and high effectiveness. Symbols: 0 = ineffective, at the highest possible concentrations less than 3% of the flies react; + = effective, but no threshold data available; * = extrapolated values obtained by using extremely hungry flies. All threshold values from Dethier (1955) (*Phormia regina,* Ph.r.), if not stated otherwise in column 3:
P: Pflumm, 1971, 1972 (*Protophormia terraenovae,* PPh.t.), E: Evans, 1963 (Ph.r.), G: Goldrich, 1973; Shiraishi and Kuwabara, 1970 (Ph.r.), W: Wieczorek (unpublished observations) (PPh.t.). Column 4—6: Parameter of concentration—response curves obtained electrophysiologically from the largest labellar taste hairs.

Column 4: K_b values (mM) obtained from the fleshfly *Boettcherisca peregrina* (B.p.) (Hanamori *et al.,* 1972, 1974; Morita and Shiraishi, 1968; Shiraishi and Kuwabara, 1970).

Column 5: Relative maximal responses (R_{max}) measured by using high concentrations (0.8 and 1.0M) except 45 and 48 (15, 20 mM). All values from largest hairs of PPh.t. (Wieczorek and Köppl, unpublished observations), except those marked:* Jakinovich *et al.,* 1971 (*Sarcophaga bullata,* S.b.), + Hanamori *et al.,* 1972 (B.p.).

Column 6: Hill coefficients, all values from B.p. (Morita and Shiraishi, 1968; Hanamori *et al.,* 1972, 1974).

Column 7: Inhibition of the sugar receptor response of B.p. by *p*-mercuribenzoate (*p*-Mb), as described in Section 8.3.5. 1.0: response not influenced by pretreatment with *p*-Mb. 0: complete inhibition (Shimada *et al.,* 1972, 1974; Shimada, 1975a; Ninomiya and Shimada, 1976).

Column 8: Depression of the electrophysiological response to 0.1 M sugars in the *Drosophila* mutant. ++ 50—60%, + 15—35%, − no depression, respectively (Isono and Kikuchi, 1974; Kikuchi, 1975).

Column 9: Pyranose site substances are denoted P, furanose site F.

Column 10: Oligosaccharides and glycosides split (++, +) or not split (−) by glycosidases of crude extracts of tarsi; monosaccharides inhibiting (I +) or with no effect (i −) on glucosidase activity (Hansen, 1968, 1969).

receptor proteins or subunits facilitates binding of the next one. Therefore K_b is a more complex constant than in case of curves with Hill coefficients of 1.0.

Several cases of Hill coefficients greater than one are known.

(a) The pyranose site of the sugar receptor exhibits values as high as 2.0 for β-glucosides, while those for α-glucosides are nearly 1 (Hanamori *et al.,* 1972). *p*-nitrophenyl-β-glucoside (40 mM) and quinine-HCl (20 µM) behave as typical allosteric inhibitors; in the presence of those compounds, the K_b for sucrose is shifted toward higher concentrations by a factor of 4, the Hill coefficient increases from 1.1 to 2.2, while the maximal response remains unaffected (Morita *et al.,* 1977).

(b) The glycoside receptors from two different strains of *Mamestra* exhibit different Hill coefficients for naphthyl-β-glucoside. In one strain, the value is 1.0; in the other a value of 1.7 is found; the curves for sinigrin, which occupies another site on the same receptor membrane, are the same in both strains ($n_H = 0.7$) (Wieczorek, 1976).

(c) For the water receptor cell of the fly, inhibition by salt and reactivation by sugars have the same Hill coefficient of about 2 (Wieczorek and Köppl, 1978).

Hill coefficients below 1.0 raise some problems. Sinigrin binding to the glycoside receptor shows a Hill coefficient of 0.7. It is not possible to determine whether

(a) the concentration—response curve obeys a monotonic function and thus there is negative co-operativity, or

(b) the curve represents the sum of two curves generated by different sites with different K_b values (Wieczorek, 1976). A similar situation is discussed by Morita, (1972) for the sugar receptor.

8.3.5 Pharmacological studies on transduction

The use of protein-modifying reagents, various inhibitors, detergents, and membrane degrading enzymes may help

(1) to identify different sites on the same cell,

(2) to discriminate between effects at the level of stimulus binding and of ion channels, and

(3) to elucidate common properties of receptor membranes of different specificities. A general review on this topic is given by Narahashi (1974). For the study of chemosensitive sensilla it is an advantage that the reagents pass through the stimulus-conducting openings and make contact first with those membranes involved in transduction. Other membranes are about 300 µm away in the long taste hairs of flies and the long olfactory hair of lepidopteran antennae, respectively. Spreading of the reagents by diffusion over the longer distance requires at least 1—3 min. Therefore interactions of the reagents with other membranes can be excluded by short periods of treatment.

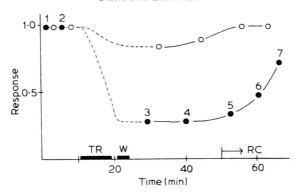

Fig. 8.9 Typical sequence of procedures for testing pharmacological agents. Here the effect of *p*-mercuribenzoate on sugar reception is shown.
1,2: Responses (spike frequency) to 0.1 M glucose (closed circle) and fructose (open circle) respectively before treatment. TR: treatment period: 3 min, 0.5 mM *p*-MB, optimized by varying time and concentration. W: washing with balanced salt medium, 3,4: response after treatment, response to glucose is reduced to 25%, that to fructose unaltered. 5−7: recovery effects. (After Shimada *et al.,* 1974).

(a) *Protein-modifying reagents (Cohen 1970, Glaser 1976).*
These reagents can be used to determine the functional importance of certain amino acid side chains in transduction.

The influence of *p*-mercuribenzoate (*p*-MB) on the electrophysiological response of the labellar sugar receptor of flies provides strong evidence for two separate sites (Fig. 8.9, Sections 8.4.1c,d,f; Shimada *et al.,* 1972, 1974; Shimada, 1975a). After pretreatment with *p*-MB, the response to glucose (or sucrose) is reduced to 25% of its original value, while there is only a slight effect on the fructose response. Depression of the glucose response is eliminated by mercaptoethanol. This demonstrates the SH-group-specificity as well as the reversibility of the *p*-MB effect. Glucose applied simultaneously with *p*-MB has no specific protecting effect. By varying the sucrose concentration it could be shown that the maximal response rather than the K_b is affected. Shimada *et al.* suggest that *p*-MB does not compete with the glucopyranose binding site, but may block the change of membrane permeability. The blocking of SH-groups inhibits the response of several other receptors too. In the fly, the salt cell is depressed by *p*-MB, but the water cell not at all (Shimada *et al.,* 1972). In the moth *Heliothis,* the EAG response (Fig. 8.7, EA 6) to *n*-pentyl acetate is inhibited by 50% after 2 min treatment with fluorescein mercuric acetate (25 μM) (Frazier and Heitz, 1975).

Tests with other modifying agents (given in brackets) revealed that tryptophan (*N*-bromo-succinimide; NBS), arginine (glyoxal) and lysine (2,4,6-trinitrobenzene sulfonic acid; TNBS) residues are involved functionally in the glucopyranose-site (Shimada, 1975a). The periods of treatment for depression of the response by NBS or mercuric chloride are remarkably short, only 0.5 s. Like *p*-MB, mercuric chloride probably reacts with SH-groups. TNBS suppresses the response to fructose more effectively than that to glucose. No effect was obtained with CMC (2-cyclohexyl-3-(2-morpholinyl-4-ethyl) carbondiimide) (metho-*p*-toluene sulfonate) indicating that carboxyl groups are not functionally involved.

(b) *Other inhibitors*

Little data are available. Sucrose solutions which contain higher aliphatic alcohols ($C_6 - C_8$) in millimolar concentrations are rejected by flies in behavioral tests. This observation led to the erroneous conclusion that there should be a receptor cell responsible for rejection (Dethier and Chadwick, 1950; Dethier, 1953), but it was later demonstrated electrophysiologically that the sugar receptor itself contains a hydrophobic site which inhibits the sugar response. Alcohols and amines reacting at this site inhibit the sugar response in a pattern that corresponds formally to competitive inhibition. The best ligands are octanol and octylamine (Steinhardt *et al.,* 1966). Many known natural feeding inhibitors (Chapman, 1974, Meinwald *et al.,* 1978; Navon and Bernays, 1978) might act in a similar manner, inhibiting receptors responsible for feeding activity.

A further type of inhibition is observed with quinine hydrochloride and *p*-nitrophenyl-β-glucoside. The substances are chemically unrelated but inhibit the sugar receptor in a similar manner. K_b values and Hill coefficients for both types of sugar sites increase while the maximal responses remain constant. Both reagents inhibit the salt receptor but only nitrophenylglucoside affects the water receptor (Morita *et al.,* 1977).

There is one somewhat perplexing report that cAMP (5×10^{-4} M) and aminophylline (2 mM, an inhibitor of phosphodiesterase) depress the response of the sugar receptor to 0.2 M sucrose to 32%, while cGMP (1 mM) elicited an increased response (140%) (Daley and Vande Berg, 1976).

(c) *Inorganic ions*

The spike response of the water receptor cell of flies is reduced to 50% by 30 mM Na^+, 2 mM Ca^{2+} or 0.4 mM La^{3+} (Rees, 1970, 1972). The inhibition of the salt cell by Ca^{2+} is complex. Ca^{2+} totally supresses the spontaneous frequency of spikes at concentrations above 0.05 mM. In the presence of alkali ions as stimuli, the calcium concentration required for inhibition increases with stimulus concentration. Calcium itself elicits no spikes during stimulation. But after removal of the stimulating pipet a characteristic volley of spikes is observed (off-discharge, rebound effect) (Rees, 1968). In the sugar receptor cell of flies, Ca^{2+} (5–10 mM) inhibits the response to 0.2 M sucrose to 50% (Morita, 1967). In the presence of 1 M NaCl the K_b values for sucrose, glucose and fructose are increased by the factor 8 in the tarsal D-hairs of flies; the maximal response is not affected at all, and the Hill coefficient only slightly increased (Shiraishi and Miyachi, 1976).

(d) *Proteases and phospholipases*

Proteases and phospholipases do not always destroy membranes (Jain, 1973). Application of pronase, a rather aggressive bacterial protease, to the taste hair tip for at least 10 min reduces the response to sucrose to half the initial value. Other proteases such as nagarse and trypsin produce a weaker or no effect, respectively. Phospholipases A and D were ineffective (Shimada, 1975a). The often observed phenomena of recovery, especially after irreversible destruction, (e.g. pronase) suggest a renewal mechanism. The action of this mechanism should include synthesis of replacements for the destroyed protein in the cell body and transport of the protein through the dendrite to the tip (Shimada, 1975a).

(e) *Detergents*

Detergents such as sodium dodecylsulfate (SDS, 5%) immediately eliminate the sugar response. A few seconds later a high spike discharge from several cells is observed, indicating an injurious increase of conductance. Despite this high concentration of SDS, the sugar receptor cell is able to recover from a 2 min treatment with SDS within 20 min.

(f) *Tetrodotoxin*

The substances cited above inhibit by decreasing the stimuli-specific conductance change. Receptor current and spike frequency are thereby reduced. The shape of active potentials remains unchanged. In contrast, tetrodotoxin, a potent blocker of Na-channels in excitable membrane, reduces the negative phase of the biphasic action potentials even at the extremely low concentration of 10^{-8} M. This effect reflects the inhibition of action potentials which normally spread over the proximal parts of the dendritic outer segment antidromically. Therefore the dendritic outer segment should contain at least patches of conductile membrane (Wolbarsht and Hanson, 1965).

(g) *Agents without influence*

Attempts to incorporate macrocyclic antibiotics as artificial pores in the membrane have been without success. Tests were performed with the K-specific neutral ionophore valinomycin, the carboxylic ionophore nigericin and gramicidin D which forms quasi-ionophore channels (Shimada, 1975a).

For the water receptor cell no effects were observed with the following agents: physostigmine (an acetylcholinesterase inhibitor of the carbamate-type), acetylcholinchloride, ATP, ouabain (an ATP-ase inhibitor) (Rees, 1970).

8.4 SELECTED EXAMPLES OF SPECIFICITY

8.4.1 Sugar and amino acid receptors

(a) *Special features of sugars*
Sugars have several special properties as stimulating substances:

(1) They are uncharged; this is an important advantage for the experimenter since they do not influence electrical events at the membrane directly, but only by their binding to receptor proteins.

(2) Binding to the receptor protein occurs by means of a set of hydrogen bonds. Therefore only the hydroxyl groups of the sugar are of interest; the puckered furan or pyran rings are not distinguished by the receptor protein and serve only as backbone for the three-dimensional arrangement of the hydroxyl groups.

(3) A broad pattern of test substances is available which differ only in the steric arrangement of hydroxyl groups. Therefore it is possible to test a series of systematically altered sugars.

(4) The mixture of several conformational states like pyranose and furanose forms, different chair types in pyranoses and still more complex forms in furanoses or α- and β-anomeres, is a disadvantage which complicates the elucidation of structure— activity relationships. The conformations of several of the sugars of interest are shown in Fig. 8.10.

(b) *The general specificity of the sugar receptor*
In flies sugar receptor cells are localized in taste hairs on the distal segments of the legs, the tarsi, and on the distal lobes of the proboscis, the labella. Altogether about 200 substances have been tested for their stimulating effectiveness. A selection of them is listed in Table 8.2. Before analysing the spectrum in detail we can make the following generalizations:

(1) Only pentoses, hexoses, di- and oligosaccharides and glycosides are effective; trioses, tetroses, heptoses and polysaccharides are ineffective (Dethier, 1955).

(2) Only certain members of each group are effective and others not.

(3) Behavioral threshold values range over three orders of magnitude, (*p*-nitro-phenyl-α-glucoside (45) exhibits the lowest threshold of 1 mM, mannose (15) the highest, 4 M.

(4) Disaccharides and glycosides with an α-glycosidic linkage and glucose as the non-reducing monosaccharide unit are much more effective than sugars with a β-linkage.

(5) Two linear hexitols are slightly effective (49, 50).

(6) Two of the existing nine isomers of cyclitols are effective (51, 52) (Jakinovich *et al.,* 1971, Jakinovich and Agranoff, 1972).

(7) Amino acids, several derivatives and certain fatty acids are stimulating (Shiraishi and Kuwabara, 1970; Goldrich, 1973; Shimada, 1975a, 1978).

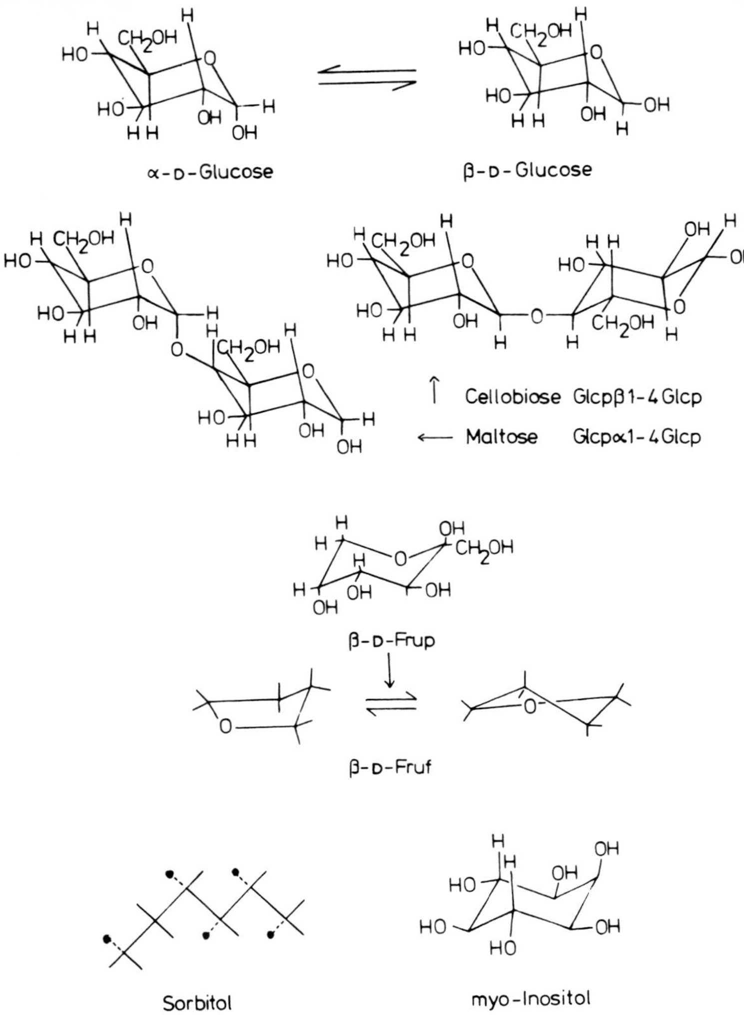

α-D-Glucose ⇌ β-D-Glucose

Cellobiose Glcpβ1-4Glcp
Maltose   Glcpα1-4Glcp

β-D-Frup

β-D-Fruf

Sorbitol   myo-Inositol

Fig. 8.10 Conformation of essential mono- and disaccharides and of related compounds. α-D-glucopyranose best fullfills the principle requirements of the pyranose site of the fly's sugar receptor (see Section 8.4.1(d)). Maltose and cellobiose (> 10 times less sweet than the former) differ in α- resp. β-linkage which correspond to an axial resp. equatorial position of the glycosidic oxygen, and in the spatial orientation of the reducing glucose units. In fructose solution, an equilibrium exists between the β-D-pyranose and the β-D-furanose. The furanose form itself is present in the 'envelope' (left) and the 'twist' (right) conformation. For sorbitol, the preferred bent-chain conformation is shown; hydroxyl groups are marked by point. (Rao and Foster, 1963; Angyal, 1972; Jeffrey and Kim, 1970).

(8) The cardenolide ouabain (*g*-strophantidine-L-rhamnoside), which is known as a potent ATPase inhibitor stimulates the sugar receptor with the extraordinarily low K_b of 5×10^{-7} M, but is inhibitory if applied together with glucose at higher concentration (Elizarov and Gritsai, 1975).

(9) The following artificial sweeters have been found to be completely ineffective: saccharine, dulcin, cyclamate, glycyrrhicine and the sweet-tasting protein thaumatine (von Frisch, 1935; Schoonhoven, 1974).

The threshold values in column 2 of Table 8.2 are based on the quantification of a behavioral reaction. Water-satiated, but hungry, flies, bees and butterflies extend their proboscida after bringing their legs or mouthparts into contact with a sucrose solution (Minnich, 1921; von Frisch, 1935). Dethier tested about 100 flies individually with a series of solutions containing logarithmically scaled sugar concentrations to determine the minimal concentration which elicits proboscis extension. He defined the threshold as that sugar concentration which elicits a response in 50% of the flies (Hassett *et al.*, 1950; Dethier, 1955). Because thresholds depend on the period of food deprivation (Haslinger, 1935), they are often normalized to the sucrose (Pflumm, 1971, 1972) or glucose (Evans, 1963) threshold.

Recent electrophysiological studies by Shiraishi and Tanabe (1974) indicate that the behavioral threshold values can be used as a first approximation for the actual K_b values of the D-hairs (terminology according to Grabowski and Dethier, 1954) of the lower side of the foreleg tarsi, since there was a correlation between the concentration of sugar that elicited proboscis extension and the concentration that produced half maximal spike frequency. Although D-hairs are only 5% of the taste hair population they displayed the lowest K_b values for sucrose, glucose and fructose and the highest maximal spike frequencies and thus it is probably their reactions that exert the primary influence on the behavioral response. The only reservation about this important correlation between behavioral and electrophysiological data is that it rests on the assumption that all the sugars stimulate D-hairs, and that the maximal responses are similar.

(c) *The existence of two sites*
Difficulties (von Frisch, 1935; Dethier, 1955) in defining a single site recognizing an hydroxyl group arrangement common to both glucose and fructose were overcome by the idea that two separate sites might exist (Evans, 1963). This suggestion is based on the observation that the poor stimulant mannose considerably elevated the behavioral threshold for fructose, but not for glucose, sucrose and maltose (Dethier, 1955a). This effect has been confirmed electrophysiologically. Mannose inhibits the fructose response at concentrations below those where it itself is stimulating (Morita and Shiraishi, 1968; Omand and Dethier, 1969). In the same manner, *p*-nitrophenyl-α-mannoside shifts the concentration—response curve for fructose, but not that for sucrose, to ten-fold higher concentrations without affecting the maximal response (Morita *et al.*, 1977). But the two sites are not completely

independent since glucose and fructose responses are not additive for responses near maximum which are nearly maximal (Morita and Shiraishi, 1968); however, such interactions may occur at the level of receptor current electrogenesis (Morita *et al.*, 1977). Shimada *et al.* (1972) developed an excellent tool for differentiating between the two sites. Pretreatment with *p*-mercuribenzoate (see Section 8.3.5a and column 7 of Table 8.2) reversibly suppresses response to glucose and several structurally related sugars (e.g. α-glucosidic disaccharides) without affecting response to fructose, galactose or amino acids (Shimada *et al.*, 1972; 1974; Shimada, 1975). Separate sites for glucose and fructose have also been demonstrated in *Drosophila* by selection of mutants defective in response to the former but not to the latter (Isono and Kikuchi, 1974; Kikuchi, 1975, Table 8.2, column 8). The mutants exhibit a depressed electrophysiological response to glucose and related sugars, but normal response to fructose, raffinose, palatinose and trehalose. This might indicate a third site in *Drosophila* for trehalose, since that sugar does not contain fructose.

(d) *The pyranose site*
Sugars interacting with the pyranose site are marked in column 9 by the symbol P. The structural requirement of this site for monosaccharides is well-defined. Inversion of the hydroxyl groups of glucose at C–2, C–3 or C–4 from the equatorial into the axial position (mannose, allose, gulose) or substitution of the same hydroxyl groups by H (desoxy-glucoses) or by groups bulkier than hydroxyl groups ($-OCH_3$) produces less effective or ineffective compounds (behavioral data from Evans, 1963; Pflumm, 1971, 1976; maximal responses obtained electrophysiologically, from Jakinovich *et al.*, 1971). Therefore, these three equatorial hydroxyl groups are necessary for hydrogen bonds. Jakinovich *et al.* showed that the ring oxygen is less important since replacement by a C-atom having an equatorial hydroxyl group to yield myo-inositol (Fig. 8.10) does not drastically influence stimulating effectiveness. Without the ring oxygen there is no difference between the C1 and 1C chair conformations. L-sugars of 1C conformation can now be superimposed by rotation over the C1 conformation. Therefore, it is understandable how L-sorbose, L-glucose and L-xylose react with the pyranose site. Consequently, the initial concept of the importance of equatorial hydroxyl groups at the C–2, C–3 and C–4 of a C1 pyranose was superceded by the more general statement that a pyranose with three adjacent equatorial hydroxyl groups is required for recognition (Shimada *et al.*, 1974; Hanamori *et al.*, 1974). The hydrogen atoms of these hydroxyl groups should be involved as donors in hydrogen bonds.

All effective di- and oligosaccharides contain an α-glucosidic group and therefore react with the pyranose site. The thresholds of these disaccharides are ten times lower that for glucose. This is correlated with the fact that the oxygen of the glycosidic linkage acts as a hydrogen acceptor, while the corresponding hydroxyl group in the glucose is a hydrogen donor.

The structural basis of the stimulating effectiveness of disaccharides is discussed in detail by Pflumm (1972), Hanamori *et al.* (1972), Hansen (1974) and Ninomiya and Shimada (1976). Briefly, in the glycosidic glucose moiety, alterations are tolerated only at the C—6; for disaccharides the nature of the non-glycosidic sugar only slightly influences the thresholds; trehalose with its more stable 1—1 linkage shows an elevated threshold.

(e) *The glucosidase hypothesis*
Hassett *et al.* (1950) noted that the specificity of the sugar receptor cell for disaccharides might parallel the substrate specificity of α-glucosidases. Later, Dethier (1955b) and Wiesmann (1960) observed that the legs of flies contain a sucrose-splitting enzyme. The specific activities of this enzyme as determined with sucrose was 3—5 times higher in extracts of taste hair-rich segments (tarsi and labella) than in extracts of taste hair-poor parts (tibiae, femora, proximal parts of the proboscis) (Hansen 1964, 1968, 1969). Extracts of tarsi split α-glucosidic di- and trisaccharides and glucosides (sucrose, maltose, turanose, melezitose; *p*-nitrophenyl-α-glucoside, methyl-α-glucoside, see Table 8.2 column 10); thus this enzyme was identified as a typical α-glucosidase of broad specificity (E.C. 3.2 1.20). The tarsal sugar receptor cells respond to the same disaccharides with particularily low thresholds (see Table 8.2). Other saccharides or glycosides (cellobiose, lactose, raffinose, gentiobiose, methyl-β-glucoside) are not hydrolysed by the tarsal extracts; correspondingly, they are perceived poorly (cellobiose, raffinose, gentiobiose, methyl-β-glucoside) or not at all (lactose). Moreover, the threshold for *p*-nitrophenyl-α-glucoside was found to be ten times lower than that for sucrose (Pflumm, 1972); correspondingly glycosidases generally have lower dissociation constants for nitrophenylglycosides than for disaccharides. On the other hand, trehalose seems to be an exception in both systems; it exhibits a higher threshold than all other α-glucosides, and is not split by α-glucosidases, but by a specific trehalase. These correlations led to the working hypothesis that an α-glucosidase may act as a receptor protein of the sugar receptor cell for substrate-like sugars (Hansen, 1969). Certain monosaccharides also interact with glucosidases. Typical sugars of the pyranose site, such as glucose, sorbose and xylose inhibit the glucosidase activity of tarsal extracts, while fructose is ineffective (Hansen, 1968). Thus the hypothesis can be reduced to the simple formula: The pyranose site may be identical with an α-glucosidase. The idea that the glucosidase is not the receptor protein, but functions analogously to acetylcholine esterase by inactivating stimulating disaccharides does not seem very probable, because the receptor protein exhibits an affinity for glucose and fructose, the products of disaccharide splitting.

Further supporting evidence for the hypothesis was the demonstrations of glucosidase activities

(a) on the outside of tarsi and labella *in vivo* (Koizumi *et al.*, 1973),
(b) in pieces of labellar integuments with intact taste hairs (Amakawa *et al.*, 1975),
(c) at the tip of labellar taste hairs (Kijima *et al.*, 1973; Koizumi *et al.*, 1974) and
(d) in isolated hairshafts (Amakawa *et al.*, 1975).

The enzyme activity of the taste hair tips splits sucrose, turanose, maltose, trehalose and nitrophenyl-α-glucoside. Its apparent K_m for sucrose is about 50 mM. The enzyme is not released into the incubation medium during the incubation period and is therefore assumed to be bound to the dendritic membranes. If the hair tip is cut off, a thirty-times more active, soluble glucosidase of low K_m emerges from the hair shaft. It has been proposed that the soluble enzyme is identical to P-III (Fig. 8.10, peak V) (Kijima *et al.*, 1973).

Attempts to localize glucosidases on the cellular level by histochemical methods have not been successful; always the whole area of the sensilla were stained (Hansen, 1966, 1968; Amakawa *et al.*, 1975).

Glucosidases have also been observed in taste hair-rich segments of other insects and spiders: in the tarsi of the butterfly *Vanessa io*, the bugs *Picromerus* and *Rhaphigaster* and the grass hopper *Stenobothrys*, in the legs of the spider *Araneus sclopetarius* (Hansen, 1968), in the palps of cockroaches (Wieczorek, 1978), and in the maxillae of the caterpillar of the butterfly *Mamestra* (Wieczorek, 1976). Gaffal (1977) detected a maltose-specific glucosidase in the distal segments of the antennae of the bug *Dysdercus* by gel chromatography.

Initial chromatographic fractionation of glucosidases from taste hair-rich tarsi and labella of flies revealed three different enzymes (Hansen and Kühner, 1972; Morita, 1972; Amakawa *et al.*, 1972: P–I, P–II, P–III). Later five glucosidases were separated from tarsi (Kühner and Hansen, 1975; I = P–I (Amakawa *et al.*, 1972; III + IV = P–II, V = P–III). A further separation was obtained by reducing the steepness of the KCl-gradient and/or by a subsequent stepwise gel chromatography. Using these techniques peak III was resolved into three further peaks (III_1, III_2, III_3 (Hansen, 1974)). Fig. 8.10 demonstrates clearly that all peaks differ in their substrate specificities and are therefore not multiple forms of one and the same enzyme.

Chromatographic separations were performed on material from three species of flies (*Boettcherisca peregrina, Phormia regina* and *Protophormia terraenovae*). The main labellar and tarsal glucosidases of each species are the same, but they differ in activity. The enzymes of the fly *Boettcherisca* deviate in some respects from those of *Protophormia* (Amakawa *et al.*, 1972; Kühner and Hansen, 1975; Kijima, 1976). A rather different pattern is obtained from the tarsi of *Calliphora* (Hansen, unpublished observations). The intestinal glucosidases of *Protophormia,* being 10^3 times more active, show a completely different elution profile.

There have been several attempts to identify one or more glucosidases with a sugar receptor protein. Morita (1972) compared the K_b values of the labellar taste hairs for sucrose (60 mM) and *p*-nitrophenyl-α-glucoside (3 mM) with the corresponding K_m values of the three enzymes P–I, P–II and P–III. As he had determined theoretically earlier, the dissociation constants of the sugar − receptor protein complex must always be greater than the respective K_b values (see Section 8.3.5). In this regard, the glucosidase P–II (K_m (nitrophenylglucoside) = 10–25 mM; K_m (sucrose) = 50–100 mM) could act as receptor protein. A similar value was obtained for the enzyme of the hair tip (K_m (sucrose) = 20–100 mM). On the other hand, the glucosidases P–I and P–III were excluded because of their low K_m values. A second approach is provided by a comparison of the glucosidase activities of taste hair-rich (tarsi, labella) with those of taste hair-poor segments (tibia, femora) (Hansen, 1974; Hansen *et al.*, 1976). The tibiae and femora contain high activities of glucosidases I and V; therefore neither could be a receptor protein. The activities of enzymes III and IV are strongly reduced in tibiae and femora. These observations correlate well with the number of taste hairs in the respective segments. Comparison of glucosidases in tarsomeres 2–5 (= segments of the tarsi), tarsomere 1, and the tibia, which differ in the number and/or type of taste hairs, reveals hair-type specific glucosidases. From this respect, the enzymes III_2 and a membrane-bound component of peak IV might be receptor proteins (Hansen *et al.*, 1976; Hansen, unpublished observations).

A third approach has recently been worked out by Amakawa *et al.* (1975) and Kijima *et al.* (1977). They prepared membrane-bound glucosidases which consisted mainly of the enzyme P–II by differential centrifugation. Subsequent gel chromatography revealed three peaks (P–II M, P–II D, P–II T) of rather similar specificity and substrate affinity, but of different molecular weights. At present the relation of these species to the enzymes $III_1 - III_3$ remains unclear.

P–II D, molecular weight 200 000, is assumed to be identical with the enzyme localized in the hair tip (Kijima *et al.*, 1973). This has been questioned recently: Morita *et al.* (1977) reported that a potent inhibitor of glucosidases, the *N*-analogue of D-glucose (norijimycin, 5-amino-5-desoxy-glucose) inhibits P–II D with a K_I of $10^{-5} - 10^{-6}$ M. In contrast, the sugar receptor cell is influenced only at much higher concentration of 40 mM. Surprisingly, the hair tip glucosidase seems to be less sensitive to the inhibitor; in the presence of 0.1 M sucrose 1 mM norijimycin results in only a 50% inhibition. All correlations of *in vivo* properties of glucosidases depend on reliable characterizations of the glucosidase activity of the intact hair tip. The usual one hour incubation time of substrate and tips may cause difficulties in this respect since during that period substrates have been shown to diffuse to the inner compartments of the sensillum. ^{14}C-glucose applied to the hair tip for 20 min was detected in both canals I and II, which were laterally pierced by glass capillaries (Hanamori, 1976). Therefore during determinations of tip glucosidase activity sucrose might well come into contact with the soluble, highly active enzyme of low K_m observed by Kijima *et al.* (1973) directly after cutting off the hair tips. Consequently, activities of glucosidases other than the tip enzyme may be included in these determinations.

In corresponding *in vivo* experiments with the short taste hairs of the maxillary palps of the cockroach *Periplaneta,* Wieczorek (1978) observed more glucosidase activity in intact hairs bathed in substrate than in homogenates of the cut-off integuments and found that the concentration dependence of the two activities differed. Once again, inner compartments of the palps seemed to be involved in the hydrolysis observed at the outside.

The unequal effect of norijimycin on the sugar receptor and on P–II D seems to be an argument against the glucosidase hypothesis. But it should not be forgotten

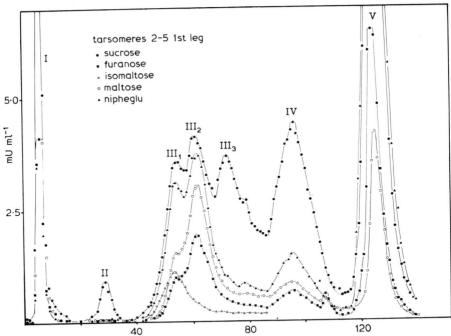

Fig. 8.11 Chromatographic separation of α-glucosidases from taste-hair-rich tarsomeres 2—5 of the first legs of the fly *Protophormia terraenovae.*
1950 tarsomeres 2—5 (2.1 mg protein, 470 000 taste hairs) were homogenized for 30 min at $0°C$ in 400 μl barbital-Na-buffer pH 7.6 (40 mM, 100 mM KCl, 1% Triton X-100) in a conical Duall glass homogenizer, the homogenate was stirred for 7 h at $5°C$ and centrifuged for 30 min at 20 000 g after addition of mannitol to 0.2 M. The supernatant containing more than 97% of the total activity was dialysed against elution buffer (20 mM barbital-Na, pH 6.0, 0.1% Triton X-100) and applied to a DEAE-cellulose column (0.6 x 27 cm). The KCl gradient was formed by the LKB ultrograd and recorded by a flow through conduction monitor. Fraction volume was 0.5 ml. The glucosidase activities were determined as nmol glucose liberated per min and ml eluate (glucose oxidase-peroxidase method); in the case of nitrophenyl-α-glucoside (nipheglu) the liberated nitrophenol was determined at pH 10. The specific activities with sucrose as substrate are in the range of 0.2 U mg^{-1} protein for the peaks I, III and IV and 10 U mg^{-1} for peak V. Maltose, isomaltose and melezitose have been purified by large scale gel chromatography on Sephadex G 10. (Hansen, unpublished.)

that the causal connection between response of the receptor and rate of hydrolysis of the glucosidase is not clear. The maximal responses upon stimulation by sucrose, maltose, melezitose and palatinose are nearly the same in all labellar hairtypes of

Protophormia (Wieczorek and Köppl, in press). This is not the case for any known glucosidase (compare Fig. 8.11). Therefore it is possible that inhibitors of the catalytic reaction might not inhibit conductance changes.

In summary there are several suggestive parallels between the pyranose site of the sugar receptor cell and glucosidases. However, experimental investigations of those parallels have revealed many complex features in the two systems while leaving the role of glucosidases in sugar reception unresolved. If the glucosidase hypothesis were true, such an enzymatically-active receptor protein would have one exceptional property. The recognition site could be investigated by using the enzymatic reaction as a tool for studying its kinetics. This approach would represent an additional method independent of the concentration-response curves obtained electrophysiologically.

(f) *The furanose site*

The highly effective stimulant fructose does not possess the three adjacent equatorial hydroxyl groups necessary for interactions with the pyranose site. Furthermore, the response of sugar receptor cells to fructose exhibits several unusual features discussed in Section 8.4.1c. Therefore several authors postulate a separate site for fructose (Evans, 1963; Morita and Shiraishi, 1968; Omand and Dethier, 1969; Pflumm, 1971; 1976; Shimada *et al.,* 1972, 1974; Hanamori *et al.* 1974; Shimada, 1975). By comparison of concentration-response curves obtained either with freshly dissolved fructose or with equilibrium solutions, it is evident that only β-D-fructofuranose is effective, and that coexisting β-pyranose inhibits competitively (Hanamori *et al.,* 1974). This result led to the term 'furanose site'. The conformations of furanoses are much more complex than for pyranoses, because there are two furanose conformations, the 'envelope' and the 'twist' form (Fig. 8.10) which interconvert easily because of their similar energy content; furthermore, the terminology axial/equatorial does not describe the position of the hydroxyl groups sufficiently. Galactose and D-fucose may be recognized by the furanose site since response to those sugars is not drastically affected by pretreatment with *p*-mercuribenzoate. Galactose is as effective a stimulant as β-D-pyranose or furanose, but not effective as α-D-pyranose (Hanamori *et al.,*1974; Shimada *et al.,* 1974). If the ring oxygen of furanoses is not essential for recognition then rotation of the three sugars reveals a common conformation of hydroxyl groups in the upper position at $C-1$ and $C-2$ which might be essential for effectiveness (Shimada *et al.,* 1974).

(g) *The sugar specificity of the water receptor*

The response of the water receptor cell (Section 8.4.5a) is completely suppressed in the presence of 100 mM NaCl. In this state the water cell behaves like a typical sugar receptor cell upon stimulation by sugars. Response increases with sugar concentration, and the receptor shows a distinct specificity for the same sugars that stimulate the furanose site: D-fructose, D-fucose and D-galactose; sugars which are typical stimulants for the pyranose site have little or no effect (Wieczorek and Köppl, 1978).

(h) *Amino acid reception*

In marine animals (crustaceans, molluscs and fishes) reception of amino acids is the most prominent chemical sense (Bardach, 1975), but in insects it plays a less important role. Most studies have focused on the sensitivity of the fly's sugar receptor for amino acids. It responds only to valine, leucine, isoleucine, methionine and phenylalanine. Phenylalanine exhibits the surprisingly low K_b of 0.6 mM; therefore it is about 100 times 'sweeter' than sucrose. Because of interactions between responses for fructose and phenylalanine, it is assumed that amino acids bind to the furanose site (Shiraishi and Kuwabara, 1970). This is supported by the observation that the response to phenylalanine is not inhibited by a pretreatment with p-MB (Shimada, 1975). Further investigations revealed a rather broad specificity pattern (Shimada, 1978). Alteration of the carboxyl group eliminates effectiveness but modifications and substitutions at the α-amino group are tolerated. Several fatty acids (butyrate, isovalerate, caproate) stimulate the receptor; rather similar effects are known to occur at higher concentrations at the 'fifth cell' of the same taste hair (Dethier and Hanson, 1968; see Section 8.4.5c). The sugar receptor of mosquitoes also responds to amino acids but with a different specificity: alanine, histidine, arginine, lysine and valine are effective (Elizarov and Sinitsina, 1974). Still a different patterns is known from an amino acid receptor of the caterpillar of *Pieris.* This cell responds to proline, cysteine, methionine, serine and leucine (Schoonhoven, 1969b).

(i) *Sugar receptors in other insects*

Sugar receptors are common in most orders of insects (Frings and Frings, 1949). All known receptors are sensitive to glucose and sucrose. Those sugars play a decisive role as nutrients for plant-dependent insects and thus would strongly influence selection of receptor specificity. Other sugar are less significant for the insect, but are useful for the investigator in characterizing particular receptor proteins. The following examples may illustrate the situation:

(1) In the light of the differentiated pyranose and furanose sites in flies, it is remarkable that fructose does not stimulate sugar receptor cells of the bug *Dysdercus* (Pflumm, 1976; Bresch, 1973), and elicits no feeding response in the Colorado potato beetle (Hsiao and Fraenkel, 1968).

(2) p-Nitrophenyl-α-glucoside, the most effective glycoside in flies (Pflumm, 1972), does not stimulate certain receptors of *Dysdercus* (Bresch, 1973) or of the fly *Drosophila* (Isono and Kikuchi, 1974).

(3) In the ants *Lasius* and *Myrmica rubra,* raffinose is more effective than sucrose (Schmidt, 1938).

(4) Lactose, ineffective for the flies *Protophormia* (Pflumm, 1972) and *Phormia* (Dethier, 1955), is an effective stimulus for the labellar receptors of *Calliphora* (Haslinger, 1935), for mosquitoes (*Salama,* 1966), and is a feeding stimulant for *Locusta* (Cook, 1977).

(5) A particular diversity of different sugar spectra has been observed in the

maxillary sensilla styloconica of lepidopterous larvae (Schoonhoven, 1969a, 1973). There are receptors responding (a) to sucrose and glucose, but not to other sugars (*Dendrolimus*; Ma, 1972), or (b) to sugars which are ineffective in flies, as e.g. rhamnose (silkmoth; Ishikawa, 1963, 1967) or ribose (*Dendrolimus*; Ma, 1972), or (c) more strongly to mannose than glucose (*Spodoptera*; Khalifa *et al.,* 1974).

8.4.2 Receptors for secondary plant substances

Insect contact chemoreceptors respond not only to nutrients but also to a variety of so-called secondary plant substances (for reviews see Schoonhoven, 1968, 1969a,b, 1972, 1973; Swain, 1977). This class includes about 10 000 structurally complex compounds which exhibit a scattered distribution in higher plants; some occur in a single plant species, others are restricted to closely related taxa. The functions of secondary plant substances are heterogeneous or often unknown. Several of them are involved in the primary metabolism of plants (Seigler and Price, 1976); others developed during insect–plant co-evolution; still others are present independent of any co-evolution, but insects have developed appropriate receptors for them in connection with oligophagy.

(a) *Deterrent receptors*

Many secondary plant substances are poisonous for insects (Schoonhoven, 1972; Table 5). Thus it is now generally accepted that plants have developed such substances as protective agents: 'without such compounds the majority of species of higher plants could not long withstand the voracious and destructive appetites of the various guilds of herbivorous insect pests' (Swain, 1977, p. 491); Feeny, 1975). As an effective counter-weapon, insects developed special gustatory chemoreceptors for the detection of such poisonous agents. Stimulation of these receptors during a probing bite inhibits subsequent ingestive feeding. These inhibitory agents are called deterrents. A catalogue of deterrents is given by Schoonhoven (1972), Table 2); further data are found in Chapman (1974), Navon and Bernays (1978) and Meinwald *et al.* (1978).

Deterrent receptors of several lepidopteran larvae have been investigated by electrophysiological methods. The single receptor cell responds to a variety of deterrents with drastically different chemical structures (Fig. 8.12).

All alkaloids are highly toxic. Ecdysterone represents a special case; it is not only an intermediate of plant steroid metabolism but also an insect hormone controlling ecdysis. Therefore the deterrent receptor protects the caterpillar from disturbances of its metamorphosis. The number of sites involved in reception of the whole deterrent spectrum is unknown. The 'bitter receptor' of the silkworm *Bombyx* exhibits a comparable pattern with threshold concentrations of 10^{-7}M for strychnine and 10^{-6}M for salicine, brucine, pilocarpine and berberine (Ishikawa, 1966).

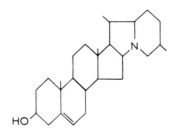

Atropine

Nicotine

Ecdysterone

Colchicine

Solanidine

Fig. 8.12 Chemical structures of secondary plant substances which stimulate the deterrent receptor cell of the maxillary taste sensilla of the cabbage caterpillar (*Pieris brassicae*). Other effective compounds are: berberine, conessine, pilocarpin, quinine, morphine, picrotoxinin, sparteine, strychnine, brucine, scopolamine, azadirachtin and tomatidine (Ma, 1972; Schoonhoven, 1972).

(b) *Receptors responsible for monophagy*

In phytophagous insects preference for a certain host plant (monophagy, oligophagy) is widespread. Monophagy allows adaptation to the phenology of a particular species of plant and its microhabitat. Probably monophagy developed in conjunction with detoxication mechanisms by turning earlier deterrent agents into phagostimulating key substances for host plant recognition (Feeny, 1975). Therefore in the central nervous system interpretation of information from plant substance receptors may have been remodeled from an avoidance into an acceptance behaviour.

There are only a few electrophysiological data available from this type of receptor. In several lepidopterous larvae, which are monophagous feeders on cruciferous plants, certain receptor cells respond to glucosinolates (mustard oil glycosides), which occur only in the Cruciferae (Schoonhoven, 1972; Ma, 1972). One case in which the specificity pattern was studied more intensively and quantitatively, is the glycoside receptor of the *Mamestra* larvae (Wieczorek, 1976; Fig. 8.13). However, unfortunately this caterpillar is not monophagous, but, more precisely, polyphagous with the tendency to prefer cruciferous plants. Another uncertainty is introduced by the fact that two deterrents, convallatoxin and strychnine, are stimulants. The beetle *Chrysolina* possesses tarsal receptor cells which respond specifically to hypericin, a constituent of its host plant *Hypericum* (Rees, 1969).

In the African armyworm *Spodoptera* which feeds exclusively on Gramineae, a receptor cell responds to adenosine and adenine, but not to other purines, pyrimidines, nucleosides and nucleotides; adenosine is present in sufficient concentrations in the maize plants to serve as a stimulant (Ma, 1977).

In lepidopterous larvae, receptor cells are frequently found which respond to myo- and epi-inositol (Jakinovich and Agranoff, 1971; Ma, 1972) with thresholds as low as 10^{-7}M (Ishikawa, 1967). Further phagostimulating substances have been compiled by Schoonhoven (1972, Table 1).

Another mechanism by which oligophagy is obtained occurs in the strictly graminivorous *Locusta*. The Gramineae contain rather low concentrations of deterrents and thus are preferred to dicotyledonous plants containing higher concentrations (Bernays and Chapman, 1977).

8.4.3 Food odor receptors

Food odors play a dominant role in the search phase of orientation of insects toward food sources. The following is a selection of representative receptor cells. See also reviews of Kaissling (1971), Schoonhoven (1968, 1972) and Städler (1977).

(1) The pine weevil *Hylobius* possesses receptors which react to the monoterpenes α- and β-pinen; these terpenes emanate from coniferous trees and act as attractants for the beetles (Mustaparta, 1975).

(2) The sensilla coeloconica on the antennae of the graminiphagous locust *Locusta* contain 'green odor' receptors. They react most effectively to hexenal

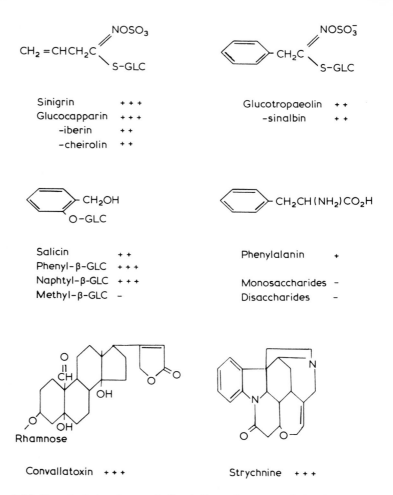

Fig. 8.13 Chemical structures of stimulating substances of the glycoside receptor of the larvae of *Mamestra brassicae* (Lepidoptera, Noctuidae). Effective stimulants are alkyl- and aryl-glucosinolates, aryl-β-glycosides, convallatoxin and strychnine; the amino acids phenylalanine, methionine and norleucine are only slightly effective; ineffective compounds are mono- and disaccharides, inorganic salts and the amino acids glycine, alanine and serine. The existence of at least two sites has been suggested: the 'glucosinolate' site reacts with glucosinolates and *p*-nitrophenyl-β-glucoside, the 'aryl glycoside' site with arylglycosides, convallatoxin and strychnine (Wieczorek, 1976).

which is released by many plants. The strucutural requirements of these receptors have been studied using large numbers of chemically related substances (Boeckh, 1967; Kafka, 1970). Maximal receptor activity is obtained by an aliphatic chain of 5—7 C-atoms with an terminal carbonyl or carboxyl group together with a double bond in the middle of the chain. Terpenoids and flower scents are ineffective.

(3) Olfactory receptors on the antennae of the carrion beetle *Necrophorus* and the fly *Calliphora* respond to odors of carrion and putrefying meat. The chemical components of these odors have not been identified. However, the receptors respond to several compounds that may be constituents of such odors, for example H_2S, NH_3, acetic acid, as well as aliphatic aldehydes, ketones and alcohols of carbon chain length 5—6 (Boeckh, 1962; Waldow, 1973; Kaib, 1974).

(4) Bees (and many other insects) visit flowers and are rewarded for pollination with sugar-containing nectar. In the course of the co-evolution of this bee—plant relationship plants must have developed flower scents as attractants for bees, and bees developed the corresponding receptors. Early electrophysiological investigations of the antennal sensilla placodea revealed overlapping specificity patterns which varied from cell to cell (Lacher, 1964). Later several distinct types of receptor cells with slightly overlapping specificity patterns were described (Vareschi, 1971); among these, one type responds to linear monoterpenoids, typical components of flower scents such as geranial, neral, geraniol, citronellol, nerol and eugenol. Receptor cells with similar specificity are also known in butterflies and flies (Boeckh *et al.*, 1965; Kaib, 1974). It is appropriate to mention that research in insect chemoreception began in 1919 with behavioral experiments on bee olfaction by von Frisch.

(5) Basiconic sensilla on antennae of the omnivorous cockroach *Periplaneta* contain receptor cells responding to odors of fruits, cheese and meat. The receptors can be characterized by concentration—response curves ($n_H = 1$, equal R_{max} values) for particular compounds occuring in the natural odors (Sass, 1976); the most effective stimulant for each cell type is pentanol, hexanol, octanol, formic and butyric acid, respectively. The spectrum of sensitivity for a given cell type is quite constant in contrast to the variability observed in several other olfactory receptors (Lacher, 1964; Vareschi, 1971; Mustaparta, 1975). The spectra of the three cells reacting to aliphatic alcohols overlap considerably thus providing a basis for central discrimination of odors (Boeckh, 1977; Boeckh *et al.*, 1976). Several theoretical concepts have been offered as bases for an explanation of the variety of odors perceived by insect olfactory receptors (Kafka and Neuwirth, 1975; Kafka, 1976; Kaissling, 1976, 1977; Diesendorf *et al.*, 1974; Callahan, 1975, 1977; Diesendorf, 1977a,b; Wright, 1966; Amoore *et al.*, 1969).

8.4.4 Nucleotide receptors

Nucleotides play an important role as phagostimulants in many blood sucking insects: the bugs* *Rhodnius* and *Reduvius,* the mosquitoes, the tsetse-flies

---

* In this paper the term 'bug' always means a member of the hemipterous insect group Heteroptera.

Table 8.3 Pattern of response of the blood sucking bug *Rhodnius prolixus* to phagostimulatory nucleotides (after Smith and Friend, 1976). ED_{50} is the concentration causing 50% of third instar larvae, starved for 40 days, to gorge.

ED_{50}	Purine bases			Pyrimidine bases		
4 μM	ATP, A (tetra) P					
30–70 μM	ADP, dATP	GTP	ITP	CTP, CDP		
120–200 μM	cAMP, dADP	GDP	IDP		UTP	
600 μM	AMP					
> 1500 μM	dibutyryl-cAMP	GMP	IMP	CMP	UMP	dTMP

Glossina, the black flies *Simulium* and the rat flea *Xenospylla* (Galun, 1977; Friend and Smith, 1977). In the bug *Rhodnius,* the responsible sense organs may be eleven very small epipharyngeal sensilla in the food channel, similar to those described by Moulins (1968) in the hypopharyngeal area of the cockroach. Behavioral tests with nucleotides are essentially similar to those described for the sugar receptor (see Section 8.4.1b) and have been used to determine nucleotide concentrations which elicit gorging responses in 50% of a test population. The natural phagostimulant is ATP. It is assumed to be released from blood platelets which aggregate in the region penetrated by the stylets (Galun, 1977). The pattern of response to various nucleotides is shown in Table 8.3.

For highest effectiveness, the NH_2 group on the C–6 position of the adenine moiety, three or four phosphate groups and the OH group on the C–2 of the ribose are important. The phosphodiesterase inhibitor theophylline (1, 3-dimethyl-2, 6-dioxopurine 1 mM) enhances sensitivity to ATP 2–4 times; therefore involvement of cAMP in the reception mechanism was suggested (Smith and Friend, 1972); however, the situation has become less clear by the ineffectiveness of dibutyryl-cAMP which was expected to increase intracellular cAMP level because of its ability to penetrate membranes (Smith and Friend, 1976). Electrophysiological investigations have been possible in the ATP-sensitive labellar taste hairs of the tsetse fly *Glossina* (Mitchell, 1976).

8.4.5 Water, CO_2 and inorganic salt receptors

It is typical for the reception of these small molecules that only one subsite-like interaction with the receptor is involved in binding.

(a) *Water receptors*

Thirsty flies extend their proboscides upon tarsal stimulation by pure water. Tarsal as well as labellar taste hairs contain a separate receptor cell for water. The cell responds quite normally with a high initial frequency of about 170 impulses per second decreasing to a steady-state frequency of about 40 impulses per second (similar to Fig. 8.5e) (Evans and Mellon, 1962; Rees, 1970b, 1972). The problem is how to explain induction of a membrane depolarization by water. Rees (1970b) developed the streaming potential hypothesis: Stimulation by water results in a decrease of osmotic pressure and ion concentration in the medium surrounding the dendrite. Under the influence of the osmotic pressure difference at the receptor cell membrane, a water- and cation-flow through negatively lined pores occurs. The cation flow constitutes the receptor current.

Response to water is completely depressed by low cation concentrations (100 mM Na^+, 10 mM Ca^{2+}) and by high non-electrolyte concentrations (e.g. 2–5 M urea, glycerol or sugars). For re-activation of the salt-inhibited water cell activity by furanoses see Section 8.4.1g. Narcotics, such as halothane (1, 1, 1-trifluor-2-chlor-2-brom-ethane) and chloroform, are stimulants of the water receptor (Dethier and Goldrich-Rachman, 1976). In the fly *Calliphora* more than one cell responds on stimulation by water (van des Starve, 1972).

(b) CO_2 *receptor*

Recognition of CO_2 occurs in rather varied biological situations.

(1) The searching behavior of haematophagous insects is activated by CO_2 produced by their hosts (Galun, 1977; Friend and Smith, 1977).

(2) Many phytophageous larvae recognize CO_2 produced by roots (Klinger, 1966).

(3) Bees measure the CO_2 concentration in the hive and keep it low by wing buzzing at the entrance.

The receptors in bees have been investigated electrophysiologically. They are localized in antennal pit sensilla and react after a latency of 3 ms with a high phasic response. Numerous other olfactory stimuli are ineffective. Anesthetics, such as N_2O and xenon, are inhibitory and elicit off-responses (Lacher, 1964; Stange, 1973, 1975). The response is strongly affected by acetazolamide if applied orally in an amount providing a 1 μM concentration with respect to the total volume of the bee. This substance is a common non-competitive inhibitor of the carbonic anhydrases which hydrate CO_2 to bicarbonate in connection with active transport. Therefore the CO_2-binding sites of the bee receptor may be similar to those of carbonic anhydrases (Stange, 1974).

(c) *Salt receptors*

The salt receptor cell (type 1 cell, Rees, 1968; 'cation' receptor, Steinhardt, 1965; Hodgson, 1974; L-spikes, Hodgson and Roeder, 1956) of the labellar taste hairs of the blowfly *Phormia regina* is differentially sensitive to various alkali halides. Potassium is most effective, sodium slightly less, lithium, rubidium and cesium relatively ineffective. Thus electrostatic, as well as steric parameters must be involved. The effectivity of the anion increases monotonically with atomic number (I^- Br^- Cl^- F^-) (Gillary, 1966 a,b). The salt receptor exhibits an unstimulated response of 3–4 impulses per second, which is depressed by low Ca^{2+} concentrations (> 50 μM); Ca^{2+} itself is not stimulating, but elicits an off-response (Rees and Hori, 1968). On the other hand, salt cells of the interpseudotracheal papillae of the fly, and of the labellar hairs of the mediterranean fruit fly *Ceratitis,* respond to stimulation with $CaCl_2$ (Dethier and Hanson, 1968; Gothilf *et al.,* 1971).

The absolute response and the concentration-response curve of the salt cell of *Phormia* depend on the age of the fly. It reaches its maximal response three days after emergence; at an age of 15 days, 50% of the life expectancy, response to 1 M NaCl is reduced to 60% and that to 0.1 M to 30% of the maximal value (Rees, 1970a).

A theory regarding the mechanism of salt reception was developed by Rees (1968). According to his model, the ion activity-response curves are explained in terms of activity-dependent diffusion potentials considering the ion-specific permeability coefficients of the membrane.

There have been several observations of a second salt-sensitive cell in the taste hairs of *Phormia* which exhibited a smaller spike amplitude and a different anion specificity than type I cells ('anion cell', Steinhardt, 1965; Hodgson, 1974; fifth cell, Dethier and Hanson, 1968; type 4 cell, Rees, 1968).

In the labellar hairs of *Calliphora,* as many as three cells respond to salt stimulation; the absolute responses of one tarsal salt receptor differ from hair to hair, while the rank of stimulating effectiveness of the alkali cations remains fairly constant (references in den Otter, 1972). On the ovipositor of *Lucilia* a salt cell is reported to have an electrophysiological threshold of 1 mM for NaCl; this value being about 100 times lower than that for labellar salt receptors of *Phormia* (Rice, 1977). The biological functions of salt receptors are still a matter of discussion (Fredman and Steinhardt, 1974).

8.5 CONCLUDING REMARKS

This review outlines the present state of insect chemoreception (except pheromone reception, see Kramer, this volume). Insect chemoreceptor cells provide a useful model for the study of basic sensory processes, that is stimulus conduction, membrane transduction and permeability change and generation of receptor currents and action potentials.

(1) The chemosensory organs (sensilla) show a simple morphological construction; those selected for experimental work consist of 2–5 receptor cells and three sheath cells.

(2) There exists a broad diversity of stimulating substances (sugars, amino acids, secondary plant substances, food odors, nucleotides, CO_2, salts and water); therefore various structure-activity relationships can be studied.

(3) The insect chemoreceptors are accessible to several technical methods; the response of a single receptor cell can be recorded electrophysiologically; biochemical approaches regarding the nature of receptor proteins are in progress; the use of mutants has begun.

Future research will help to develop our molecular understanding of recognition mechanisms by intensifying the study of identification of receptor and pore proteins as well as of receptor kinetics.

REFERENCES

Adam, G. and Delbrück, M. (1968), Reduction of dimensionality in biological diffusion processes. In: *Structural Chemistry and Molecular Biology* (Rich, A., Davidson, N. eds), pp. 198—215, Freeman, San Francisco.

Altner, H. (1977a), Insektensensillen: Bau und Funktionsprinzipein. *Verh. Dtsch. Zool. Ges.*, 139—153, Gustav Fischer Verlag, Stuttgart.

Altner, H. (1977b), Insect sensillum specificity and structure: an approach to a new typology. In: *Proc. VI. Int. Symp. Olfaction and Taste.* (le Magnen, J. and MacLeod, P. eds), Paris 1977, Inform. Retrieval London, pp. 295—304.

Altner, H. and Thies, G. (1973), A functional unit consisting of an eversible gland with neurosecretory innervation and a proprioreceptor derived from a complex sensillum in an insect. *Z. Zellforsch,* **145**, 503—519.

Amakawa, T., Kawabata, K., Kijima, H. and Morita, H. (1972), Isozymes of α-glucosidase in the proboscis and legs of flies. *J. Insect Physiol.,* **18**, 541—553.

Amakawa, T., Kijima, H. and Morita, H. (1975), Insoluble α-glucosidase: possible pyranose site of the sugar receptor of the labellar hairs of the blowfly, *Phormia regina. J. Insect Physiol.,* **21**, 1419—1425.

Amoore, J.E., Palmieri, G., Wanke, E. and Blum, M.S. (1969), Ant alarm pheromone activity: correlation with molecular shape by scanning computer. *Science,* **165**, 1266—1269.

Angyal, S.J. (1972), Conformation of sugars. In: *The Carbohydrates,* (Pigman, W. and Horton, D. eds), Vol. 1A, pp. 195—216, 2nd edn., Academic Press, New York.

Bardach, I.E. (1975), Chemoreception of aquatic animals. In: *Proc. V. Int. Symp. Olfaction and Taste* (Denton, D.A. and Coghlan, I.P. eds), Melbourne, 1974, Academic Press, New York, 1975, pp. 121—132.

Beidler, L.M. (1961), Taste receptor stimulation. In: *Progress in Biophysics and Biophysical Chemistry,* Vol. **12**, Pergamon Press, London, pp. 107—151

Beidler, L.M. (ed.) (1971a), Chemical senses, olfaction and taste. In: *Handbook of Sensory Physiology,* Vol. IV, part 1, 518 pp., part 2, 410 pp., Springer Verlag, Berlin, Heidelberg, New York.

Beidler, L.M. (1971b), Taste receptor stimulation with salts and acids. In: *Handbook of Sensory Physiology,* Vol. IV, Chemical senses-taste, p. 200—220.

Benz, G., (ed.) (1976), Structure-activity relationships in chemoreception. *Proc. Symp. Eur. Chemoreception Res. Org.* Information Retrieval, London, 232 pp.

Bernays, E.A., Blaney, W.M. and Chapman, R.F. (1972), Changes in chemoreceptor sensilla on the maxillary palps of *Locusta migratoria* in relation to feeding. *J. exp. Biol.,* **57**, 745—753.

Bernays, E.A., Blaney, W.M. and Chapman, R.F. (1975), The problems of perception of leaf-surface chemicals by locust contact chemoreceptors. *Proc. V. Int. Symp. Olfaction and Taste* (Denton, D.A. and Coghlan, J.P. eds), Melbourne 1975, Academic Press, New York, pp. 227—229.

Bernays, E.A., Blaney, W.M., Chapman, R.F. and Cook, A.G. (1976), The ability of *Locusta migratoria* L. to perceive plant surface waxes. In: *The Host-plant in relation to Insect Behaviour and Reproduction.*, (Jermy, T. ed), *Proc. Symp. Biol. Hung.*, **16**, 35—40.

Bernays, E.A. and Chapman, R.F. (1972), The control of changes in peripheral sensilla associated with feeding in *Locusta migratoria* (L.). *J. exp. Biol.*, **57**, 755—763.

Bernays, E.A. and Chapman, R.F. (1977), Deterrent chemicals as a basis of oligophagy in *Locusta migratoria*. *Ecol. Ent.*, **2**, 1—18.

Blaney, W.M., Chapman, R.F. and Cook, A.G. (1971), The structure of the terminal sensilla on the maxillary palps of *Locusta migratoria* (L.) and changes associated with moulting. *Z. Zellforsch.*, **121**, 48—68.

Boeckh, J. (1962), Elektrophysiologische Untersuchungen an einzelnen Geruchs-rezeptoren auf den Antennen des Totengräbers (*Necrophorus*, Coleoptera). *Z. vergl. Physiol.*, **46**, 212—248.

Boeckh, J. (1967), Reaktionsschwelle, Arbeitsbereich und Spezifität eines Geruchsrezeptors auf der Heuschreckenantenne. *Z. vergl. Physiol.*, **55**, 378—406.

Boeckh, J. (1969), Electrical activity in olfactory receptor cells. *Proc. III. Int. Symp. Olfaction and Taste,* New York 1968 (Pfaffmann, C., ed), Rockefeller University Press, pp. 34—51.

Boeckh, J. (1977), Aspects of nervous coding of sensory quality in the olfactory pathway of insects. *Proc. XV. Int. Congr. Entomol.,* Washington 1976, pp. 308—322.

Boeckh, J., Ernst, K.D., Sass, H. and Waldow, U. (1976), Zur nervösen Organisation antennaler Sinneseingänge bei Insekten unter besonderer Berücksichtigung der Riechbahn. *Verh. Dtsch. Zool. Ges.* 1976, 123—139, Gustav Fischer Verlag, Stuttgart.

Boeckh, J., Kaissling, K.-E. and Schneider, D. (1965), Insect olfactory receptors. *Cold Spring Harbor Symp. Quant. Biol.*, **30**, 263—280.

Bownds, D. and Gaide-Huguinin, A.C. (1970), Rhodopsin content of frog photo-receptor outer segments. *Nature*, **225**, 870—872.

Bresch, W.-E. (1973), Der Zuckerrezeptor eines Rüsselhaares der Baumwollwanze *Dysdercus intermedius*, eine electrophysiologische Untersuchung. Dissertation Universität Heidelberg 1973.

Brown, B.L. and Hodgson (1962), Electrophysiological studies of arthropod chemoreception. IV. Latency, independence and specificity of labellar chemo-receptors of the blowfly *Lucilia*. *J. cell comp. Physiol.*, **59**, 187—202.

Broyles, J.L. and Hanson, F.E. (1976), Ion-dependence of the tarsal sugar receptors of the blowfly *Phormia regina*. *J. Insect Physiol.*, **22**, 1587—1600.

Callahan, P.S. (1975), Insect antennae with special reference to the mechanism of scent detection and the evolution of the sensilla. *Insect Morphol. Embryol.*, **4**, 381—430.

Callahan, P.S. (1977), Comments on Mark Diesendorf's critique of my review paper. *Insect Morphol. Embryol.*, **6**, 111—122.

Changeux, J.P. (1972), Studies on the molecular mechanism of the response of an excitable membrane to cholinergic agents. In: *Proc. IV. Int. Symp. Olfaction and Taste,* Starnberg 1971, (Schneider, D. ed.), Wiss Verlagsges, Stuttgart, pp. 81–87.

Chapman, R.F. (1974), The chemical inhibition of feeding by phytophagous insects: a review. *Bull. ent. Res.,* **64,** 339–363.

Chu, I.-W. and Axtell, R.C. (1971), Fine structure of the dorsal organ of the house fly larva, *Musca domestica* L. *Z. Zellforsch.,* **117,** 17–34.

Chu-Wang, I.-W. and Axtell, R.C. (1972), Fine structure of the terminal organ of the house fly larva, *Musca domestica* L. *Z. Zellforsch.,* **127,** 287–305.

Cohen, L.A. (1970), Chemical modifications as a probe of structure and function. In: *The Enzymes,* Vol. I (Boyer, P.D. ed), 3rd edn., pp. 148–211.

Colquhoun, D. (1973), The relation between classical and cooperative models for drug action. In: *Drug receptors, a symposium* (Rang, H.P., ed), MacMillan London, pp. 149–182.

Cone, R.A. (1973), The internal transmitter model for visual excitation: some quantitative implications. In: *Biochem. Physiol. Visual Pigments* (Langer, H. ed), Springer Heidelberg, pp. 275–282.

Cook, A.G. (1977), Nutrient chemicals as phagostimulants for *Locusta migratoria* (L.). *Ecol. Ent.,* **2,** 113–121.

Daley, D.L. and Vande Berg, J.S. (1976), Apparent opposing effects of cyclic AMP and dibutyryl-cyclic GMP on the neuronal firing of the blowfly chemoreceptors. *Biochem. biophys. Acta,* **437,** 211–220.

Denton, D.A. and Coglan, J.P. (eds.), (1975), *Proc. V. Int. Symp. Olfaction and Taste,* Academic Press, New York.

Dethier, V.G. (1953), Summation and inhibition following contralateral stimulation of the tarsal chemoreceptors of the blowfly. *Biol. Bull.,* **105,** 257–268.

Dethier, V.G. (1955a), The physiology and histology of the contact chemoreceptors of the blowfly. *Q. Rev. Biol.,* **30,** 348–371.

Dethier, V.G. (1955b), Mode of action of sugar-baited fly traps. *J. Econ. Ent.,* **48,** 235–239.

Dethier, V.G. (1963), *The Physiology of Insect Senses.* Methuen, London.

Dethier, V.G. (1976), *The Hungry Fly.* Harvard University Press, Cambridge, Massachusetts.

Dethier, V.G. and Chadwick, L.E. (1950), An analysis of the relationship between solubility and stimulating effect in tarsal chemoreception. *J. gen. Physiol.,* **33,** 589–599.

Dethier, V.G. and Goldrich-Rachman, N. (1976), Anesthetic stimulation of insect water receptors. *Proc. natn. Acad. Sci. U.S.A.,* **73,** 3315–3319.

Dethier, V.G. and Hanson, F.E. (1968), Electrophysiological response of the chemoreceptors of the blowfly to sodium salts of fatty acids. *Proc. natn. Acad. Sci. U.S.A.,* **60,** 1296–1303.

Diesendorf, M. (1977a), Insect sensilla: are dielectric aerials for scent detection? Comments on a review by P.S.P. Callahan. *Insect Morph. Embryol.,* **6,** 105–110.

Diesendorf, M. (1977b), The 'dielectric waveguide theory' of insect olfaction: a reply to P.S.P. Callahan. *Insect Morphol. Embryol.,* **6**, 123—126.

Diesendorf, M., Stange, G. and Snyder, A.W. (1974), A theoretical investigation of radiation mechanisms of insect chemoreception *Proc. R. Soc. Lond. ser. B* **185**, 33—49.

Eldefrawi, A.T., Eldefrawi, M.E., Albuquerque, E.X., Oliveira, A.C., Mansour, N., Adler, M., Daly, J.W., Brown, G., Burger-Meister, W. and Witkop, B. (1977), Perhydrohistrionicotoxin: a potential ligand for the ion conductance modulator of the acetylcholine receptor. *Proc. natn. Acad. Sci. U.S.A.,* **74**, 2172—2176.

Elizarov, Yu.A. and Gritsay, O.B. (1975), The effect of ouabain on the sugar receptor of an contact chemoreceptor of *Protophormia terraenovae. Zh. Evol. Biokhim. Fiziol.,* **11**, 164—170.

Elizarov, Yu.A. and Sinitsina, E.E. (1974), Contact chemoreception in *Aedes aegypti. Zool. Zhurnal,* **53**, 577—584.

Ernst, K.-D. (1969), Die Feinstruktur von Riechsensillen auf der Antenne des Aaskäfers *Necrophorus* (Coleoptera), *Z. Zellforsch.,* **94**, 72—102.

Ernst, K.-D. (1972), Die Ontogenie der basiconischen Riechsensillen auf der Antenne von *Necrophorus* (Coleopt.). *Z. Zellforsch.,* **129**, 217—236.

Esslen, J. and Kaissling, K.-E. (1976), Zahl und Verteilung antennaler Sensillen bei der Honigbiene (*Apis mellifera* L.), *Zoomorphologie,* **83**, 227—251.

Evans, D.R. (1963), Chemical structure and stimulation by carbohydrates. In: *Proc. I. Int. Symp. Olfaction and Taste* (Zotterman, I.Y., ed), Stockholm 1962, Pergamon Press, Oxford, pp. 165—176.

Evans, D.R. and Mellon, D. (1962), Electrophysiological studies of a water receptor associated with the taste sensilla of the blowfly. *J. gen. Physiol.,* **45**, 487—500.

Feeny, P., (1975), Biochemical coevolution between plants and their insect herbivores. In: *Co-evolution of Animals and Plants* (Gilbert, L.E. and Raven, P.H., eds). University of Texas Press, Austin, pp. 3—19.

Felt, B.T. and Vande Berg, J.S. (1976), Ultrastructure of the blowfly chemoreceptor sensillum (*Phormia regina*), *J. Morphol.,* **150**, 763—784.

Frazier, J.L. and Heitz, J.R. (1975), Inhibition of olfaction in the moth *Heliothis virescens* by the sulfhydryl reagent fluorescein mercuric acetate. *Chem. Senses and Flavour,* **1**, 271—281.

Fredman, S.M. and Steinhardt, R.A. (1973), Mechanism of inhibitory action by salts in the feeding behaviour of the blowfly, *Phormia regina. J. Insect Physiol.,* **19**, 781—790.

Friend, W.G. and Smith, J.J.B. (1977), Factors affecting feeding by bloodsucking insects. *A. Rev. Entomol.,* **22**, 309—331.

Frings, H. and Frings, M. (1949), The loci of contact chemoreceptors in insects. *Am. Midland Naturalist,* **41**, 602—658.

Frisch, K. von (1919), Über den Geruchssinn der Biene und seine blütenbiologische Bedeutung. *Zool. Jb. (Allg. Zool.),* **37**, 1—238.

Frisch, K. von (1935), Über den Geschmackssinn der Biene. *Z. vergl. Physiol.,* **21**, 1—156.

Gaffal, P. (1973), Die Feinstruktur von Sensillen auf Antennen- und Rüsselspitze der Baumvollwanze *Dysdercus intermedius* Dist. (Pyrrhocoridae). Dissertation der Universität Heidelberg, 1973.

Gaffal, P. (1977), Changing distribution patterns of α-glucosidase isoenzymes in extracts of antennal segments and in the haemolymph of the cotton stainer *Dysdercus intermedius* Dist. *Comp. Biochem. Physiol.*, **58B**, 71–79.

Gaffal, K.-P. and Bassemir, U. (1974), Vergleichende Untersuchung modifizierter Cilienstrukturen in den Dendriten mechano- und chemosensitiver Rezeptorzellen der Baumwollwanze *Dysdercus* und der Libelle *Agrion. Protoplasma,* **82**, 177–202.

Gaffal, K.-P., Tichy, H., Theiss, J. and Seelinger, G. (1975), Structural polarities in mechanosensitive sensilla and their influence on stimulus transmission (Arthropoda). *Zoomorphologie,* **82**, 79–103.

Galun, R. (1977), The physiology of hematophagous insect, animal host relationships. *Proc. XV. Int. Cong. Entomol.* Washington, 1976, pp. 257–265, Ent. Soc. Am.

Gillary, H.L. (1966a), Stimulation of the salt receptor of the blowfly. I. NaCl. *J. gen. Physiol.,* **50**, 351–358.

Gillary, H.L. (1966b), Stimulation of the salt receptor of the Blowfly. III. The alkali halides. *J. gen. Physiol.,* **50**, 359–368.

Glazer, A.N. (1976), The chemical modification of proteins by group-specific and site-specific reagents. In: *The Proteins* Vol. II, (Neurath, H. and Hill, R.L., eds), 3rd edn. Academic Press New York, pp. 1–103.

Goldrich, N.R. (1973), Behavioral responses of *Phormia regina* (Meigen) to labellar stimulation with amino acids. *J. gen. Physiol.,* **61**, 74–88.

Gothilf, S., Galun, R. and Bar-Zeev, M. (1971), Taste reception in the Mediterranean fruit fly: Electrophysiological and behavioural studies. *J. Insect Physiol.,* **17**, 1371–1384.

Grabowski, C.T. and Dethier, V.G. (1954), The structure of the tarsal chemoreceptors of the blowfly, *Phormia regina* Meigen, *J. Morph.,* **94**, 1–20.

Greaves, M.F. (1976), Cell surface receptors, a biological perspective. In: *Receptors and Recognition,* Series A, Vol. 1 (Cuatrecasas, P. and Greaves, M.F., eds), p. 1–32, Chapman and Hall, London.

Hanamori, T. (1976), Penetration of sugars from the chemosensory hairtip in the fleshfly. *Chem. Senses and Flavour,* **1**, 229–239.

Hanamori, T., Shiraishi, A., Kijima, H. and Morita, H. (1972), Stimulation of labellar sugar receptor of the fleshfly by glycosides. *Z. vergl. Physiol.,* **76**, 115–124.

Hanamori, T., Shiraishi, A., Kijima, H. and Morita, H. (1974), Structure of effective monosaccharides in stimulation of the sugar receptor of the fly. *Chem. Senses and Flavour,* **1**, 147–166.

Hansen, K. (1964), Über Carbohydrasen in den Tarsen von *Calliphora* und *Phormia. Verh. Deutsch. Zool. Ges. München,* 1963, Zool. Anz. Suppl. **27**, 628–634.

Hansen, K. (1966), Zum histochemischen Nachweis der Trehalase in den Mitochondrien von Insekten-Flugmuskeln. *Histochemie,* **6**, 290–300.

Hansen, K. (1968), Untersuchungen über den Mechanismus der Zucker-Perzeption bei Fliegen. Habilitationsschrift der Universität Heidelberg.

Hansen, K. (1969), The mechanism of insect sugar reception, a biochemical investigation. *Proc. III Int. Cong. Olfaction and Taste,* (Pfaffmann, C., ed.), pp. 382–391, Rockefeller University Press, New York.

Hansen, K. (1974), α-Glucosidases as sugar receptor proteins in flies. 25 Mosbacher Colloquium Ges. biol. Chem. (Jaenicke, L., ed), Springer Verlag, Heidelberg, pp. 207–232.

Hansen, K., Bührer, H. and Wieczorek, H. (1976), α-Glucosidases as sugar receptor proteins in flies. In: (Benz, G., ed), *Structure–Activity Relationships in Chemoreception.* Inform. Retrieval London, pp. 79–88, Proc. Symp. Europ. Chemorec. Res. Organ, Zürich, 1975.

Hansen, K. and Heumann, H.-G. (1971), Die Feinstruktur der tarsalen Schmeckhaare der Fliege *Phormia terraenovae* Rob.-Desv. *Z. Zellforsch., 117*, 419–442.

Hansen, K. and Kühner, J. (1972), Properties of a possible receptor protein of the fly's sugar receptor. In: *Proc. IV. Int. Symp. Olfaction and Taste, IV,* (Schneider, D., ed.), pp. 350–356. Wiss. Verlagsges, Stuttgart.

Happ, G.M. and Happ, Chr. M. (1977), Cytodifferentiation in the accessory glands of *Tenebrio molitor.* III. Fine structure of the spermathecal accessory gland in the pupa. *Tissue and Cell, 9,* 711–732.

Harbach, R.E. and Larsen, J.R. (1976), Ultrastructure of sensilla on the distal antennal segment of adult *Oncopeltus fasciatus* (Dallas) (Hemiptera Lygaeidae). *Insect Morphol. Embryol., 5,* 23–33.

Haslinger, F. (1935), Über den Geschmackssinn von *Calliphora erythrocephala* Meigen und die Verwertung von Zuckern und Zuckeralkoholen durch diese Fliege. *Z. vergl. Physiol., 22,* 614–640.

Hassett, C.C., Dethier, V.G. and Gans, J. (1950), A comparison of nutritive values and taste thresholds of carbohydrates for the blowfly. *Biol. Bull., 99,* 446–453.

Hayashi, T. (ed.) (1967), *Proc. II Int. Symp. on Olfaction and Taste.* Pergamon Press, Oxford, 835 pp.

Henke, K. (1953), Über Zelldifferenzierungen im Integument der Insekten und ihre Bedingungen. *J. Embryol. exp. Morph., 1,* 217–226.

Hodgson, E.S. (1965), The chemical senses and changing viewpoints in sensory physiology. In: *Viewpoints in Biology* (Carthy, J.D. and Duddington, C.L., eds), Vol. 4, 83–124, Butterworths, London.

Hodgson, E.S. (1968), Taste receptors of arthropods. *Symp. Zool. Soc. Lond.,23,* 269–771.

Hodgson, E.S. (1974), Chemoreception. In: *The Physiology of Insecta* (Rockstein, M., ed.), Vol. 2, 2nd edn., pp. 127–165, Academic Press, New York.

Hodgson, E.S. and Roeder, K.D. (1956), Electrophysiological studies of arthropod chemoreception. I. General properties of the labellar chemoreceptors of Diptera. *J. cell comp. Physiol., 48,* 51–76.

Hsiao, T.H. and Fraenkel, G. (1968), The influence of nutrient chemicals on the feeding behavior of the Colorado potato beetle, *Leptinotarsa decemlineata* (Coleopt: Chrysom.), *Ann. Ent. Soc. Am., 61,* 44–54.

Ishikawa, S. (1963), Responses of maxillary chemoreceptors in the larva of the silkworm *Bombyx mori* to stimulation by carbohydrates. *J. cell comp. Physiol., 61,* 99–107.

Ishikawa, S. (1966), Electrical response and function of a bitter substance receptor associated with the maxillary sensilla of the larva of the silkworm *Bombyx mori* L. *J. Cell Physiol., 67,* 1–12.

Ishikawa, S., (1967), Maxillary chemoreceptors in the silkworm. In: *Proc. II. Int. Symp. Olfaction and Taste* (Hayashi, ed.). Pergamon Press, Oxford, pp. 761–777.

Isono, K. and Kikuchi, T. (1974), Autosomal recessive mutation in sugar response of *Drosophila. Nature,* **248**, 243–244.

Jain, M.K. (1973), Enzymic hydrolysis of various components in biomembranes and related systems. In: *Current topics Memb. Transp.,* **4**, 176–255.

Jakinovich, W. Jr. and Agranoff, B.W. (1971), The stereospecificity of the inositol receptor of the silkworm *Bombyx mori. Brain Res.,* **33**, 173–180.

Jakinovich, W. and Agranoff, B.W. (1972), Taste receptor response to carbohydrates. *Proc. IV. Int. Symp. Olfaction and Taste,* (Schneider, D., ed.), pp. 371–377, Wiss verlagsges, Stuttgart.

Jakinovich, W. Jr., Goldstein, I.J. and Baumgarten, R.J.v., Agranoff, B.W. (1971), Sugar receptor specificity of the fleshfly *Sarcophaga bullata. Brain Res.,* **35**, 369–378.

Jeffrey, G.A. and Kim, H.S. (1970), Conformation of the alditols. *Carbohydrate Res.,* **14**, 207–216.

Kafka, W.A. (1970), Analyse der molekulaten Wechselwirkungen bei der Erregung einzelner Riechzellen. *Z. vergl. Physiol.,* **70**, 105–143.

Kafka, W.A. (1976), Energy transfer and odor recognition. In: *Structure—Activity Relationships in Chemoreception* (Benz, G., ed.), Proc. Symp. Europ. Chemoreception Res. Org. Inform. Retrieval London, pp. 123–136.

Kafka, W.A. and Neuwirth, J. (1975), A model of pheromone molecular acceptor interaction. *Z. Naturforsch.,* **30c**, 278–282.

Kaib, M. (1974), Die Fleisch- und Blumenduftrezeptoren auf der Antenne der Schmeissfliege *Calliphora vicina. J. comp. Physiol.,* **95**, 105–121.

Kaissling, K.-E. (1969), Kinetic of olfactory receptor potentials. *Proc. III. Int. Symp. Olfaction and Taste* (Pfaffmann, C., ed.), pp. 52–70. Rockefeller University Press, New York.

Kaissling, K.-E. (1971), Insect Olfaction. In: *Handbook of Sensory Physiology,* Vol. IV. Chemical senses, Olfaction (Beidler, ed.), Springer Verlag, Berlin, Heidelberg, New York, pp. 351–431.

Kaissling, K.-E. (1974), Sensory transduction in insect olfactory receptors. 25. Mosbacher Colloquium Ges. biol. Chem. (Jaenicke, L., ed.), Springer Verlag, Heidelberg, pp. 243–271.

Kaissling, K.-E. (1975), Sensorische Transduktion bei Riechzellen von Insekten. *Verh. Dtsch. Zool. Ges.,* 1974, Fischer Verlag, Stutggart, pp. 1–11.

Kaissling, K.-E. (1976), The problem of specificity in olfactory cells. In: *Structure—Activity Relationships in Chemoreception* (Benz, G., ed.), Proc. Symp. Eur. Chemoreception Res. Org. Information Retrieval London, pp. 137–148.

Kaissling, K.-E. (1977), Structure of odor molecules and multiple activities of receptor cells. *Proc. VI. Int. Symp. Olfaction and Taste* (le Magnen, J. and MacLeod, P., eds), pp. 9–16, Information Retrieval London.

Kaissling, K.E. and Priesner, E. (1970), Die Riechschwelle des Seidenspinners, *Naturwissenschaft,* **57**, 23–28.

Kerjaschki, D. (1977), Some-freeze-etching data on the olfactory epithelium. *Proc. IV. Int. Symp. Olfaction and Taste,* (le Magnen, J. and MacLeod, P., eds), pp. 75–86, Information Retrieval, London.

Kerjaschki, D. and Hörandner, H. (1976), The development of mouse olfactory vesicles and their cell contacts: A freeze etching study. *J. Ultrastruct. Res.*, **54**,, 420–444.

Khalifa, A., Salama, H.S., Azmy, N. and El-Sharaby, A., (1974), Taste sensitivity of the cotton leafworm, *Spodoptera littoralis,* to chemicals. *J. Insect Physiol.*, **20**, 67–76.

Kijima, H. (1976), Specificity of two receptor sites and identification of receptor molecules in sugar receptor of flies. In: *Structure–Activity Relationships in Chemoreception*, (Benz, G., ed.), pp. 87–97, Eur. Chemorec. Res. Organ. Symp. Zürich, Inform. Retrieval London.

Kijima, H., Amakawa, T., Nakashima, M. and Morita, H. (1977), Properties of membrane-bound α-glucosidases: possible sugar receptor protein of the blowfly, *Phormia regina. J. Insect Physiol.,* **23**, 469–479.

Kijima, H., Koizumi, O. and Morita, H. (1973), α-Glucosidase at the tip of the contact chemosensory seta of the blowfly, *Phormia regina. J. Insect Physiol.,* **19**, 1351–1362.

Kikuchi, T. (1975), Genetic alteration of insect sugar reception. *Proc. V. Int. Symp. Olfaction and Taste* (Denton, D.A. and Coghland, J.P., eds), Melbourne 1975, Academic Press, New York, pp. 27–31.

Klingler, J., (1966), Über den Sitz der CO_2-Rezeption der Larve von *Otiorrhynchus sulcatus. Ent. exp. appl.,* **9**, 271–277.

Koizumi, O., Kijima, H., Kawabata, K. and Morita, H. (1973), α-Glucosidase activity on the outside of labella and legs of the fly. *Comp. Biochem. Physiol.,* **44B**, 347–356.

Koizumi, O., Kijima, H. and Morita, H. (1974), Characterization of a glucosidase at the tips of the chemosensory setae of the fly, *Phormia regina. J. Insect Physiol.,* **20**, 925–934.

Korenbrot, J.I. (1977), Ion transport in membranes: Incorporation of biological ion translocating proteins in model membrane systems. *Ann. Rev. Physiol.,* **39**, 19–49.

Kühner, J. and Hansen, K. (1975), Chromatographic isolation of α-glucosidases from the taste hair rich tarsi of the fly *Protophormia terraenovae.* Their possible role as sugar receptor proteins. *J. comp. Physiol.,* **99**, 257–270.

Küppers, J. (1974), Measurement on the ionic milieu of the receptor terminal in mechanoreceptive sensilla of insects. Symposium: *Mechanoreception.* Abh. Rhein.-Westf. Akad. Wiss. **53**, 387–393.

Kurihara, K. (1972), Inhibition of cyclic $3'$, $5'$-nucleotide phosphodiesterase in bovine taste paillae by bitter taste stimuli. *FEBS Letters,* **27**, 279–281.

Lacher, V. (1964), Elektrophysiologische Untersuchungen an einzelnen Rezeptoren für Geruch, Kohlendioxyd, Luftfeuchtigkeit und Temperatur auf den Antennen der Arbeitsbiene und der Drohne. *Z. vergl. Physiol.,* **48**, 587–623.

Larsen, J.R. (1962), The fine structure of the labellar chemosensory hairs of the blowfly, *Phormia regina* Meig. *J. Insect Physiol.,* **8**, 683–691.

Lawrence, P.A. (1966), Development and determination of hairs and bristles in the milkweed bug *Oncopeltus fasciatus* (Lygaeidae, Hemiptera), *J. Cell Sci.,* **1**, 475–498.

Loewenstein, W.R. (1971), Mechano-electric transduction in the Pacinian corpuscle. Initiation of sensory impulses in mechanoreceptors. In: *Handbook of Sensory Physiology*, **1**, Principles of receptor physiology (Loewenstein, W.R., ed.), Springer Verlag, Berlin, pp. 269–290.

Ma, W.Ch. (1972), Dynamics of feeding responses in *Pieris brassicae* Linn. as a function of chemosensory input: a behavioural, ultrastructural and electro-physiological study. *Meded. Landbouwhogesch. Wageningen*, **72**, 1–162.

Ma, W.Ch. (1977), Electrophysiological evidence for chemosensitivity to adenosine, adenine and sugars in *Spodoptera exempta* and related species. *Experientia*, **33**, 356–358.

Maes, F.W. (1977), Simultaneous chemical and electrical stimulation of labellar taste hairs of the blowfly *Calliphora vicina*. *J. Insect Physiol.*, **23**, 453–460.

Le Magnen, J. and MacLeod, P., (eds) (1977), *Proc. VI. Int. Symp. Olfaction and Taste*. Information Retrieval, London.

Mankin, R.W., Mayer, M.S. and Callahan, P.S. (1977), Odorant deposition onto insect antennal sensilla. In: *Proc. VI. Int. Symp. Olfaction and Taste* (Le Magnan, J. and MacLeod, P., eds), Paris 1977, Information Retrieval London, p. 356 (Abstract).

McIver, S. and Siemicki, R. (1978), Fine structure of tarsal sensilla of *Aedes aegypti* (Dipt. Culic.), *J. Morphol.*, **155**, 137–156.

Meinecke, C.-Ch. (1975), Riechsensillen und Systematik der Lamellicornia (Ins. Coleopt.), *Zoomorph.*, **82**, 1–42.

Meinwald, J., Prestwich, G.D., Nakanishi, K. and Kubo, I. (1978), Chemical ecology: Studies from East Africa. *Science*, **199**, 1167–1173.

Minnich, D.E. (1921), An experimental study of the tarsal chemoreceptors of two nymphalid butterflies. *J. exp. Zool.*, **33**, 173–203.

Mitchell, B.K. (1976), Physiology of an ATP receptor in labellar sensilla of the tsetse fly *Glossina morsitans morsitans* Westw. (Diptera: Glossinidae). *J. exp. Biol.*, **65**, 259–271.

Moncrieff, R.W. (1967), *The Chemical Senses.* Hill, London, 3rd edn.

Montal, M., Darszon, A. and Trissl, H.W. (1977), Transmembrane channel formation in rhodopsin-containing bilayer membranes. *Nature*, **267**, 221–225.

Morita, H. (1967), Effects of salts on the sugar receptor of the fleshfly. *Proc. II. Int. Symp. Olfaction and Taste* (Hayashi, T. ed.), pp. 787–798, Pergamon Press, Oxford.

Morita, H. (1969), Electrical signs of taste receptor activity. In: *Proc. III. Int. Symp. Olfaction and Taste*, New York, 1968 (Pfaffmann, C., ed.), pp. 370–381, Rockefeller University Press, New York.

Morita, H. (1972), Properties of the sugar receptor site of the blowfly. *Proc. IV. Int. Symp. Olfaction and Taste.* (Schneider, D., ed.), pp. 357–363, Wiss. Verlagsges, Stuttgart.

Morita, H., Enomoto, K.I., Nakashima, M., Shimada, I. and Kijima, H. (1977), The receptor sites for sugars in chemoreception of the fleshfly and blowfly. *Proc. VI. Int. Symp. Olfaction and Taste*, pp. 39–46, (le Magnen, J. and MacLeod, P., eds), Information Retrieval London 1977.

Morita, H. and Shiraishi, A. (1968), Stimulation of the labellar sugar receptor of the fleshfly by mono- and disaccharides. *J. gen. Physiol.*, **52**, 559–583.

Morita, H. and Takeda, K. (1957), The electrical resistance of the tarsal chemosensory hair of the butterfly *Vanessa indica*. *J. Fac. Sci. Hokkaido Univ. Ser.* VI, *Zool*, **13**, 465–469.

Morita, H. and Yamashita, S. (1959), Generator potential of insect chemoreceptor. *Science*, **130**, 922.

Moulins, M. (1968), Les sensilles de l'organe hypopharyngien de *Blabera craniifer* Burm. (Insecta, Dictyoptera). *J. Ultrastruct. Res.*, **21**, 474–513.

Mustaparta, H. (1975), Responses of single olfactory cells in the pine weevil *Hylobius abietis* (Col. Curcul.). *J. comp. Physiol.*, **97**, 271–290.

Narahashi, T. (1974), Chemicals as tools in the study of excitable membranes. *Physiol. Rev.*, **54**, 813–889.

Navon, A. and Bernays, E.A. (1978), Inhibition of feeding in acridids by non-protein amino acids. *Comp. Biochem. Physiol.*, **53A**, 161–164.

Neher, E. and Stevens, C.F. (1977), Conductance fluctuations and ionic pores in membranes. *Ann. Rev. Biophys. Bioeng.*, **6**, 345–381.

Ninomiya, M. and Shimada, I. (1976), Steoreospecificity for oligosaccharides of two receptor sites in a labellar sugar receptor of the fleshfly. *J. Insect Physiol.*, **22**, 483–487.

Noirot, Ch. and Quennedey, A. (1974), Fine structure of insect epidermal glands. *Ann. Rev. Entomol.*, **19**, 61–80.

Norris, D.M. (1976), Physico-chemical aspects of the effects of certain phytochemicals on insect gustation. In: *The host-plant in Relation to Insect Behaviour and Reproduction* (Jermy, T., ed.), *Proc. Symp. Biol. Hung.*, **16**, 197–201.

Norris, D.M. and Chu, H.M. (1974), Chemosensory mechanism in *Periplaneta americana*: electroantennogram comparison of certain quinone feeding inhibitors. *J. Insect Physiol.*, **20**, 1687–1697.

Oakley, B. and Benjamin, R.M. (1966), Neural mechanisms of taste. *Physiol. Rev.*, **46**, 173–211.

Omand, E. and Dethier, V.G., (1969), An electrophysiological analysis of the action of carbohydrates on the sugar receptor of the blowfly. *Proc. natn. Acad. Sci. U.S.A.*, **62**, 136–143.

Den Otter, C.J. (1972), Interactions between ions and receptor membrane in insect taste cells. *J. Insect Physiol.*, **18**, 389–402.

Peper, K., Dreyer, F., Sandri, C. and Akert, K. (1974), Structure and ultrastructure of the frog motor endplate, a freeze etching study. *Cell Tiss. Res.*, **149**, 437–455.

Pfaffmann, C. (ed.) (1969), *Proc. III Int. Symp. on Olfaction and Taste*. Rockefeller University Press, New York.

Pflumm, W. (1971), Zur Reizwirksamkeit von Monosacchariden bei der Fliege *Phormia terraenovae*. *Z. vergl. Physiol.*, **74**, 411–426.

Pflumm, W. (1972), Molecular structure and stimulating effectiveness of oligosaccharide and glycosides. *Proc. IV. Int. Symp. Olfaction and Taste* (Schneider, D. ed.), pp. 364–370.

Pflumm, W. (1976), Molekülstruktur von Zuckern und ihre Reizwirksamkeit bei Insekten. *Naturwiss. Rdsch.*, **29**, 73–81.

Poynder, T.M. (ed.) (1974), Transduction mechanisms in chemoreception. *Proc. Symp. Eur. Chemoreception Res. Organ.* Egham England 1973, Information Retrieval, London, pp. 366.

Price, S. (1974), Chemoreceptor proteins in taste cell stimulation. In: *Transduction Mechanisms in Chemoreception* (Poynder, T.M., ed.), Proc. Symp. Eur. Chemoreception Res. Organ, Information Retrieval, London, pp. 177−188.

Price, S. and Desimone, J.A. (1977), Models of taste receptor cell stimulation. *Chem. Senses and Flavour*, **2**, 427−456.

Priesner, E. (1973), Artspezifität und Funktion einiger Insektenpheromone. *Fortschr. Zool.*, **22**, 49−135.

Rao, V.S.R. and Foster, J.F. (1963), On the conformation of the α-glucopyranose ring in maltose and in higher polymers of D-glucose. *J. Phys. Chem.*, **67**, 951−952.

Raftery, M.A., Bode, J., Vandlen, R., Chao, Y., Deutsch, J., Duguid, J.R., Reed, K. and Moody, T. (1974), Characterization of an acetylcholine receptor. 25. *Mosbacher Coll. Ges. Biol. Chem.* (Jaenicke, L., ed.), pp. 541−562.

Reed, J.K. and Raftery, M.A. (1976), Properties of the tetrodotoxin binding component in plasma membranes isolated from *Electrophorus electricus. Biochem.*, **15**, 944−953.

Rees, C.J.C. (1967), Transmission of receptor potential in dipteran chemoreceptors. *Nature* **215**, 301−302.

Rees, C.J.C. (1968), The effect of aqueous solutions of some 1:1 electrolytes on the electrical response of the type 1 (salt) chemoreceptor cell in the labella of *Phormia. J. Insect Physiol.*, **14**, 1331−1364.

Rees, C.J.C. (1969), Chemoreceptor specificity associated with choice of feeding site by the beetle *Chrysolina brunsvicensis* on its foodplant, *Hypericum hirsutum. Ent. exp. expl.*, **12**, 565−583.

Rees, C.J.C. (1970a), Age dependency of response in an insect chemoreceptor sensillum. *Nature*, **227**, 740−742.

Rees, C.J.C. (1970b), The primary process of reception in the type 3 ('water') receptor cell of the fly *Phormia terranovae. Proc. R. Soc. London ser. B*, **174**, 463−490.

Rees, C.J.C. (1972), Responses of some sensory cells probably associated with the detection of water. *Proc. IV. Int. Symp. Olfaction and Taste* (Schneider, D., ed.), pp. 88−94. Wiss. Verlagsges, Stuttgart.

Rees, C.J.C. and Hori, N. (1968), The effect of electrolytes of the general formula XCl_2 on the response of the type 1 labellar chemoreceptor of the blowfly, *Phormia. J. Insect Physiol.*, **14**, 1499−1513.

Rice, M.J. (1977), Blowfly ovipositor receptor neuron sensitive to monovalent cation concentration. *Nature*, **268**, 747−749.

Salama, H.S. (1966), The function of mosquito taste receptors. *J. Insect Physiol.*, **12**, 1051−1060.

Sass, H. (1976), Zur nervösen Codierung von Geruchsreizen bei *Periplaneta americana. J. comp. Physiol.*, **107**, 49−65.

Schmidt, A. (1938), Geschmacksphysiologische Untersuchungen an Ameisen. *Z. vergl. Physiol.*, **25**, 351−378.

Schneider, D. (1957), Elektrophysiologische Untersuchungen von Chemo- und Mechanorezeptoren der Antenne des Seidenspinners *Bombyx mori* L. *Z. vergl. Physiol.*, **40**, 8–41.

Schneider, D. (1964), Insect antennae. *A. Rev. Ent.*, **9**, 103–122.

Schneider, D. (1971), Molekulare Grundlagen der chemischen Sinne bei Insekten. *Naturwissenschaften*, **58**, 194–200.

Schneider, D. (ed.) (1972), *Proc. IV. Int. Symp. on Olfaction and Taste.* Wiss. Verlagsges. Stuttgart.

Schneider, D. and Steinbrecht, R.A. (1968), Checklist of insect olfactory sensilla. *Symp. Zool. Soc. Lond.*, **23**, 279–297.

Schoonhoven, L.M. (1968), Chemosensory bases of host plant selection. *A. Rev. Ent.*, **13**, 115–136.

Schoonhoven, L.M. (1969a), Gustation and food plant selection in some lepidopterous larvae. *Ent. exp. expl.*, **12**, 555–564.

Schoonhoven, L.M. (1969b), Amino-acid 'receptor' in larvae of *Pieris brassicae* (Lepid.). *Nature*, **221**, 1268.

Schoonhoven, L.M. (1972), Secondary plant substance and insects. *Recent Adv. Phytochem.*, **5**, 197–224.

Schoonhoven, L.M. (1973), Plant recognition by lepidopterous larvae. In: *Insect-Plant Relationships* (Emden, H.F. von, ed.). *Symp. R. Ent. Soc. Lond.*, **6**, Blackwell Scientific Publishers, Oxford, pp. 87–100.

Schoonhoven, L.M. (1974), Comparative aspects of taste receptor specificity. In: *Transduction Mechanisms in Chemoreception.* Proc. Symp. Eur. Chemoreception Res. Org. (Poynder, T.M., ed.), Egham 1973, Information Retrieval, London.

Seiger, D. and Price, P.W. (1976), Secondary compounds in plants: primary functions. *Am. Nat.*, **110**, 101–105.

Shimada, I. (1975a), Chemical treatment of the labellar sugar receptor of the fleshfly. *J. Insect Physiol.*, **21**, 1565–1574.

Shimada, I. (1975b), Two receptor sites and their relation to amino acid stimulation in the labellar sugar receptor of the fleshfly. *J. Insect Physiol.*, **21**, 1675–1680.

Shimada, I. (1978), The stimulating effect of fatty acids and amino acid derivatives on the labellar sugar receptor of the fleshfly. *J. gen. Physiol.*, **71**, 19–36.

Shimada, I., Shiraishi, A., Kijima, H. and Morita, H. (1972), Effects of sulphydryl reagents on the labellar sugar receptor of the fleshfly. *J. Insect Physiol.*, **18**, 1845–1855.

Shimada, I., Shiraishi, A., Kijima, H. and Morita, H. (1974), Separation of two receptor sites in a single labellar sugar receptor of the flshfly by treatment with *p*-chloromercuribenzoate. *J. Insect Physiol.*, **20**, 605–621.

Shiraishi, A. and Kuwabara, M. (1970), The effects of amino acids on the labellar hair chemosensory cells of the fly. *J. gen. Physiol.*, **56**, 768–782.

Shiraishi, A. and Miyachi, N. (1976), The peripheral inhibition of the tarsal sugar receptor by sodium chloride in the proboscis extension response of the blowfly, *Phormia regina* M. *J. comp. Physiol.*, **110**, 97–109.

Shiraishi, A. and Tanabe, Y. (1974), The proboscis extension response and tarsal and labellar chemosensory hairs in the blowfly. *J. comp. Physiol.*, **92**, 161–179.

Slifer, E.H. (1970), The structure of arthropod chemoreceptors. *A. Rev. Ent.*, **15**, 121–142.

Smith, J.J.B. and Friend, W.G. (1972), Chemoreception in the blood feeding bug *Rhodnius prolixus*: a possible role of cyclic AMP. *J. Insect Physiol.,* **18**, 2337—2342.

Smith, J.J.B. and Friend, W.G. (1976), Further studies on potencies of nucleotides as gorging stimuli during feeding in *Rhodnius prolixus. J. Insect Physiol.,* **22**, 607—611.

Sreng, L. and Quennedey, A. (1976), Role of a temporary ciliary structure in the morphogenesis of insect glands. *J. Ultrastruct. Res.,* **56**, 78—95.

Städler, E. (1977), Sensory aspects of insect plant interactions. *Proc. XV. Int. Cong. Ent.* Washington 1976, pp. 228—248.

Stange, G. (1973), The response of the honeybee antennal CO_2-receptors to N_2O and Xe. *J. comp. Physiol.,* **86**, 139—158.

Stange, G. (1974), The influence of a carbonic anhydrase inhibitor on the function of the honeybee antennal CO_2-receptors. *J. comp. Physiol.,* **91**, 147—159.

Stange, G. (1975), Linear relation between stimulus concentration and primary transduction process in insect CO_2-receptors. *Proc. V. Int. Symp. Olfaction and Taste* (Denton, D.A. and Coghlan, J.P., eds), Academic Press, New York, pp. 207—211.

van der Starre, H. (1972), Tarsal taste discrimination in the blowfly, *Calliphora vicina* Robineau-Desvoidy. *Netherlands J. Zool.,* **22**, 227—282.

Steinbrecht, R.A. (1969), Comparative morphology of olfactory receptors. In: *Proc. III. Int. Symp. Olfaction and Taste.* (Pfaffmann, C., ed.), Rockefeller University Press, New York, pp. 3—21.

Steinbrecht, R.A. (1973), Der Feinbau olfaktorischer Sensillen des Seidenspinners (Insecta, Lepidoptera), Rezeptorfortsätze und reizleitender Apparat. *Z. Zellforsch.,* **139**, 533—565.

Steinbrecht, R.A. and Kasang, G. (1972), Capture and conveyance of odour molecules in an insect olfactory receptor. *Proc. IV. Int. Symp. Olfaction and Taste* (Schneider, Ed.), Starnberg 1971. Wiss. Verlagsges, Stuttgart, pp. 193—199.

Steinhardt, R.A. (1965), Cation and anion stimulation of electrolyte receptors of the blowfly, *Phormia regina. Am. Zool.,* **5**, 651, (Abstract).

Steinhardt, R.A., Morita, H. and Hodgson, E.S. (1966), Mode of action of straight chain hydrocarbons on primary chemoreceptors of the blowfly, *Phormia regina. J. Cell Physiol.,* **67**, 53—62.

Stürckow, B. (1967), Occurence of a viscous substance at the tip of the labellar taste hair of the blowfly. *Proc. II. Int. Symp. Olfaction and Taste* (Hayashi, T., ed.), pp. 707—720, Pergamon Press, Oxford.

Stürckow, B. (1970' Responses of olfactory and gustatory cells in insects. In: *Communication by Chemical Signals,* Vol. 1 (Johnston, J.W., Moulton, D.G. and Turk, A., eds), pp. 107—159, Appleton-Century-Crofts, New York.

Stürckow, B. (1971), Electrical impedance of the labellar taste hairs of the blowfly, *Calliphora erythrocephala* Mg. *Z. vergl. Physiol.,* **72**, 131—143.

Stürckow, B., Holbert, P.E., Adams, J.R. and Anstead, R.J. (1973), Fine structure of the tip of the labellar taste hair of the blowflies, *Phormia regina* (Mg.) and *Calliphora vicina* R.-D. (Diptera, Calliphoridae). *Z. Morph. Tiere,* **75**, 87—109.

Swain, T. (1977), Secondary compounds as protective agents. *A. Rev. Plant Physiol.,* **28**, 479—536.

Tateda, H. and Morita, H. (1959), Initiation of spike potentials in contact chemosensory hairs of insects. I. The generation site of the recorded spike potentials. *J. cell comp. Physiol.,* **54**, 171–176.

Thurm, U. (1963), Die Beziehungen zwischen mechanischen Reizgrössen und stationären Erregungszuständen bei Borstenfeld-Sensillen von Bienen. *Z. vergl. Physiol.,* **46**, 351–382.

Thurm, U. (1970), Untersuchungen zur funktionellen Organisation sensorischer Zellverbände. *Verh. Dtsch. Zool. Ges.,* **64**, Köln 1970, (Rathmayer, ed.), 79–87.

Thurm, U. (1974a), Mechanisms of electrical membrane responses in sensory receptors, illustrated by mechanoreceptors. 25. Mosbacher Colloquium Ges. biol. Chem. (Jaenicke, L. ed.), Springer Verlag Heidelberg, pp. 367–389.

Thurm, U. (1974b), Basics of the generation of receptor potentials in epidermal mechanoreceptors of insects. Symposium: *Mechanoreception.* Abh. Rhein.-westf. Akad. Wiss. **53**, 355–384.

Tominaga, Y. (1975), The taste pore of the fleshfly labellar hair. *J. elect. Micros.,* **24**, 171–174.

Ulbricht, W. (1974), Ionic channels through the axon membrane (a review). *Biophys. Struct. Mech.,* **1**, 1–16.

Van der Wolk, (1977), The morphology of insect taste hairs. *Proc. VI. Int. Symp. Olfaction and Taste* (Le Magnen, J. and MacLeod, P., eds), Paris 1977, Information Retrieval London, p. 363 (Abstract).

Vareschi, E. (1971), Duftunterscheidung bei der Honigbiene: Einzelableitungen und Verhaltensreaktionen. *Z. vergl. Physiol.,* **75**, 143–173.

Waldow, U. (1973), Elektrophysiologie eines neuen Aasgeruchsrezeptors und seine Bedeutung für das Verhalten des Totengräbers (*Necrophorus*). *J. comp. Physiol.,* **83**, 415–424.

Wieczorek, H. (1976), The glycoside receptor of the larvae of *Mamestra brassicae* L. (Lepidoptera, Noctuidae). *J. comp. Physiol.,* **106**, 153–176.

Wieczorek, H. (1978), Biochemical and behavioral studies of sugar reception in the cockroach. *J. comp. Physiol.,* **124**, 353–356.

Wieczorek, H. and Köppl, R. (1978), Effect of sugars on the labellar water receptors of the fly. *J. comp. Physiol.,* in press.

Wiesmann, R. (1960), Zum Nahrungsproblem der freilebenden Stubenfliegen *Musca domestica* L. *Z. angew. Zool.,* **47**, 159–182.

Wolbarsht, M.L. (1958), Electrical activity in the chemoreceptors of the blowfly; II. Responses to electrical stimulation. *J. gen. Physiol.,* **42**, 413–428.

Wolbarsht, M.L. (1965), Receptor sites in insect chemoreceptors. *Cold Spring Harbor Symp. Quant. Biol.,* **30**, 281–288.

Wolbarsht, M.L. and Hanson, F.E. (1965), Electrical activity in the chemoreceptors of the blowfly. III. Dendritic action potentials. *J. gen. Physiol.,* **48**, 673–683.

Wright, R.H. (1966), Primary odors and insect attraction. *Can. Ent.,* **98**, 1083–1093.

Zottermann, Y. (ed.) (1963), *Proc. I Int. Symp. Olfaction and Taste.* Pergamon Press, Oxford.

9 Leucocyte Chemotaxis

P. C. WILKINSON

Taxis and Behavior
(*Receptors and Recognition,* Series B, Volume 5)
Edited by G.L. Hazelbauer
Published in 1978 by Chapman and Hall, 11 New Fetter Lane, London EC4P 4EE
© Chapman and Hall

9.1 INTRODUCTION

Leucocytes are cells with an important role in the defence of the body against pathogenic micro-organisms and in maintaining the *status quo* by removing damaged cells and tissues. They achieve these tasks by locomotion towards and phagocytosis of such objects; thus they require to be able to respond to chemotactic gradients. In the developing vertebrate embryo many cells are motile; however, in the adult, most cells have interacted with their neighbours to form organs and tissues, and show little movement. Leucocytes do not organize in this way. The individual cells remain free. They show invasive behaviour both *in vivo* and *in vitro,* and can penetrate into spaces between other cells to reach sites of inflammation. Many leucocytes are professional phagocytes with an armoury of microbicidal mechanisms and hydrolytic enzymes. Others (lymphocytes) mount specific immune responses on contact with antigen.

The leucocytes serve the interest of the body as a whole, not their own interests. It is possible, but not certain, that their chemotactic and phagocytic functions have evolved from a requirement for food-seeking in free-living amoebae. Whatever their origins, these functions are quite different from those of the other cells considered in this volume. Many readers of this book, whose primary interest is not in this chapter, may be unfamiliar with mammalian leucocytes. For that reason, I shall devote some space to a brief account of these cells, their functions and their mode of locomotion before beginning to consider the possible recognition mechanisms which they may use to serve these functions.

9.2 THE LEUCOCYTES

The leucocytes are the 'white cells' of the blood of vertebrate species. There are a number of different types, all of which almost certainly originate from a single population of precursor stem cells in the bone marrow as shown in Fig. 9.1. The cells which we wish to consider belong to three cell lines, the myeloid line, the mononuclear phagocyte line and the lymphoid line. After maturation in the bone marrow (or in the thymus in the case of T-lymphocytes), the functionally mature cells of these lines appear in the blood, in which they circulate, and from which they can migrate into tissues. Chemotactic reactions are especially important at this stage of migration of leucocytes from the blood into the tissues. The granulocytes (myeloid line) and mononuclear phagocytes are phagocytic cells and play an important role at sites inflammation in ingesting, killing and digesting foreign micro-organisms and damaged tissue cells. Lymphocytes are not phagocytic. They mediate specific immune reactions by virtue of their possession of surface receptors for antigen. On appropriate

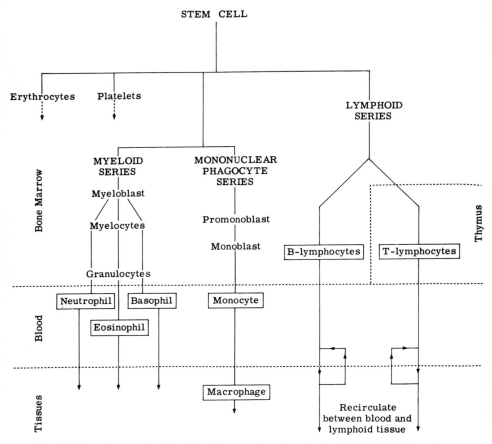

Fig. 9.1 Development of the blood leucocytes (much simplified). The boxed forms are those which are seen in inflammatory sites and show chemotactic reactions.

stimulation by antigen, lymphocytes differentiate into effector cells, i.e. B lympho-cytes differentiate to form cells with the capacity to make and secrete antibody specific for the inducing antigen, and T-lymphocytes differentiate to form a number of subsets some of which are directly cytotoxic for target cells or which release soluble mediators of immune function, others of which may act as helpers or suppressors of B lymphocyte function.

9.2.1 Granulocytes

The neutrophil granulocytes (polymorphonuclear leucocytes or PMN) are the most numerous of the white blood cells, and the majority of studies of leukocyte chemotaxis have been carried out using this cell type. Neutrophils are the classical cells of acute inflammation and respond immediately to injury by migrating from the blood into the injured tissue. The other granulocytes (eosinophil and basophil) are less numerous and have a more specialized function in defence against infestations with metazoan parasites and in immediate hypersensitivity. Granulocytes are short-lived cells. There is a considerable pool of mature forms normally present in the bone marrow which are released rapidly in response to infection or injury by a mechanism which is not understood. There is also a pool of non-circulating granulocytes marginated in capillaries in the bloodstream and capable of rapid mobilization on demand. Granulocytes circulate in the blood probably only for a few hours, then may leave the blood for the tissues where they do not survive for more than a few days. All granulocyte differentiation takes place in precursor cells in the bone-marrow. The mature granulocyte which is the typical chemotactic cell, is an end cell which has lost most of its capacity for protein synthesis and possesses few mitochondria. This in some ways simplifies the problem of understanding leucocyte chemotaxis, which is little affected by the presence of inhibitors of protein synthesis (Carruthers, 1967) or of inhibitors of oxidative phosphorylation (Bryant *et al.,* 1966; Ward, 1966), so that it is unlikely that these functions play any major part in the locomotor responses of these cells to attractants. Chemotactic responses can occur even in anucleate granulocytes (Keller and Bessis, 1975). Neutrophils have a cytoplasm which is abundant in lysosomal granules, which play a part in their microbicidal and digestive functions. They are rich in cytoplasmic actin and myosin (Tatsumi *et al.,* 1973; Stossel and Pollard, 1973), proteins of major importance for locomotion.

9.2.2 Monocytes and macrophages

Cells of the mononuclear phagocyte series also show chemotactic reactions. After leaving the bone marrow the monocytes circulate in the blood for about a day, then migrate into the tissues to become macrophages. Macrophages are not end cells, may live for considerable periods and are capable of differentiating, when appropriately stimulated, into cells which are more effective at killing bacteria than the monocytes from which they were derived. Monocytes form only about 10% of the white blood cells and are mobilized into inflammatory sites only slowly, so that in a persisting inflammation, the early wave of infiltrating neutrophil granulocytes is replaced over a period of several days by macrophages. They are therefore the classical cell type of chronic inflammation, as the neutrophils are of acute inflammation.

9.2.3 Lymphocytes

The functions and fate of the lymphocytes are much too complex to be dealt with here. Lymphocytes are mobilized into sites of inflammation more slowly than granulocytes but at the same speed as macrophages, and are therefore usually prominent in chronic inflammations. Furthermore lymphocytes recirculate continuously between blood and lymph and this requires that they leave the blood by crossing the post-capillary endothelium in lymph nodes, a process which is not shared by phagocytic cells but which may bear resemblances to the exit of leucocytes from vessels in inflammatory sites. It has only very recently been established that lymphocyt can show chemotactic reactions. One of the difficulties has been that normal lymphocytes form morphologically indistinguishable but functionally extremely heterogeneous populations, some of which are poorly adherent to substrata and not all of which show typical locomotor reactions. Another difficulty is that the small lymphocytes of blood, when stimulated with monoclonal activators (antigen) or polyclonal activators (for instance lectins or bacterial endotoxin) differentiate into large lymphoblasts, which behave differently from their small lymphocyte precursors. It has proved easier to demonstrate typical chemotactic reactions *in vitro* in these lymphoblasts after a day or two of *in vitro* culture than in lymphocytes fresh from blood (Russell *et al.*, 1975). After such a period of culture in the presence of an activator — or even in its absence — lymphocytes locomote in a relatively predictable manner in the presence of attractants.

9.3 ROLE OF LEUCOCYTE CHEMOTAXIS *IN VIVO*

At a site of inflammation observed directly under the microscope, the first changes seen include vasodilatation and the slowing of blood flow through small vessels (capillaries and post-capillary venules) draining the inflamed site. The leucocytes, which normally flow through such vessels without sticking, become marginated and adhere to the endothelial cells lining the vessel. This increased adhesion between leucocyte and endothelial cell is of extreme interest but almost nothing is known about it at the molecular level. Some preliminary experiments suggest that chemotactic substances might be involved since such substances were noted to increase leucocyte-endothelial cell adhesions *in vitro* (Hoover, 1978) and *in vivo* (Atherton and Born, 1972). Following adhesion, the leucocytes migrate out of the vessel between the endothelial cells and through the vascular basement membrane into the tissue. It is usually assumed that their subsequent locomotion through the tissues to the inflamed site is chemotactic in response to a gradient, but it is extremely difficult to demonstrate this directly *in vivo*, and the assumption is based on the behaviour of the same cells in analogous but simplified situations *in vitro*.

The inflamed site is usually taken as the *locus classicus* for leucocyte chemotaxis, probably because it is morphologically obvious to the histologist and involves large numbers of migrating cells. However, anyone who has observed the behaviour of leucocytes *in vitro* will be impressed with the rapidity with which they detect injury in one of their members or in erythrocytes and other cells surrounding them. Damage to any single isolated cell is followed immediately by the rapid locomotion of surrounding leucocytes towards the damaged cell, followed by phagocytosis of its remnants, the whole process being over in a minute or two. This behaviour has been studied in detail by Bessis (1974) who used laser beams to damage a single erythrocyte and watched the immediate chemotactic locomotion of nearby leucocytes towards the injured cell, and who used the word 'necrotaxis' to describe it. As Bessis point out, this scavenger function of chemotactically responsive leucocytes may play an important role in clearing effete cells, and may happen so rapidly that it does not result in an obvious inflammatory response because, once the dead cell is removed, there is no further inflammatory stimulus. Thus leucocytes act as scavengers under physiological conditions as well as in pathological inflammatory states.

9.4 CHEMOTACTIC FACTORS

There is now a large list of chemotactic factors which have been reported as attracting one or other type of leucocyte, and there is general agreement about the activity of many of those. It would not be appropriate to review them in detail here and this has been done elsewhere (Wilkinson, 1974b). Chemotactic factors which present interesting features from the point of view of recognition will be discussed later. Chemotactic factors can be classified according to the situation in which they occur as shown in Table 9.1. Many are proteins or peptides and vary in size from large proteins to dipeptides. A number of lipid attractants have also been described. No sugar or polysaccharide has been shown to possess chemotactic activity for leucocytes.

9.5 THE NATURE OF LEUCOCYTE LOCOMOTION IN THE PRESENCE OF CHEMO-ATTRACTANTS

Leucocytes move by crawling on surfaces and movement is associated with, and dependent on, changes in cell shape, as in amoebae and many other motile eukaryotic cells. The cell at rest is usually rounded or flattened. Movement is preceded by the adoption of an oriented morphology. A hyaline membrane or 'lamellipodium' extends forwards in the direction in which movement will take place, and the cell adopts an elongated shape (Fig. 9.2). There may be a posterior tail or uropod. This feature is especially obvious in lymphocytes (Fig. 9.3) and has been said to give the cells the appearance of a hand-mirror. As movement occurs, the cytoplasmic contents flow into the anterior lamellipodium and the cell slides along on the surface. Locomotion is obviously dependent on the adhesive forces binding the cell to its substratum. If such forces are too strong, the cell will be tethered and unable to move. Cells on

Table 9.1 Functional classification of leucocyte chemotactic factors

---

1. Products of specific immune reactions.

   (a)   Antigen—antibody reactions lead to activation of complement and liberation of chemotactic peptides e.g. C5a.
         These peptides can also be released by direct (alternative pathway) activation of complement by surf̝e polysaccharides of micro-organisms without a requirement for antibody.

   (b)   Lymphocytes can be stimulated by antigen to release chemotactic 'lymphokines'.

   (c)   If a leucocyte carries surface antibody e.g. as an integral membrane protein as in lymphocytes, or as 'cytophilic' fluid phase antibody which becomes attached to the cell, that cell may migrate in gradients of the appropriate antigen.

2. Products of non-specific reactions.

   (a)   Products of micro-organisms

   (b)   Products of cell injury
         Denatured proteins

   (c)   Products released under physiological conditions from healthy cells as a response to injury e.g. leucocytes engaged in phagocytosis may release products that attract other leucocytes.
         Eosinophil chemotactic factors (ECF-A) are released from mast cells when mast-cell-bound IgE antibody reacts with antigen.
         Chemotactic lipids e.g. HETE (*vide infra*) may be released from platelets.

3. Synthetic chemotactic factors, e.g. formyl peptides; proteins modified by conjugation of synthetic groups.

4. Physiological proteins outside their normal environment α_s-casein and β-casein.

---

untreated glass in protein-free media are tethered in this way. Addition of a protein such as serum albumin allows the cells to move on a surface of albumin instead of on the glass and thus permits movement. On the other hand cells whose attachments to surfaces are very weak show changes in morphology typical of locomotion but do not move effectively and are passively carried around by currents. Locomotion obviously requires a balance between forces promoting attachment and those allowing the cell to detach itself, and during locomotion, some areas of the cell in contact with the substratum presumably require to be attached at the same time as other areas are detached. The nature of the adhesions made by rabbit neutrophil leucocytes on protein-coated glass were examined by Armstrong and Lackie (1975) using interference-reflection microscopy. These adhesions were rather light and transient, fluctuating from second to second as the cell moved.

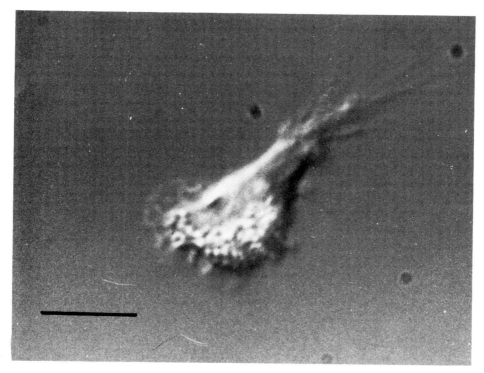

Fig. 9.2 Locomoting human blood neutrophil leucocyte. Note the anterior hyaline veil or lamellipodium with the granule-containing cell body behind it. The cell has a tail with a number of retraction fibres radiating from it. Nomarski phase contrast. Bar represents 10 μm.

These events are controlled by the contraction and relaxation of actin- and myosin-containing microfilaments. Obviously the behaviour of the microfilaments is responsive to signals from outside the cell, thus the problem of stimulus-response coupling in leucocyte locomotion and chemotaxis is how such signals regulate the behaviour of intracellular actin and myosin. This behaviour is itself not understood in detail at a molecular level, still less its control. There are a number of reviews about actin and myosin in non-muscle cells and a recent review which deals specifically with leucocytes (Stossel, 1978) is recommended to the reader.

Leucocyte chemo-attractants influence both chemotaxis and chemokinesis. *Chemotaxis* is here defined as a reaction by which chemical substances determine the direction of locomotion or the angle of turn of cells (McCutcheon, 1946; Keller *et al.*, 1977), and *chemokinesis* as a reaction by which chemical substances determine the rate of locomotion or the frequency of turning of cells (Keller *et al.*, 1977). If, for instance, a chemo-attractant such as casein is added to neutrophil leucocytes at

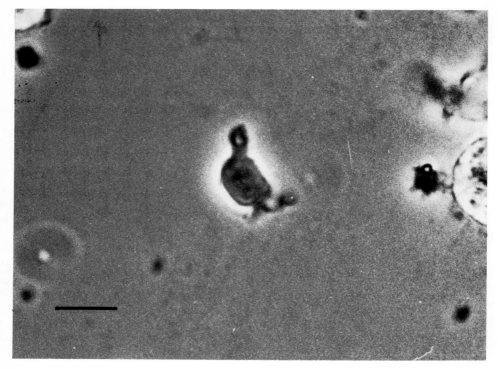

Fig. 9.3 A locomoting lymphocyte. The anterior lamellipodium is not clearly seen, but ruffling is present. Note the large nucleus and the prominent tail (below). Phase contrast. Bar represents 10 μm.

increasing absolute concentrations without a gradient, a concentration-dependent increase in speed of the cells is observed (Allan and Wilkinson, 1978). However, if the same attractant is allowed to diffuse from a source to form a concentration gradient, the cells respond by directional locomotion towards the source. Thus the reaction of leucocytes to attractants is not purely chemotactic (as defined above) and the cells are responsive both to gradients and to changes in absolute concentration. Cells moving in gradients show narrow angles of turn and, if they deviate more than 30° from the line between the cell and the gradient source, they are highly likely to correct by making their next turn towards the source (Zigmond, 1974).

It was mentioned earlier that leucocytes show morphological polarization before translocating. When placed in chemotactic gradients the direction of polarization is determined by the gradient so that the head of the cell points up-gradient towards the source and the tail away from the source (Zigmond, 1974). This orientation is quite accurate and indicates that the cell has detected the gradient before moving in it. Thus the cell probably detects differences in attractant concentration between its head and its tail. This argues in favour of a spatial gradient-detection mechanism rather than for a temporal mechanism in which the cell reads the concentration around it at different times as in bacteria. An elongated leucocyte may be 15–20 μm long and is capable of such spatial sensing. From recent studies using an assay of cell orientation in carefully chosen gradients, Zigmond (1977) has calculated that leucocytes can detect differences in concentration of 1% across their length. The spatial system of detecting gradients, of course, suggests the presence of multiple receptors on the cell surface. A single receptor would be inadequate unless it were moving rapidly between the front and back of the cell.

9.6 RECOGNITION IN LEUCOCYTE CHEMOTAXIS: GENERAL CONSIDERATIONS

Based on many paradigms for cell behaviour in response to environmental influences, an intuitive model for the control of locomotor reactions in leucocytes would suggest that discriminative functional activation is achieved when a ligand in the environment (the chemotactic factor) binds selectively to a receptor on the cell surface. This binding initiates a change in the membrane which allows passage of a signal to the interior of the cell, which in turn, and possibly through a number of steps, activates the appropriate cytoplasmic locomotor machinery i.e. the actin-containing micro-filaments. The study of chemotactic recognition by leucocytes has only just begun and it is by no means clear yet how well models of the above type describe it. Experiments are now replacing speculation but there is still a long way to go before it will be possible to propose elegant models for stimulus-response coupling in leucocytes such as are now current for the chemotactic responses of bacteria.

One of the most approachable problems ought to be how leucocytes recognize chemotactic factors. We have already seen that there are a large number of these factors. Many are fairly complex molecules but there are structural physicochemical data available for some of them which may suggest models for their action.

A successful approach to the study of ligand–receptor interactions is based on the concept of stereospecificity. The idea that enzyme–substrate interactions (Fischer, 1894, 1895) and antigen–antibody reactions (Ehrlich, 1957) owed their high degree of specificity to the exactness of the three-dimensional fit between the reactants, and to the correct spacing of chemical groupings which would attract one another, led to the 'lock-and-key' concept of cell surface recognition (Weiss, 1947). Intuitively, it seems probable that many cell functions demand specificity of this high degree, e.g. sperm–ovum recognition, hormone–target cell interactions, activation of antigen-sensitive lymphocytes. However, in other situations e.g. the sorting-out of heterotypic cell types in development, the demand for high specificity is less obvious. Leucocytes function in non-specific defence against a wide variety of infections, and are also frequently seen in sites of non-specific damage. Since in their chemotactic reactions, they respond to a wide variety of attractant molecules which are dissimilar from each

other in detailed structure, it might be argued *a priori* that these functions would not
be best served by a highly specific, and therefore highly restrictive recognition system.
Leucocytes might function best by possessing membrane recognition sites able to bind
a wide range of molecules. On the other hand, it is true that in many cases, leucocytic
recognition is indirect. Many bacteria are able to activate serum complement either by
classical antibody-mediated complement fixation or by alternative pathway fixation
in the absence of antibody. Likewise non-specific tissue injury may lead to complement
activation. Thus, in many reactions to tissue injury, chemotactic complement peptides
such as C5a are a common end product, and the leucocytes may often simply require
to recognize these peptides and not the bacterium or other injurious agent itself. This
is an indisputably important mechanism, but it is also clear that there are many situations where it does not operate. I have argued elsewhere that there could be a number
of possible explanations for the versatility of recognition by phagocytic cells as
follows (Wilkinson, 1976a)

(1) They may recognize general physicochemical characteristics which are shared
by 'abnormal' substances, but are not determined by the detailed geometric structure
of any substance.

(2) They may possess stereospecific receptors for all, or at least some, of the
substances to which they respond.

(3) Recognition may be indirect as discussed above and also in recognition of
phagocytosable objects. Since leucocytes possess binding sites for the Fc fragment of
immunoglobulin and for activated complement components (e.g. C3b), they can bind
molecules or particles which have become attached to ('opsonized' by) antibody or
complement. The onus of recognition is thus removed from the phagocyte itself to
'borrowed' molecules attached to its surface. This still leaves the problem of the
nature of the leucocyte binding site for Fc and for complement. This type of
recognition is important in phagocytosis. Its role in chemotaxis has been less studied.

(4) Since (1), (2) and (3) are not mutually exclusive, each of them may operate
in individual circumstances.

The distinction between (1) and (2) above may not be sharp. Cell surface receptors
may vary between those with very exacting binding requirements for a single ligand
or a few closely related ligands and those which can bind a very wide range of ligands,
which are not closely related structurally to each other. A good example of the latter
is provided by the very versatile binding sites of serum albumin for a wide variety of
amphipathic ligands. (Tanford, 1972; McMenamy, 1977). The latter binding sites
have quite a high affinity ($10^4 - 10^8 1\ mol^{-1}$) for many ligands and are saturable, so
have the general characteristics which would be expected of a receptor.

It has been argued that high binding affinity of a receptor for a ligand implies
stereospecific binding. This is often the case, but may not always be true, and will
vary depending on the nature of the chemical bonds between receptors and ligand.
For example, hydrogen bonds are highly directional and require the correct spatial
alignment of the reactant groups and so are of great stereochemical significance.

However, to take the example of the hydrophobic interaction, which is not strictly speaking a chemical bond at all, yet probably provides the major source of energy stabilizing the native structure of globular proteins in aqueous solution, such interactions are not directional and the structural geometry of the reactant molecules is of less importance. From an energetic point of view nevertheless, these are comparatively strong interactions. It requires the expenditure of 3.4 kcal mol^{-1} to transfer the phenylalanine sidegroup from an organic solvent to water (Nozaki and Tanford, 1971). This is comparable to the electrostatic interaction between carboxyl and ammonium ion side-chain amino acid residues (4.5 kcal mol^{-1}) or to hydrogen bonds between for instance oxygen and nitrogen (5 kcal mol^{-1}). The point is that receptor—ligand interactions which are chiefly hydrophobic will be energetically stable, but will lack steric complementarity. If the interaction involves coulombic interactions and hydrogen bonding to a considerable degree, then stereochemistry assumes major importance.

A first requirement for the study of chemotactic recognition is that chemotactic factors of good purity and defined structure be available. A lack of these until recently has held up work somewhat but there are now a number of factors which fulfil these requirements. An account is given below of work with some of these. Many of the factors listed in Table 9.1 are not discussed because they have not yet been helpful in the study of recognition. A further account of them is given in Wilkinson (1974b).

9.6.1 Formylated and other peptides

Since, during the last two or three years, these have become the most popular chemotactic factors used in receptor studies, we shall begin with them. Schiffmann *et al.,* (1975) reported that a number of *N*-formyl-methionyl dipeptides showed chemotactic activity, and this was followed by a more extended study of a series of formylated di- and tri-peptides (Showell *et al.,* 1976). The findings can be summarized as follows. Formylated methionyl peptides were active, as were a number of formyl leucyl peptides. Blockage of the *N*-terminal amino group was necessary. Thus formyl peptides were much more active than analogous unblocked peptides. Blockage of the amino groups by methods other than formylation has not been extensively studied. There was a requirement for hydrophobic residues at the C-terminal end e.g. tripeptides in which phenylalanine was in the third position were especially active. The most active tripeptides (e.g. f-Met-Leu-Phe) gave maximal responses at low concentrations (c 10^{-10} M). Dipeptides were maximally effective at higher concentrations (c 10^{-5} — 10^{-6} M). The peptides activated leucocyte functions other than chemotaxis, e.g. exocytosis. Since small changes in structure caused large changes in the effective concentration and since the peptides were active at very low doses, the authors suggested that the peptides acted by binding to a stereospecific receptor on the cell surface. More recently the binding of two peptides has been measured. Formyl ^{3}H norleu-leu-phe binds to the leucocyte surface with an association

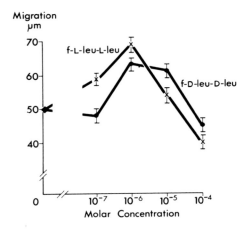

Fig. 9.4 Dose—response curves for human neutrophils migrating in the micropore filter assay towards formyl-L-leucyl-L-leucine and formyl D-leucyl-D-leucine. The differences in migration were not significant except at 10^{-7} M peptide.

constant of 10^9 l mol^{-1} and there are 10^5 binding sites per cell (Aswanikumar *et al.*, 1977). Binding can be displaced by other peptides e.g. f-Met-Leu-Phe. It has also been suggested that the receptors are freed by proteolytic cleavage of the bound peptide by neutrophil-derived enzymes (Aswanikumar *et al.*, 1976). Binding of f-Met-Leu-Phe has been measured by another group (Williams *et al.*, 1977) who obtained a K_a of c 10^8 with 2×10^3 binding sites per cell. It has been suggested that, since N-formylation of methionine is necessary to initiate protein synthesis in *E. coli* but not in eukaryotic cells, recognition by leucocytes of N-formyl methionyl peptides might act as a mechanism whereby leucocytes distinguish a 'foreign' product of prokaryotic cells which is not shared by eukaryotic cells.

The studies reported so far certainly suggest that leucocytes possess a limited number of defined surface binding sites for formyl peptides. These binding sites have not yet been characterized. It is my view that the evidence for stereospecificity of binding is at present insecure. All the peptides studied in the papers cited above were in a narrow range, i.e. formyl-methionyl or formyl-leucyl peptides, and other peptides were not looked at. They were all composed of L-aminoacids although Aswanikumar *et al.* (1977) reported that f-D-phe-D-met failed to affect chemotaxis or interact with peptide chemotactic receptors, while its enantiomer, f-L-Phe-L-met, did have such effects. We have looked at L and D forms of f-Leu-Leu and find that chemotactic activity is about the same for both configurations (Fig. 9.4). This is clearly an important point and deserves further study. We have also examined a variety of peptides other than methionyl or leucyl peptides. Fig. 9.5 shows dose—response curves for formyl di-tyrosine and formyl tri-tyrosine. These peptides act at

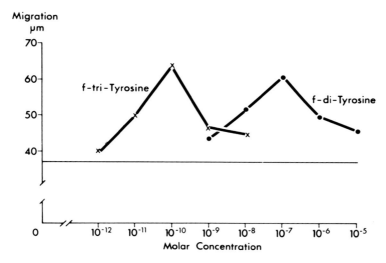

Fig. 9.5 Dose—response curves for human neutrophils migrating in the micropore filter assay towards formyl dityrosine and formyl trityrosine.

similar molar concentrations to analogous methionyl peptides. We have obtained similar curves with phenylalanyl peptides. The conclusion from study of these and related peptides is that very many peptides are chemotactically active to varying degree. There is a requirement for a blocked N-terminal amino group (thus making the peptide anionic) and for hydrophobicity. Activity increases with increasing length of peptide up to 3 residues. Other than this, specificity may not be strict* and I am inclined at present to believe that the receptor for formyl peptides is a very catholic one, possibly a conformationally flexible site which undergoes ligand-induced shape changes and can thus bind a wide range of ligands. Furthermore the anionic, amphipathic nature of the active peptides is shared by some of the other chemotactic factors discussed later. It is only fair to add that other workers in the field do hold the view that the receptors for these peptides are stereospecific. There is a good recent review on the peptides and on behavioural studies of locomotion by Zigmond (1978b).

There is a second group of peptides, the eosinophilotactic tetrapeptides (ECF-A or eosinophil chemotactic factors of anaphylaxis), Val-Gly-Ser-Glu and Ala-Gly-Ser-Glu (Goetzl and Austen 1975). These attract eosinophils, but also, under suitable conditions, neutrophils and monocytes. Their activity requires a negative charge at the C-terminal end and a nonpolar residue at the N-terminal end. Relationships between these and the formyl-peptides have not been explored.

* However, Showell *et al.* (1976) observed that, while f-Met-Leu-Phe is maximally active at around 10^{-10} M, f-Met-Phe-Leu is only active at around 10^{-7} M. Likewise we have observed that for instance f-Tyr-Phe is effective at lower concentrations (10^{-7} – 10^{-8} M) than f-Phe-Tyr (10^{-5} – 10^{-6} M).

9.6.2 Lipids

Lipids and fatty acids have chemo-attractant activity for leucocytes. Many are weak attractants but some act more strongly. Lipid fractions of bacteria e.g. *Corynebacterium parvum* (Russell *et al.*, 1976) and *Escherichia coli* (Tainer *et al.*, 1975; Sahu and Lynn, 1977) have activity. Sahu and Lynn (1977) found that 75% of the leucocyte chemotactic activity of *E. coli* was due to lipid. The most active fractions were anionic and an active 12-hydroxy fatty acid was identified. Oxidised forms of prostaglandins PGA_2 and PGE_2 were active and malonaldehyde was shown to react with phosphatidylethanolamine to produce an active lipid. Activity could be destroyed by catalytic reduction or by methylation.

Platelets may be another physiologically important source of lipids. Platelet aggregation is one of the earliest events in the inflammatory response and it has been shown that platelet-derived arachidonic acid is acted on by an aggregation-activated lipoxygenase to form 12-hydroxy-5, 8, 10, 14-eicosatetranoic acid (HETE) (Turner *et al.*, 1975), one of the most active of the chemotactic lipids yet identified. It seems difficult to visualize a stereospecific receptor for lipid attractants, although amphipathic lipids could integrate into the bilayer or bind to hydrophobic sites on membrane proteins in a way similar to the binding of fatty acids to albumin. Some structural specificity is suggested by the fact that anionic lipids are more active than others, and that hydroxylation or oxidation of unsaturated fatty acids increases their activity. The fact that these fatty acids are unstable and tend to oxidise (and thus gain activity) on storage, together with their poor solubility and difficulty in setting up good gradients makes their study rather difficult.

9.6.3 Complement

Considering that, in inflammatory lesions, activated complement is probably the most important chemo-attractant of human leucocytes, there is remarkably little information about the interactions of complement-derived attractants with the leucocyte membrane. There is not even general agreement about which moieties of activated complement are chemotactic, although there is a consensus that peptides derived by cleavage of the fifth component of complement, C5, do have major activity. Perhaps one of the most useful studies, which has been rather ignored, was that of Wissler and colleagues (Wissler, 1972a,b; Wissler *et al.*, 1972a) who carried out a very detailed fractionation of dextran-activated rat or pig serum and obtained active peptides in a state of high purity. They did not discuss the relation of these peptides to C5 or to other possible precursors. Two peptides were isolated, one named 'classical anaphylatoxin' or CAT (mol.wt. 9500) and the other 'co-cytotaxin' or CCT (mol.wt. 8500). When these peptides were isolated from one another, neither was active. When both were present they acted together as chemotactic factors. By varying the concentration ratios between the peptides, selective chemotaxis of neutrophils or of eosinophils could be obtained (Wissler *et al.*, 1972b). These observations are extremely interesting because one of the unsolved problems with leucocytes is how cell specificity in chemotaxis is regulated, and what relation chemotaxis has with the influx of cells of one or other type into inflammatory lesions. Many chemotactic factors attract several different types of leucocyte but act more strongly on one type than on another. Kay *et al.* (1973) showed that the ability of eosinophilotactic peptides to attract either eosinophils or neutrophils is related to the proportion of each cell type in the test sample, and showed synergistic effects between ECF-A and C5a. Two-peptide systems like that of Wissler might provide an explanation for cell specificity. Such systems would certainly present intriguing problems for receptor studies.

9.6.4 Succinyl-melittin

Melittin is a surface-active amphipathic peptide from bee venom which is known to interact strongly with lipid bilayers, including those of liposomes and of cell membranes, and which is strongly cytotoxic. It contains 26 residues, the first 20 of which are chiefly non-polar and the remaining C-terminal portion of the peptide is strongly basic. Habermann and Krowallek (1970) showed that cytotoxicity could be reduced considerably by succinylating that α and ϵ-amino groups of melittin, thus reducing the positive charge. Following succinylation, melittin retained surface activity. I have shown that pure succinyl melittin is chemotactic for leucocytes at concentration of $10^{-5}-10^{-6}$ M although the unsuccinylated form is cytotoxic and has no chemotactic activity (Wilkinson, 1977a). Succinyl-melittin shares general features in common with many of the chemotactic factors mentioned above, i.e. it is anionic and amphipathic, though its detailed structure is different from that of the lipid attractants or from that of peptides such as f-Met-Leu-Phe; melittin contains no methionine or phenylalanine.

9.6.5 Requirement for protein for chemotactic activity of low-molecular-weight chemotactic factors

Most of the low-molecular-weight chemotactic factors listed above do not induce locomotion of leucocytes in the absence of protein. However, if the cells are suspended in human serum albumin (HSA), a response is seen (Wilkinson, 1976c). The presence of protein does not affect the binding affinity of these factors to the cells. Rather, it appears to be necessary because, for locomotion, cells require to move on surface-bound attractant molecules. Protein attractants (*vide infra*) bind well to surfaces such as glass, plastic, or micropore filters but the low-molecular-weight attractants do not. However, if the surface is first coated with serum albumin, small peptides and lipids can bind to the serum albumin and thus the cell moves on a surface of protein-bound attractant (Wilkinson and Allan, 1979) (see Fig. 9.8).

9.6.6 Protein attractants: recognition of altered conformation

For several years our laboratory has been interested in the effects of alterations of protein structure on recognition by leucocytes. If leucocytes possess a mechanism for distinguishing ordered or 'normal' structure from disordered or 'abnormal' structure, this might help explain their function in removal of damaged or effete cells and tissues. Physiologically important proteins can be obtained in a state of high purity and their structure can be modified easily in a controlled way.

Native haemoglobin and myoglobin are not chemotactic for leucocytes. A reversible denaturation can be induced in these molecules if the haem group is removed from the globin molecule. The α-helix content of globin drops from 70% to about 55% when this is done, the molecule unfolds, becomes poorly soluble in aqueous media and tends to aggregate. This denaturation can be completely reversed by adding haem back to the globin, until, at the molar ratio of one haem group per globin dimer, the globin is completely restored to its native state. I showed that, on removal of haem, globin became chemotactic for leucocytes (Wilkinson, 1973) and that, when the haem was allowed to rebind, the globin refolded and completely lost chemotactic activity (Fig. 9.6).

The effect of conformational changes in serum albumin has been studied in detail. Native human serum albumin (HSA) has a chemokinetic effect on leucocyte loco-motion but is not chemotactic. On denaturation e.g. with alkali or by reduction-alkylation, the protein becomes chemotactic. Acquisition of chemotactic activity can be shown to be correlated with an increase in viscosity (Wilkinson and McKay, 1971), surface activity (Wilkinson, 1974a) and with a change in the absorption spectrum of HSA evidenced by a peak in the difference spectrum against native HSA at 287nm. Although HSA may polymerize when denatured, gel filtration to separate polymerized from monomeric forms shows that denatured monomeric albumin is active, thus the cells recognize the conformational change in the monomer rather than simply the presence of aggregates. Binding of ^{125}I alkali-denatured HSA to leucocytes has been studied (Wilkinson and Allan, 1978). Denatured protein binds much more strongly than native HSA. The K_a for alkali-denatured HSA was around 10^6 l mol^{-1} and the number of binding sites about 10^6. In other studies, we con-jugated a wide variety of small synthetic molecules to serum albumin (Wilkinson and McKay, 1972). Non-polar molecules containing aromatic groups or alkyl chains frequently conferred chemotactic activity on the protein, whereas polar molecules had less effect.

The major force maintaining globular proteins in the native state in aqueous solution is provided by the hydrophobic interactions between non-polar side-chains packed into the interior of the protein molecule, thus when the protein becomes denatured these side-chains are forced into contact with solvent water molecules. Hence, a possible mechanism for chemotactic recognition might be based on the increased hydrophobicity of unfolded, denatured proteins. These proteins, being thermodynamically unstable in aqueous solution, will find their lowest free energy

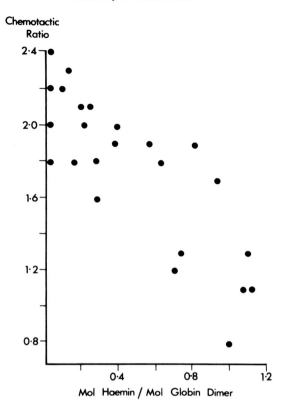

Fig. 9.6 Effect of binding of haemin on the chemo-attractant activity of globin for human neutrophil leucocytes. Chemotactic ratio = migration towards test sample/migration towards native myoglobin. Note that haem-free globin is active but that as the haem: globin ratio is increased (and the protein renatures), activity is progressively lost. From Wilkinson (1973) by courtesy of *Nature*.

state at relatively hydrophobic surfaces, of which the lipid bilayer of the cell membrane may be one. Thus the exposed hydrophobic side-chains might integrate into the bilayer rather like an intrinsic membrane protein. If this is so, probably the integration of such proteins would initially require polar interactions with extrinsically placed polar groups on the membrane in order for the non-polar groups to appose sufficiently to interact with non-polar areas of the membrane. Thus, these chemotactic factors require to be amphipathic rather than purely hydrophobic. The same kind of considerations would apply were binding to hydrophobic membrane protein sites rather than to lipid. This kind of recognition would allow stimulus—response coupling by a wide range of structurally different molecules based not on steric

criteria but on common physico-chemical properties of chemotactic molecules as a
class. Nevertheless the binding studies cited above suggested that denatured proteins
do bind to defined sites on cell membranes and do not simply partition non-specifically
into the membrane. Those studies also suggested that the binding sites are saturable.
Thus it could be said that there are receptors for such proteins but these seem unlikely
to be of the lock-and-key type because of the wide variety of structurally altered
proteins which can be chemotactic. Probably as discussed earlier, binding which was
predominantly due to hydrophobic interactions would lack the directionality which
is a prerequisite for stereospecificity, but might nevertheless show fairly high affinity.

Another strongly chemotactic protein is milk casein. Some of the activity of
casein is due to lipid (Lynn *et al.,* 1974). However, if pure lipid-free α_s, β- and
κ-casein are examined, it can be shown that α_s- and β-caseins have chemotactic
activity but κ-casein does not (Wilkinson, 1974a). κ-casein is a glycoprotein which
does not resemble α_s- or β-caseins closely. α_s-Casein and β-casein, however, are very
similar. Both are phosphoproteins with an acidic moiety at one end of the molecule
and a non-polar moiety at the other. If the acidic portion of β-casein is separated by
cyanogen bromide cleavage from the hydrophobic portion, neither has chemotactic
activity alone, but when they are combined, chemotactic activity is regained (Suzue
et al., 1976). Casein is, of course, a protein of physiological importance in milk. The
Ca^{2+} concentration is high in milk and casein is present in the form of large macromolecular complexes stabilized by Ca^{2+}. These are presumably poorly diffusible and
have little chemotactic activity. If the Ca^{2+} concentration is lowered to that of other
body fluids, the casein complexes dissociate and chemotactic activity appears.

9.6.7 Deactivation

One approach to the problem of specificity of binding of various chemotactic
factors might be to pretreat cells with one factor and to see if they could still respond
to a second factor, or to a further dose of the same factor. Becker (1972) reported
that chemotactic factors could 'de-activate' to themselves i.e. that pretreatment with
a factor caused cells to fail to locomote in a gradient of that factor. It is certainly
true that, for instance, formyl-peptides, complement peptides or denatured albumin
de-activate to themselves (author's unpublished observation with Dr. Susanna Spisani).
However, they also de-activate to a variable extent to each other and to other factors.
It is difficult to interpret these findings in terms of receptor occupancy or saturation
and there may be some other limiting step which causes de-activation. Ward and
Becker (1968) have suggested that it may follow irreversible activation of an
'activatable esterase' which is involved at some stage of the chemotactic response.

9.6.8 Recognition of chemotactic factors by lymphocytes

The activity of the chemotactic factors discussed above was studied chiefly using
neutrophil leucocytes. Lymphocytes can also be shown to recognize most of these

factors. However, lymphocytes are known to possess surface receptors e.g. for antigen-binding, not possessed by phagocytes. It is therefore of interest to know whether this type of receptor is involved in chemotactic reactions in lymphocytes. That this might be so was suggested by some studies we carried out using phytohaemagglutinin (PHA) a lectin from the kidney bean *Phaseolus vulgaris,* which binds to surface glycoproteins on lymphocytes and stimulates mitogenic activity. We found that PHA at doses a hundred to a thousandfold lower than the mitogenic dose would induce moderate chemotactic reactions in lymphocytes (Wilkinson *et al.,* 1976). Another polyvalent ligand, staphylococcal Protein A, which binds to lymphocyte surface immunoglobulin, had a similar effect in stimulating locomotor responses in lymphocytes. These ligands bind to surface proteins or glycoproteins, are not amphipathic and presumably activate chemotactic responses in quite a different way from that discussed above. Neutrophil leucocytes have been reported to respond chemotactically to a fucose-binding lectin (van Epps and Tung, 1977) so they also presumably use this type of recognition system in appropriate situations.

As stated earlier, phagocytic cells possess a binding site for the Fc fragment of immunoglobulin and, if they are coated with immunoglobulin, can recognize antigen at 'second-hand'. Jensen and Esquenazi (1975) coated neutrophils with cytophilic antibody against selected antigens, placed the antigen below the filter, and showed that these neutrophils, but not uncoated neutrophils, would migrate towards the specific antigen but not to other proteins. In recent experiments to explore antigen recognition in lymphocyte chemotaxis, we (Wilkinson *et al.,* 1977) primed mice with antigen (serum albumin or ovalbumin), challenged the mice and examined lymphocytes taken 3–10 days later from the lymph nodes draining the site of challenge. These primed lymphocytes showed chemotactic responses to antigen, but control unprimed lymphocytes did not. We have not established whether these responses were due to binding of antigen to intrinsic membrane immunoglobulin combining sites or to soluble immunoglobulin attached to Fc binding sites as in the phagocytes used in Jensen's study quoted above. Lymphocyte populations are very heterogeneous and contain numerous subsets which differ in their surface structure. A good deal more work will be needed to sort out the possibilities for chemotactic recognition offered by this diversity.

9.7 EFFECTS OF SPECIFIC ENZYMES AND BACTERIAL TOXINS ON CHEMOTACTIC RESPONSES OF LEUCOCYTES

In trying to define the membrane sites responsible for initiating chemotactic reactions, it is useful to modify the membrane with enzymes which attack known substrates. One can also use a number of bacterial toxins which affect membrane function by a non-enzymatic action at specific sites.

We have examined the effects of proteases, glycosidases and lipid-specific enzymes and toxins on locomotion of leucocytes towards a number of chemotactic factors.

Table 9.2 Effects of membrane-active enzymes and toxins on the locomotion of human blood neutorphils and monocytes in chemotaxis chambers

Agent used	Concentration range	Locomotion to casein (1 mg ml^{-1}) or alkali-denatured HSA (1 mg ml^{-1}) as per cent locomotion of control untreated cells ± S.E.M.			
		Neutrophils		Monocytes	
		No. of experiments	Locomotion per cent control	No. of experiments	Locomotion per cent control
Lipid-specific agents					
Phospholipase C	50–200 mU ml^{-1}	7	101 ± 6	7	64 ± 4
Sphingomyelinase C	10^2–10^3 HU ml^{-1}	9	96 ± 3	13	58 ± 5
θ-toxin	0.5–1 HU ml^{-1}	14	62 ± 4	9	92 ± 3
Proteases					
Pronase	100 µg ml^{-1}	4	103 ± 5	4	108 ± 4
Trypsin	100–200 µg ml^{-1}	4	94 ± 8	3	103 ± 9
Glycosidases					
α-Fucosidase	0.66 u ml^{-1}	3	102 ± 0.6	3	112 ± 4
α-Mannosidase	3 u ml^{-1}	2	97 ± 13	3	105 ± 8
Neuraminidase	4 u ml^{-1}	9	90 ± 3	9	104 ± 4

(From Wilkinson, 1977b).

The results are somewhat complex and vary from one leucocyte-type to another and also from one species to another. Some results for the responses of human leucocytes to casein and to denatured HSA are shown in Table 9.2. The response of human, rabbit, and mouse leucocytes to these factors was abolished or reduced by pre-treatment of the cells with lipid-specific agents but not with proteases or glycosidases. In human monocytes, phospholipase C and sphingomyelinase C were most effective; in human neutrophils, the oxygen-labile toxins, — i.e. *Clostridium perfringens* θ-toxin and Streptolysin-O, acted most strongly (van Epps and Andersen, 1974; Wilkinson, 1975a). Similarly, chemotactic responses of leucocytes to succinyl-melittin and to formyl peptides were reduced after treatment of the cells with lipid-specific agents, but not with pronase (unpublished).

It is possible that these results were obtained because the receptor for these chemotactic factors is, at least in part, lipid. Recent studies of the author have shown that leucocytes treated with θ-toxin or phospholipases C bind ^{125}I-denatured HSA in lower amounts than control leucocytes (Wilkinson and Allan, 1978). It could also be argued that, since such toxins are known to initiate a re-organization of membrane lipids (Freer and Arbuthnott, 1976) and since a defined lipid environment is crucial to the action of some membrane proteins, the toxins are simply disrupting the environment of a protein or glycoprotein receptor. If such a receptor is present, it is resistant to pronase and trypsin. However, if it lay within the bilayer rather than superficially, it might not be accessible to proteolytic cleavage.

On the other hand, the ability of lymphocytes to respond by locomotion to PHA and protein A is reduced if the cells are pretreated with pronase or trypsin, but is unaffected by lipid-specific agents (Wilkinson *et al.*, 1976). Since these ligands are known to bind to membrane proteins or glycoproteins, these results are not unexpected. Nevertheless, they indicate clearly that chemotactic factors can be recognised at at least two types of site, one protease-sensitive, one sensitive to lipid-specific agents (Fig. 9.7).

There is as yet no literature on attempts to isolate or define chemotaxis receptors in leucocytes by chemical means. The modifications described above represent no more than a very preliminary approach to this important area.

9.8 ARE SIMILAR RECOGNITION MECHANISMS INVOLVED IN CHEMOTAXIS, PHAGOCYTOSIS AND OTHER LEUCOCYTE FUNCTIONS ?

I believe the answer to the above question will be 'Yes'. There are a number of suggestive parallels between some of the proposals I have outlined for chemotactic recognition and hypotheses for recognition in phagocytosis based on experiments conducted on quite independent lines.

Many years ago, Fenn (1922) and Mudd *et al.* (1934) proposed that a contact between a phagocytic cell and a particle would result in phagocytosis if the interfacial

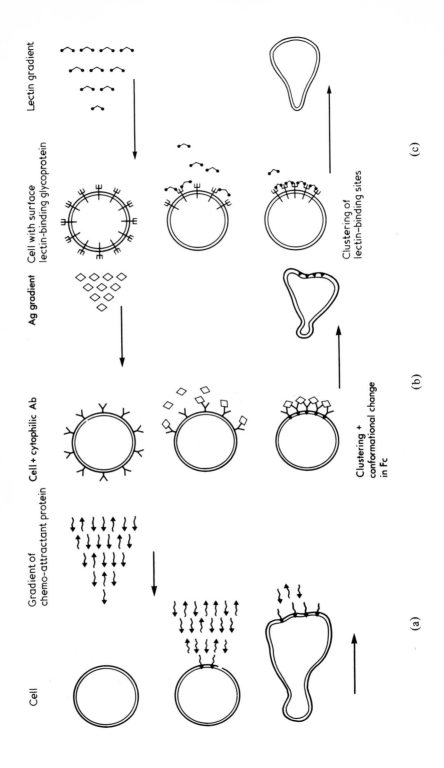

Cell

Gradient of chemo-attractant protein

Cell + cytophilic Ab

Ag gradient

Cell with surface lectin-binding glycoprotein

Lectin gradient

Clustering + conformational change in Fc

Clustering of lectin-binding sites

(a)

(b)

(c)

tension between the cell and the particle was lower than that between the cell and the medium in which the two objects were suspended, since, under these conditions, engulfment of the particle by the cell would be energetically favoured. A similar hypothesis has more recently been proposed by van Oss and colleagues who use the contact angle made by droplets of water on monolayers of cells or on lawns of bacteria (van Oss *et al.*, 1975) as a measure of the relative hydrophilicity/hydrophobicity of the surface. They related this to the ability of the cells to phagocytose and concluded that phagocytes would ingest particles or cells whose surface was more hydrophobic than their own but not particles or cells whose surface was more hydrophilic than their own. This is consistent with the greater ability of bacteria with hydrophilic polysaccharide capsules than of uncapsulated bacteria to resist phagocytosis. Opsonization of capsulated bacteria with antibody reduced their hydrophilicity and thus favoured phagocytosis.

Stendahl and Edebo (1972) observed that rough mutants of *Salmonella typhimurium*, possessing little surface polysaccharide, were phagocytosed more readily than smooth strains of the same organism in which a full complement of surface sugars was present. The same group have shown, using an aqueous two-phase polymer partition system, that rough strains separate into the hydrophobic phase (palmitoyl-polyethylene glycol) and smooth strains into the hydrophilic phase (dextran) (Magnusson *et al.*, 1977). This suggests that net hydrophobicity is an important prerequisite for attachment and particle ingestion by phagocytes. Opsonization of smooth strains of *S. typhimurium* with IgG-antibody increased their hydrophobicity and enhanced phagocytosis. It also enhanced binding of these bacteria to protein-free liposomes, allowing marker release from the liposomes (Tagesson *et al.*, 1977) as was shown earlier for IgG aggregates which also bound to and caused marker release from liposomes (Weissmann *et al.*, 1974). The Fc portion of IgG was necessary since F (ab$_2'$)-sensitized bacteria failed to show this effect. Coating of *Salmonella* with IgA antibody instead of with IgG does not lead to enhancement of phagocytosis and IgA-coated bacteria do not show an affinity for the hydrophobic phase in the two phase system (L. Edebo, personal communication). These studies suggest in broad terms that hydrophobicity is an important factor in particle—phagocyte interactions and thus that the physicochemical requirements for chemotaxis and phagocytosis are related. However, further studies are needed to unravel the details of the molecular interactions involved in phagocytosis at the level of the cell surface binding sites.

Fig. 9.7 Possible mechanisms for activation of locomotor responses in leucocytes. (a) Amphipathic molecules with exposed hydrophobic groups (represented as the heads of arrows) may penetrate directly into hydrophobic areas of the cell membrane. (b) Cell-bound antibody may provide a mechanism for activation of locomotion on binding antigen. Whether clustering then occurs as represented is not known. (c) Polyvalent ligands such as lectins may initiate locomotion by a mechanism similar to (b). (From Wilkinson, 1976a by courtesy of *Clinical and Experimental Immunology*).

Mononuclear phagocytes especially in the liver are known to clear bacteria and other particulate matter from the circulation *in vivo*. Thorbecke *et al.* (1960) showed that proteins modified by methods which increased their hydrophobicity were removed from the circulation of experimental animals more rapidly than native proteins. These proteins included alkali-denatured or acid- or urea-denatured serum albumin and were thus presumably similar to those used in the chemotaxis studies discussed in Section 9.6.6.

Data from other sources also suggest a relationship between phagocytosis and chemotaxis. Musson and Becker (1976) have shown that if chemotactic factors such as C5a and formyl peptides are presented to neutrophils at the same time as complement-coated red cells (EAC 423), they inhibit phagocytosis of the red cells. More directly, Becker (1976) has reported that f-Met-Leu-Phe-coated latex particles are ingested more rapidly by neutrophils than the same particles uncoated. Thus a molecule which is chemotactic in free solution activates phagocytosis when presented to the cell on the surface of a particle.

Griffin *et al.* (1975) have proposed that when opsonized particles (red cells) are presented to macrophages, attachment occurs by binding of ligands on one pole of the particle to cell surface receptors, but that for ingestion to follow, the whole surface of the particle must be coated with ligand (complement). Then, sequential circumferential interactions take place between receptor sites on the extending pseudopod and ligand molecules on the particle. If ligand molecules are cleared from the free side of the particle following attachment but before ingestion, no ingestion follows (Fig. 9.8a and b). This has been named the 'zipper' model for phagocytosis. We believe that something very similar happens in locomotion. Dierich *et al.* (1977) have shown that, if filters are soaked in casein, then washed thoroughly to remove all free casein, some casein molecules remain irreversibly bound to the filter, and that neutrophils migrate the same distance into such casein-coated filters as before washing. We have observed (Wilkinson and Allan, 1979) that chemotactic factors such as denatured albumin and α_s-casein bind appreciably both to the leucocyte surface and to the glass or other substrate on which they are moving but, as mentioned earlier, under conditions where chemotactic factors fail to bind to the substratum, they also fail to allow locomotion. Thus locomotion, like phagocytosis, may depend on a sequential 'zipper'-like interaction of the leucocyte with surface-bound ligand (Fig. 9.8c,d).

Other leucocyte functions may be triggered by chemotactic signals. Chemotactic factors can induce exocytosis of cytoplasmic granules from neutrophils and Showell *et al.* (1976) showed a very close parallel between the concentrations of a variety of formyl peptides which were maximally effective in inducing locomotion and in causing exocytosis. Exocytosis and hydrolase release into the medium may be an important mechanism for digestion of non-phagocytosable objects by leucocytes e.g. leucocytes attracted to aggregated immunoglobulin bound to a surface are unable to phagocytose the surface-bound aggregate, and can be seen to release hydrolases by exocytosis (Henson, 1971).

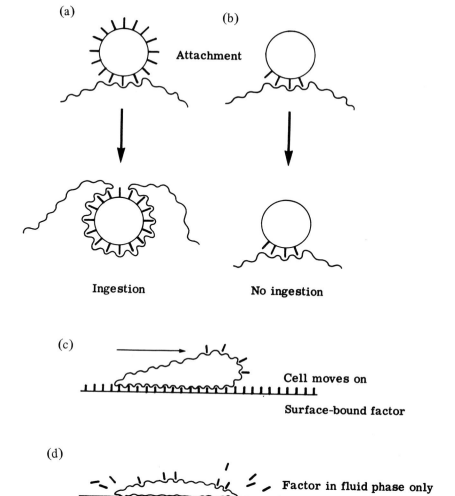

Fig. 9.8 Possible relationship between locomotion of leucocytes on surfaces and Silverstein's 'zipper' model for phagocytosis (Griffin *et al.*, 1975). In (a) phagocytosis occurs by sequential attachment of the cell membrane binding sites to particle-bound ligand. (b) If the ligand is not circumferentially distributed on the particle, phagocytosis does not occur. Similarly (c) cells may move by sequential attachment to surface-bound ligand (chemotactic or chemokinetic factor). (d) If the ligand is not surface-attached, but in fluid phase only, the cell becomes stuck to the surface, and is unable to move.

Leucocytes possess a surface-binding site for the Fc fragment of immunoglobulin, which, as mentioned earlier, probably plays an important part in the attachment and phagocytosis of opsonized particles or bacteria. It has been calculated that the approximate number of these sites on macrophages is 10^6 per cell (Phillips-Quagliata *et al.*, 1971; Leslie and Cohen, 1974). Leucocytes with immunoglobulin bound at these sites may show diminished responses to chemotactic factors (Wilkinson, 1976b; Kay *et al.* 1978; van Epps and Williams, 1976). The ability to bind Fc is abolished by treating leucocytes with the same enzymes, phospholipase C and sphingomyelinase C, that abolish chemotactic responses (Wilkinson, 1977b). It is possible, but has not been demonstrated, that the membrane sites for chemotaxis and for Fc binding may be related or identical or at least sterically hinder one another. Since leucocytes with cytophilic antibody bound to the Fc receptor recognize and migrate towards antigen (Jensen and Esquenazi, 1975; Wilkinson, 1976b), it is possible that antibody binding at this site blocks recognition of non-specific chemotactic factors and allows the cell to respond only in an immunologically specific manner i.e. to antigen. Such a switch might be immunologically useful, but there is no hard evidence at present that it exists.

It is also possible that changes in the Fc fragment of IgG may cause the IgG molecule to become chemotactic. Proteolytic digestion of a small fragment of Fc causes the IgG molecule to acquire chemotactic activity (Hayashi *et al.*, 1974). Possibly, conformational changes in cell-bound Fc play some part in the chemotactic recognition of antigen discussed earlier (Section 9.6.8).

To summarize the preceding sections, possible mechanisms for recognition of chemotactic factors at the leucocyte membrane are as follows. Lymphocytes (and possibly also phagocytic cells) may respond to ligands which bind to membrane glycoproteins, and these responses are abolished in pronase- or trypsin-treated cells (Fig. 9.7c). In the same way lymphocytes can locomote towards antigen, and this is also possible for phagocytes, provided these have specific antibody bound to their membranes by the Fc binding site (Fig. 9.7b). Further, leucocytes of all types respond to a wide variety of factors, proteins, lipids and peptides, most of which can be shown to be amphipathic, usually containing a substantial hydrophobic moiety (Fig. 9.7a). Many of these are anionic. Responses to these factors, but not to the first group, are diminished by pretreatment of the cells with one or more of a variety of lipid-binding enzymes or toxins. The precise pattern of inhibition depends on the leucocyte type and the species. It should perhaps be emphasized that the hypothesis proposed here (Fig. 9.7a) does not predict that *all* amphipathic or hydrophobic molecules will act as chemotactic factors. Detergents such as SDS, for instance, do not, although they fall into the general class of anionic, amphipathic molecules.

It is probable that chemotactic recognition takes place at a restricted number of defined and saturable binding sites and that binding is at a measurable affinity such that the association constant (K_a) is close to the optimal effective concentration for chemotactic responses. The formyl tripeptides which stimulate chemotaxis maximally at $10^{-9} - 10^{-10}$ M have K_a values around 10^9 l mol^{-1}. Denatured albumin is most effective as an attractant at $10^{-5} - 10^{-6}$ M and has a K_a of about $10^6 l \, mol^{-1}$. The generalization that chemotactic recognition works best at around the concentration of the K_a value may hold for all chemotactic factors. Zigmond (1978a) has argued that a cell which senses a gradient by detecting a different proportion of receptors bound on its two sides would be able to do this best in the concentration range of the K_a. Receptor occupancy at this concentration will be optimal for detection of differences in concentration between the two ends of the cell.

The question of whether there are multiple receptors for the varieties of chemotactic factors discussed in Section 9.6 cannot be answered at present. It is particularly embarrassing that nothing at all is known about binding of what may be physiologically the most important of chemotactic molecules, namely the peptides released by activation of complement.

9.9 HOW DOES THE CHEMOTACTIC SIGNAL ACTIVATE THE LOCOMOTOR APPARATUS ?

The leading lamellipodium of the leucocyte, which is presumably the site of activation of the cell by chemotactic factors, is characterized by the presence of a dense network of microfilaments which are believed to provide the motive force for locomotion. These actin filaments are almost certainly attached to the cell membrane and events at the outer surface of the membrane are assumed to control the arrangement and activity of these filaments. However very little is known about the mechanism of this control. There are two popular candidates for such control in eukaryotic cells. One is regulation of the intracellular levels of cyclic nucleotides by activation of membrane-bound nucleotide cyclases. The other is the regulation of intracellular cation concentrations by transmembrane ion fluxes and by the action of membrane-bound Na^+, K^+, ATPases or Ca^{2+}, ATPases which act as cation pumps. There has been a certain amount of work on the role of cyclic nucleotides in leucocyte chemotaxis but no really clear message has emerged. Although intracellular levels of cAMP and cGMP influence locomotion and are altered by addition of chemotactic factors to leucocytes, the evidence does not suggest that membrane cyclases have any direct role in signal transduction in chemotaxis (Rivkin *et al.*, 1975; Anderson *et al.*, 1976). There is certainly more enthusiasm at present for the idea that ion fluxes control motor events, especially since this is known to be the case in muscle, which consists of essentially the same proteins, actin and myosin.

The simplest model would be that chemotactic factors increase the permeability of the cell membrane to ions, thus allowing an influx of Na^+ and possibly also of Ca^{2+}, since the cytoplasmic Ca^{2+} concentration is normally low. Pumping enzymes would be required if it were necessary to move ions against a concentration gradient, and to restore the *status quo* in the cell following passive fluxes due to increases in membrane permeability. Such a model is probably too simple, since enhanced membrane permeability does not always lead to a chemotactic response, and because leucocyte locomotion is, to a considerable extent, independent of extracellular ion concentrations. Leucocytes move in the absence of extracellular calcium (Becker and Showell, 1972; Wilkinson, 1975b) and it is possible that ion movements which take place between intracellular compartments, rather than between the cytoplasm and the extracellular medium, may regulate cell locomotion. Nevertheless, amphipathic chemotactic factors are very likely to act as membrane perturbants, and polyvalent ligands which cause clustering of membrane proteins are known to have the same effect.

Direct evidence that chemotactic factors affect membrane potential in leucocytes has recently been provided since a technique has been developed for inserting microelectrodes into macrophages. Gallin *et al.* (1976) showed that slow hyperpolarizations may occur spontaneously in mouse macrophages. These could be augmented using the divalent cation ionophore A23187, and blocked with the Ca^{2+} chelator EGTA. Dos Reis and Oliveira-Castro (1977) abolished hyperpolarization in mouse macrophages with tetramethyl ammonium and induced rapid permanent hyperpolarization with valinomycin. They ascribed the development of hyperpolarization to an increased membrane permeability to K^+. Still more recently, Gallin and Gallin (1977) have shown that addition to macrophages of endotoxin-activated serum as a source of complement-derived chemotactic factors, or addition of f-Met-Leu-Phe, induced a brief depolarization followed by a more prolonged hyperpolarization and they suggested that the hyperpolarization was probably related to potassium efflux. Repeated stimulation of the cells led to desensitization.

It has also recently been shown that the same chemotactic peptide, f-Met-Leu-Phe induced a rapid and large increase in permeability of the neutrophil plasma membrane to Na^+, followed by a smaller, delayed enhancement of K^+ uptake and Na^+ efflux (Naccache *et al.,* 1977). The authors believe that a membrane-associated Na^+, K^+, ATPase (Sha'afi *et al.,* 1976) is implicated in these events. There were also fluxes of Ca^{2+} which were dependent on the extracellular Ca^{2+} concentration. If this was low (10^{-5} M) the peptide caused a decrease in the steady-state level of cell-associated Ca^{2+}. If it was high (2.5×10^{-4} M), there was an increase in steady-state Ca^{2+} level (Naccache *et al.,* 1977). While, in the electrophysiological studies, K^+ efflux is suggested as a major event, this is not emphasized by the ion flux studies. However, the two groups were using different cell types.

These results are encouraging if preliminary, and although they do not yet give a coherent picture of the role of transmembrane cation exchange in chemotaxis, they do point strongly to the conclusion that transmembrane ion fluxes do play a role, and will thus encourage further work. We can at least say that chemotactic factors do directly affect membrane permeability to ions and membrane potential, but we cannot yet say how this is related to the actin-myosin system.

9.10 CONCLUSIONS

Recognition of chemotactic factors by leucocytes may take place by a number of different mechanisms. A common feature of many chemotactic factors is that they contain a substantial hydrophobic moiety, usually together with polar sites some of which are frequently negatively charged. It is therefore possible that many amphipathic molecules are recognized at binding sites which are adapted to bind a wide range of ligands with the above physicochemical properties. These binding sites, though of high affinity, may not require strict steric complementarity. Possibly these sites are conformationally flexible to accommodate a variety of ligands. Their nature is unknown, nevertheless lipid-specific membrane-modifying agents can inhibit chemotactic reactions to these factors and reduce their binding to the cell surface. Tissue damage may lead to the release of molecules, which are thermodynamically unstable in aqueous solution e.g. denatured proteins, or chemotactic lipids released from damaged cells. Their appearance may therefore be an index of disorder in the leucocyte's environment and may thus allow a versatile form of recognition of disorder by leucocytes. In my view the formylated peptides fall into this category of chemotactic factors. There is no indication yet as to how complement peptides work.

In addition, certainly in lymphocytes and possibly in phagocytes also, polyvalent ligands which bind to membrane glycoproteins can induce chemotactic reactions. In our hands these are not such strong reactions as those discussed above. Binding of antigen to surface-bound immunoglobulin can induce chemotactic reactions, which may suggest that the 'Fc-receptor' plays a critical role in chemotaxis. Perhaps antigen-binding switches the response from a non-specific to an immunologically specific form or from an 'order-disorder' to a 'self-non-self' form of discrimination. At present this is speculation only. In any case, chemotactic reactions induced by binding of ligands to membrane glycoproteins or to antibody are clearly mediated by a different recognition system from the one involved in recognition of amphipathic or hydrophobic molecules.

Binding of chemotactic factors to the cell surface induces changes of transmembrane potential and ion fluxes. Thus a mechanism for transmitting information from outside the cell to inside can be seen in outline. What happens thereafter in the cell cytoplasm is a mystery. Whatever it is, it results in the formation of networks of actin—myosin filaments at the leading edge of the cell and at the sites of attachment to the substratum. These filaments are almost certainly the locomotor machinery of the cell. The details of the molecular interactions involved in their function are not yet understood.

REFERENCES

Allan, R.B. and Wilkinson, P.C. (1978), A visual analysis of chemotactic and chemokinetic locomotion of human neutrophil leucocytes. *Exp. Cell Res.,* **111**, 191–203.

Anderson, R., Glover, A., Koornhof, H.J. and Rabson, A.R. (1976), *In vitro* stimulation of neutrophil motility by levamisole: maintenance of cGMP levels in chemotactically stimulated levamisole-treated neutrophils. *J. Immunol.*, **117**, 428–432.

Armstrong, P.B. and Lackie, J.M. (1975), Studies on intercellular invasion *in vitro* using rabbit peritoneal neutrophil granulocytes (PMNs) I. Role of contact inhibition in locomotion. *J. Cell Biol.*, **65**, 439–462.

Aswanikumar, S., Corcoran, B., Schiffmann, E., Day, A.R., Freer, R.J., Showell, H.J., Becker, E.L. and Pert, C.B. (1977), Demonstration of a receptor on rabbit neutrophils for chemotactic peptides. *Biochem. biophys. Res. Commun.*, **74**, 810–817.

Aswanikumar, S., Schiffmann, E., Corcoran, B.A. and Wahl, S.M. (1976), Role of a peptidase in phagocyte chemotaxis. *Proc. natn. Acad. Sci. U.S.A.*, **73**, 2439–2442.

Atherton, A. and Born, G.V.R. (1972), Quantitative investigations of the adhesiveness of circulating polymorphonuclear leucocytes to blood vessel walls. *J. Physiol.*, **222**, 447–474.

Becker, E.L. (1972), The relationship of the chemotactic behaviour of the complement-derived factors, C3a, C5a and C567 and a bacterial chemotactic factor to their ability to activate the proesterase 1 of rabbit polymorphonuclear leukocytes. *J. exp. Med.*, **135**, 376–387.

Becker, E.L. (1976), Some interrelations among chemotaxis, lysosomal enzyme secretion and phagocytosis by neutrophils In: *Molecular and Biological Aspects of the Acute Allergic Reaction.* (Johansson, S.G.O., Strandberg, K. and Uvnäs B., eds), pp. 353–370, Plenum, New York.

Becker, E.L. and Showell, H.J. (1972), The effect of Ca^{2+} and Mg^{2+} on the chemotactic responsiveness and spontaneous motility of rabbit polymorphonuclear leukocytes. *Z. Immunitätsforschung*, **143**, 466–476.

Bessis, M. (1974), Necrotaxis: Chemotaxis towards an injured cell. *Antibiot. Chemother.*, **19**, 369–381.

Bryant, R.E., desPrez, R.M., van Way, M.H. and Rogers, D.E. (1966), Studies on leukocyte motility I. Effects of alterations of pH, electrolyte concentration and phagocytosis on leukocyte migration, adhesiveness and aggregation. *J. exp. Med.*, **124**, 483–499.

Carruthers, B.M. (1967), Leukocyte motility II. Effect of absence of glucose in medium: effect of presence of deoxyglucose, dinitrophenyl, puromycin, actinomycin D and trypsin on the response to chemotactic substance: effect of segregation of cells from chemotactic substance. *Can. J. Physiol. Pharmacol.*, **45**, 269–280.

Dierich, M.P., Wilhelmi, D. and Till, G. (1977), Essential role of surface-bound chemoattractant in leukocyte migration. *Nature*, **270**, 351–352.

Dos Reis, G.A. and Oliveira-Castro, G.M. (1977), Electrophysiology of phagocytic membranes I. Potassium-dependent slow membrane hyperpolarizations in mice macrophages. *Biochem. biophys. Acta*, **469**, 257–263.

Ehrlich, P. (1957), *The Collected Papers of P. Ehrlich*, Vol. 2, Pergamon, London.

Fenn, W.O. (1922), The theoretical response of living cells to contact with solid bodies. *J. gen. Physiol.*, **4**, 373–385.

Fischer, E. (1894 and 1895), Einfluss der Configuration auf die Wirkung der Enzyme II und III. *Berichte der Deutschen Chemischen Gesellschaft* **27**, 3479–3483 und **28**, 1429–1438.

Freer, J.H. and Arbuthnott, J.P. (1976), Biochemical and morphological alterations of membranes by bacterial toxins. In: *Mechanisms in Bacterial Toxinology,* (Bernheimer, A.W., ed.), pp. 169–191, Wiley, New York.

Gallin, E.K. and Gallin, J.I. (1977), Interaction of chemotactic factors with human macrophages. Induction of transmembrane potential changes. *J. Cell Biol.,* **75**, 277–289.

Gallin, E.K., Wiederhold, M.L., Lipsky, P.E. and Rosenthal, A.S. (1976), Spontaneous and induced membrane hyperpolarizations of macrophages. *J. Cell. Physiol.,* **86**, 653–661.

Goetzl, E.J. and Austen, K.F. (1975), Purification and synthesis of eosinophilotactic tetrapeptides of human lung tissue: Identification as eosinophil chemotactic factor of anaphylaxis. *Proc. natn. Acad. Sci. U.S.A.,* **72**, 4123–4127.

Griffin, F.M., Griffin, J.A., Leider, J.E. and Silverstein, S.G. (1975), Studies on the mechanism of phagocytosis I. Requirements for circumferential attachment of particle-bound ligands to specific receptors on the macrophage plasma membrane. *J. exp. Med.,* **142**, 1263–1282.

Habermann, E. and Krowallek, H. (1970), Modifikationen der Aminogruppen und des Tryptophans im Melittin als Mittel zur Erkennung von Struktur-Wirkungs Beziehungen. *Hoppe Seyler's Z. physiol. Chemie.,* **351**, 884–890.

Hayashi, H., Yoshinaga, M. and Yamamoto, S. (1974), The nature of a mediator of leucocyte chemotaxis in inflammation. *Antibiot. Chemother.,* **19**, 296–332.

Henson, P.M. (1971), The immunologic release of constituents from neutrophil leukocytes. I. The role of antibody and complement on nonphagocytosable surfaces or phagocytosable particles. *J. Immunol.,* **107**, 1535–1546.

Hoover, R. (1978), Modulations of the cell surface and the effects on cellular interactions. *Symp. Soc. exp. Biol.,* in press.

Jensen, J.A. and Esquenazi, V. (1975), Chemotactic stimulation by cell surface immune reactions. *Nature,* **256**, 213–215.

Kay, A.B., Shin, H.S. and Austen, K.F. (1973), Selective attraction of eosinophils and synergism between eosinophil chemotactic factor of anaphylaxis (ECF-A) and a fragment cleaved from the fifth component of complement (C5a). *Immunology,* **24**, 969–976.

Kay, N.E., Bumol, T.F. and Douglas, S.D. (1978), Effect of phagocytosis and Fc receptor occupancy on complement-dependent neutrophil chemotaxis *J. Lab. Clin. Med.,* **91**, 850–856

Keller, H.U. and Bessis, M. (1975), Migration and chemotaxis of anucleate cytoplasmic leukocyte fragments. *Nature,* **258**, 723–724.

Keller, H.U., Wilkinson, P.C., Abercrombie, M., Becker, E.L., Hirsch, J.G., Miller, M.E., Ramsey, W.S. and Zigmond, S.H. (1977), A proposal for the definition of terms related to locomotion of leucocytes and other cells. *Clin. exp. Immunol.,* **27**, 377–380.

Leslie, R.G.Q. and Cohen, S. (1974), Cytophilic activity of IgG 2 from sera of unimmunized guinea-pigs. *Immunology,* **27**, 577–587.

Lynn, W.S., Muñoz, S., Campbell, J.A. and Jeffs, P.W. (1974), Chemotaxis and cotton extracts. *Ann. N.Y. Acad. Sci.,* **221**, 163–173.

Magnusson, K.E., Stendahl, O., Tagesson, C., Edebo, L. and Johannson, G. (1977), The tendency of smooth and rough *Salmonella typhimurium* bacteria and lipopolysaccharide to hydrophobic and ionic interaction as studied in aqueous polymer two-phase systems. *Acta path. microbiol. scand. Ser. B.,* **85**, 212–218.

McCutcheon, M. (1946), Chemotaxis in leukocytes. *Physiol. Rev.,* **26**, 319–336.

McMenamy, R.H. (1977), Albumin binding sites. In: *Albumin Structure, Function and Uses.* (Rosenoer, V.M., Oratz, M. and Rothschild, M.A., eds), pp. 143–158, Pergamon, Oxford.

Mudd, S., McCutcheon, M. and Lucke, B. (1934), Phagocytosis. *Physiol. Rev.,* **14**, 210–275.

Musson, R.A. and Becker, E.L. (1976), The inhibitory effect of chemotactic factors on erythrophagocytosis by human neutrophils. *J. Immunol.,* **117**, 433–439.

Naccache, P., Freer, R.J., Showell, H.J., Becker, E.L. and Sha'afi, R.I. (1977), Transport of sodium, potassium and calcium across rabbit polymorphonuclear leukocyte membranes: effect of chemotactic factor. *J. Cell Biol.,* **73**, 428–444.

Nozaki, Y. and Tanford, C. (1971), The solubility of amino acids and two glycine peptides in aqueous ethanol and dioxane solutions. Establishment of a hydrophobicity scale. *J. biol. Chem.,* **246**, 2211–2217.

Phillips-Quagliata, J.M., Levine, B.B., Quagliata, F. and Uhr, J.W. (1971), Mechanisms underlying binding of immune complexes to macrophages. *J. exp. Med.,* **133**, 589–601.

Rivkin, I., Rosenblatt, J. and Becker, E.L. (1975), The role of cyclic AMP in the chemotactic responsiveness and spontaneous motility of rabbit peritoneal neutrophils. *J. Immunol.,* **115**, 1126–1134.

Russell, R.J., McInroy, R.J., Wilkinson, P.C. and White, R.G. (1976), A lipid chemotactic factor from anaerobic corynedorm bacteria including *Corynebacterium parvum* with activity for macrophages and monocytes. *Immunology,* **30**, 935–949.

Russell, R.J., Wilkinson, P.C., Sless, F. and Parrott, D.M.V. (1975), Chemotaxis of lymphoblasts. *Nature,* **256**, 646–648.

Sahu, S. and Lynn, W.S. (1977), Lipid chemotaxins isolated from culture filtrates of *Escherichia coli* and from oxidized lipids. *Inflammation,* **2**, 47–54.

Schiffmann, E., Corcoran, B.A. and Wahl, S.A. (1975), N-formylmethionyl peptides as chemoattractants for leucocytes. *Proc. natn. Acad. Sci. U.S.A.,* **72**, 1059–1062.

Sha'afi, R.I., Naccache, P., Raible, D., Krepcio, A., Showell, H. and Becker, E.L. (1976), Demonstration of (Na^+, K^+)-sensitive ATPase activity in rabbit polymorphonuclear leukocyte membranes. *Biochim. biophys. Acta,* **448**, 638–641.

Showell, H.J., Freer, R.J., Zigmond, S.H., Schiffmann, E., Aswanikumar, S., Corcoran, B. and Becker, E.L. (1976), The structure-activity relations of synthetic peptides as chemotactic factors and inducers of lysosomal enzyme secretion for neutrophils. *J. exp. Med.,* **143**, 1154–1169.

Stendahl, O. and Edebo, L. (1972), Phagocytosis of mutants of *Salmonella typhimurium* by rabbit polymorphonuclear cells. *Acta path. microbiol. scand., Ser. B.,* **80**, 481–488.

Stossel, T.P. (1978), The mechanism of leucocyte locomotion. In: *Leukocyte Chemotaxis,* (Gallin, J.I. and Quie, P.G., eds), pp. 143–160, Raven, New York.

Stossel, T. and Pollard, T.D. (1973), Myosin in polymorphonuclear leukocytes. *J. biol. Chem.*, **248**, 8288–8294.

Suzue, T., Mitsushima, A. and Inada, Y. (1976), Cooperative participation of two peptides from β-casein in leukocyte chemotaxis. *FEBS Letters*, **69**, 133–136.

Tagesson, C., Magnusson, K.E. and Stendahl, O. (1977), Physicochemical consequences of opsonization: perturbation of liposomal membranes by *Salmonella typhimurium* 395MS opsonized with IgG antibodies. *J. Immunol.*, **119**, 609–613.

Tainer, J.A., Turner, S.R. and Lynn, W.S. (1975), New aspects of chemotaxis. Specific target-cell attraction by lipid and lipoprotein fractions of *Escherichia coli* chemotactic factoɪ. *Am. J. Path.*, **81**, 401–410.

Tanford, C. (1972), Hydrophobic free energy, micelle formation and the association of proteins with amphiphiles. *J. Mol. Biol.*, **67**, 59–74.

Tatsumi, N., Shibata, N., Okamura, Y., Takeuchi, K. and Senda, N. (1973), Actin and myosin from leucocytes. *Biochim. biophys. Acta,* **305**, 433–444.

Thorbecke, G.J., Maurer, P.H. and Benacerraf, B. (1960), The affinity of the reticuloendothelial system for various modified serum proteins. *Br. J. exp. Path.*, **41**, 190–197.

Turner, S.R., Tainer, J.A. and Lynn, W.S. (1975), Biogenesis of chemotactic molecules by the arachidonate lipoxygenase system of platelets. *Nature,* **257**, 680–681.

van Epps, D.E. and Andersen, B.R. (1974), Streptolysin O inhibition of neutrophil chemotaxis and mobility. Non-immune phenomenon with species specificity. *Infect. Immun.,* **9**, 27–33.

van Epps, D.E. and Tung, K.S.K. (1977), Fucose-binding *Lotus tetragonolobus* lectin binds to human polymorphonuclear leukocytes and induces a chemotactic response. *J. Immunol.,* **119**, 1187–1189.

van Epps, D.E. and Williams, R. (1976), Suppression of leukocyte chemotaxis by human IgA myeloma components. *J. exp. Med.,* **144**, 1227–1242.

van Oss, C.J., Gillman, C.F. and Neumann, A.W. (1975), *Phagocytic Engulfment and Cell Adhesiveness.* Marcel Dekker, New York.

Ward, P.A. (1966), The chemosuppression of chemotaxis. *J. exp. Med.,* **124**, 209–226.

Ward, P.A. and Becker, E.L. (1968), The deactivation of rabbit neutrophils by chemotactic factor and the nature of the activatable esterase. *J. exp. Med.,* **127**, 693–709.

Weiss, P. (1947), Problem of specificity in growth and development. *Yale J. biol. Med.,* **19**, 235–278.

Weissmann, G., Brand, A. and Franklin, E.C. (1974), Interaction of Immunoglobulins with liposomes. *J. clin. Invest.,* **53**, 536–543.

Wilkinson, P.C. (1973), Recognition of protein structure in leukocyte chemotaxis. *Nature,* **244**, 512–513.

Wilkinson, P.C. (1974a), Surface and cell membrane activities of leukocyte chemotactic factors. *Nature,* **251**, 58–60.

Wilkinson, P.C. (1974b), *Chemotaxis and Inflammation.* Churchill-Livingstone, Edinburgh.

Wilkinson, P.C. (1975a), Inhibition of leukocyte locomotion and chemotaxis by lipid-specific bacterial toxins. *Nature,* **255**, 485–487.

Wilkinson, P.C. (1975b), Leucocyte locomotion and chemotaxis. The influence of divalent cations and cation ionophores. *Exp. Cell Res.,* **93**, 420–426.

Wilkinson, P.C. (1976a), Recognition and response in mononuclear and granular phagocytes. *Clin. exp. Immunol., 25*, 355–366.

Wilkinson, P.C. (1976b), Cellular and molecular aspects of chemotaxis of macrophages and monocytes In: *Immunobiology of the Macrophage*. (Nelson, D.S., ed.), pp. 349–365, Academic Press, New York.

Wilkinson, P.C. (1976c), A requirement for albumin as carrier for low-molecular-weight leucocyte chemotactic factors. *Exp. Cell Res., 103*, 415–418.

Wilkinson, P.C. (1977a), Succinyl bee venom melittin is a leukocyte chemotactic factor. *Nature, 267*, 713–714.

Wilkinson, P.C. (1977b), Action of sphingomyelinase C and other lipid-specific agents as inhibitors of Fc binding and locomotion in human leucocytes. *Immunology, 33*, 407–412.

Wilkinson, P.C. and Allan, R.B. (1978), Binding of protein chemotactic factors to the surface of neutrophil leukocytes and its modification with lipid specific chemotactic factors. *Mol. Cell Biochem., 20*, 25–40.

Wilkinson, P.C. and Allan, R.B. (1979), Chemotaxis of neutrophil leucocytes towards substratum-bound protein attractants. *Exp. Cell Res.*, in press.

Wilkinson, P.C. and McKay, I.C. (1971), The chemotactic activity of native and denatured serum albumin. *Int. Arch. Allergy appl. Immunol., 41*, 237–247.

Wilkinson, P.C. and McKay, I.C. (1972), The molecular requirements for chemotactic attraction of leucocytes by proteins. Studies of proteins with synthetic side groups. *Eur. J. Immunol., 2*, 570–577.

Wilkinson, P.C., Parrott, D.M.V., Russell, R.J. and Sless, F. (1977), Antigen-induced locomotor responses in lymphocytes. *J. exp. Med., 145*, 1158–1168.

Wilkinson, P.C., Roberts, J.A., Russell, R.J. and McLoughlin, M. (1976), Chemotaxis of mitogen-activated human lymphocytes and the effects of membrane-active enzymes. *Clin. exp. Immunol., 25*, 280–287.

Williams, L.T., Snyderman, R., Pike, M.C. and Lefkowitz, R.J. (1977), Specific receptor sites for chemotactic peptides on human polymorphonuclear leukocytes. *Proc. natn. Acad. Sci. U.S.A., 74*, 1204–1208.

Wissler, J.H. (1972a), Chemistry and biology of the anaphylatoxin related serum peptide system I. Purification, crystallization and properties of classical anaphylatoxin from rat serum. *Eur. J. Immunol., 2*, 73–83.

Wissler, J.H. (1972b), Chemistry and biology of the anaphylatoxin related serum peptide system II. Purification, crystallization and properties of cocytotaxin, a basic peptide from rat serum. *Eur. J. Immunol., 2*, 84–89.

Wissler, J.H., Stecher, V.J. and Sorkin, E. (1972a), Chemistry and biology of the anaphylatoxin related peptide system III Evaluation of leucotactic activity as a property of a new peptide system with classical anaphylatoxin and cocytotaxin as components. *Eur. J. Immunol., 2*, 90–96.

Wissler, J.H., Stecher, V.J. and Sorkin, E. (1972b), Biochemistry and biology of a leucotactic binary serum peptide system related to anaphylatoxin. *Int. Arch. Allergy appl. Immunol., 42*, 722–747.

Zigmond, S.H. (1974), Mechanisms of sensing chemical gradients by polymorphonuclear leukocytes. *Nature, 249*, 450–452.

Zigmond, S.H. (1977), Ability of polymorphonuclear leukocytes to orient in gradients of chemotactic factors. *J. Cell Biol., 73*, 606–616.

Zigmond, S.H. (1978a), A new visual assay of leukocyte chemotaxis In: *Leukocyte Chemotaxis* (Gallin, J.I. and Quie, P.G., eds), pp. 57–66, Raven, New York.
Zigmond, S.H. (1978b), Chemotaxis by polymorphonuclear leukocytes. *J. Cell Biol.,* **77**, 269–287.

Index

Accomodation, 44

Achlya,
   chemotropism, 176–177
   hormones, 177
   hormonal mechanisms 175
   sexual reproduction, 176

Acrasins, 103, 104
   waves of, 109

Actin, in leucocyte locomotion, 301, 321, 323

Action potentials,
   averaged, 219
   of bombykol receptor, 218–219
   of nematodes, 165
   of olfactory cells, 221
   of *Paramecium,* graded, 78

Adaption,
   bacterial, 6
     and methylation, 21–23, 24–26
     in photobehavior, 45
   in *Halobacterium,* 61
     role of methionine, 61
   in *Paramecium,* 92–94, 97
   in *Paramecium tetraurelia,* 93
   and modification of excitable membrane, 93
   mutants in, 93
   of pigments, 61

Adaption time,
   bacterial, 7, 21, 22
   of *Halobacterium,* 61

S-adenosylmethionine, 12

Adenyl cyclase, *Dictyostelium,* 119–122
   stimulation of, 123
   synthesis, 127

Adhesion, cell,
   leucocyte-endothelial, 298

neutrophil leucocyte, 300

Aggregation centers, *Dictyostelium,* 104

Aggregation-competence, *Dictyostelium,* 103
   in agitated suspension, 111–112

Aggregation, *Dictyostelium,*
   concentric rings in, 109–110
   models for, 119, 129–131
   parameters of, 110, 130
   and PDE, 118
   and PDE inhibitor, 119
   pulsatile, 104
   spiral waves, 110
   termination of, 128
   time-lapse films of, 109

Albumin, serum,
   as leucocyte attractant, 310–312

Allomyces,
   gamete chemotaxis, 172–175
   life cycle, 172
   mitosphere, meiosphere and zygote chemotaxis, 175

cAMP,
   in *Dictyostelium,*
     behavioral response to, 124
     biphasic response to, 113
     emission of, 115
     inducer of differentiation, 123
     intercellular signal, 114, 123, 131
     intracellular signal, 104
     models for generation, 129–131
     pulses, 111
     secretion of, 116
   in insect receptor cells, 243
   and leucocyte locomotion, 321
   and nematodes,
     as attractant, 144–145, 164
     temporal gradients of, 163

Amphid, nematode, 152